Therapy Techniques and Treatment Planning for Breast Cancer

Therapy Techniques and Treatment Planning for Breast Cancer

Editor: Sandra Lekin

AMERICAN
MEDICAL PUBLISHERS
www.americanmedicalpublishers.com

AMERICAN
MEDICAL PUBLISHERS
www.americanmedicalpublishers.com

Cataloging-in-publication Data

Therapy techniques and treatment planning for breast cancer / edited by Sandra Lekin.
p. cm.
Includes bibliographical references and index.
ISBN 979-8-88740-507-0
1. Breast--Cancer. 2. Breast--Cancer--Treatment. 3. Breast--Cancer--Treatment--Technological innovations.
I. Lekin, Sandra.
RC280.B8 T44 2023
616.994 49--dc23

American Medical Publishers,
41 Flatbush Avenue,
1st Floor, New York,
NY 11217, USA

ISBN 979-8-88740-507-0 (Hardback)

Contents

Preface

This book aims to highlight the current researches and provides a platform to further the scope of innovations in this area. This book is a product of the combined efforts of many researchers and scientists, after going through thorough studies and analysis from different parts of the world. The objective of this book is to provide the readers with the latest information of the field.

Breast cancer is a type of cancer that originates in the breast tissue. Changes in breast shape, fluid coming from the nipple, a newly inverted nipple, or a red or scaly patch of skin are signs of breast cancer. Risk factors associated with this type of cancer include obesity, a lack of physical activity, alcoholism, hormone replacement therapy during menopause and a family history of breast cancer. It usually develops in cells from the lining of milk ducts and the lobules, which supply milk to these ducts. A biopsy of the concerning tissue makes diagnosis possible for breast cancer. After diagnosis, treatment planning should be utilized for determining the suitable treatment options according to the personalized needs of the patients. Tamoxifen and raloxifene are the two medications that can be used to prevent breast cancer in people who are at a high risk of developing it. Another preventive measure is surgical removal of both breasts in patients with a high risk. This book includes some of the vital pieces of work being conducted across the world, on various topics related to breast cancer. The extensive content of this book provides the readers with a thorough understanding of the therapy techniques and treatment planning for this disease.

I would like to express my sincere thanks to the authors for their dedicated efforts in the completion of this book. I acknowledge the efforts of the publisher for providing constant support. Lastly, I would like to thank my family for their support in all academic endeavors.

Editor

1

New Experimental Therapies Targeting Breast Cancer Cell

Di Benedetto Melanie
INSERM U940/CSPBAT, Université P13,
France

1. Introduction

Proliferation/survival, migration and invasion are processes common to both primary tumor angiogenesis and metastases formation. Among the treatment approaches being investigated, the most developed is the use of genomics and proteomics research to assist the identification of unique targets involved in tumor angiogenesis or invasiveness. In addition, metastasis in breast cancer patients accounts for over 90% of the deaths. Preclinical studies reveal that many drugs used in the management of primary tumors are not or little effective against metastasis (Perret & Crepin, 2008). Although the mechanism by which metastases develop is still not fully understood, it is generally believed that tumor cells acquire features that affect their metastatic potential during the progression of the tumor; these features include increased survival, invasive and migratory abilities of breast cancer cells. Breast cancer progression is a complex cascade of sequential steps, none of which being fully understood. Many studies implicated stroma in the development of metastases. Stroma and cancer cell interactions were found to contribute to cell detachment from primary tumors, intravasation into the blood stream, and extravasation at distant sites where tumor cells can seed and form tumor metastases (Shekhar et al., 2003). Previously, fibroblasts, endothelial cells and macrophages and other stroma cells were reported to be implicated in the occurrence of metastases (Cunha et al., 1992; Haslam et al., 2001; Shekhar et al., 2003). In these conditions, new strategies as well as the identification of novel therapeutic targets will be needed to effectively target the interactions between stroma and tumor cells via growth factor. Thus, it is important to take into account not also the context near tumor cells (like growth factors as well as chemokines) but also the distribution of the tumor cells in the metastatic sites.

As of today, the poorly predictive preclinical models, lack of tumor target specificity, lack of effective cellular and intracellular delivery, development of resistance have slowed down the progress in anti-cancer therapy. Although the pharmaceutical industry prefers to develop small molecule therapy that can be orally administered to patients, it is now admitted that development of new drug delivery system strategy is essential to increase therapeutic index. Synthetic and natural polymers have an established role as in several biomedical applications, including their use as prosthesis or implants (Anderson, 2001). During the past decade, polymer implants have been used in cancer therapy to treat locally hormone-dependent tumors (Zoladex, Lupron depot) or brain tumors by implanting chemotherapy delivering polymer post-surgically. Over than 10 water-soluble polymer drugs conjugates have entered in phase I/II clinical trials as I.V. administrated anticancer agents. These include six conjugates based on methacrylamide polymers (HPMA). These polymers have been developed in the basis of the achieved tumor-specific targeting by the enhanced permeability and retention effect (Ducan et al., 2005; Matsumura et al., 1986). This increasing tumor retention has been observed and attributed to the better extravasation in the blood vessel of macromolecules and the absence of their drainage release (Noguchi Y et al., 1998; Seymour et al., 1995). HPMA copolymer conjugate with chemotherapeutic agents as doxorubicin has shown high retention and efficacy toward tumors without side effects (Ducan et al., 2005). The specific tumor cell targeting can also be attributed to the interaction of copolymers and heparin growth factors which are highly expressed in the tumor cell environment. Better retention is also attributed to the endocytic internalisation of conjugates which allows also to bypassing MDR efflux responsible for drug resistance. Also, another type of natural polymer interesting to be evaluated is the glycoaminoglycans analogs since it is well-known that they importantly interact with growth factors and receptors on the cell membranes. In another hand, the different type of glycosaminoglycans on the cell surface support in relation with normal or tumoral statues supported their involvement. We have recently developed the two kinds of copolymers that show interesting results in basis of the possibility to functionalize them with active biomolecules. Among active biomolecules, the interesting ones are those which inhibited the ancrage of rho/ras signaling molecules to tumor cells since this pathway plays a key role in invasion, migration and proliferation of tumor cells. The inhibition of the prenylation of ras and rho leads to the blocking of ancrage to the membrane. We have focused our attention on two types of such small molecules. The first one, phenylacetate (NaPa), comes from the metabolism (Fig. 1). NaPa, which has been originally used for urea children disorders (Samid et al., 1992, 1993) has since been demonstrated to efficiently inhibits cancer cell lines proliferation *in vitro*. The second small molecules are bisphosphonates (PBs, fig 1), which are mostly known for their efficacy in the treatment of bone disorders and are also efficient *in vitro* in inhibiting cancer cell proliferation. For both molecules, the main obstacle with their use in cancer therapy stems

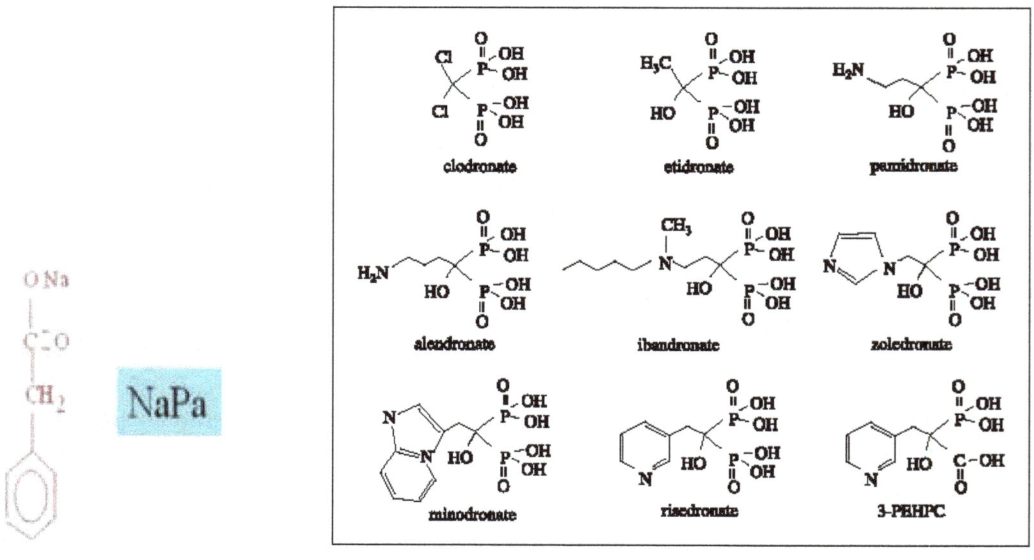

Fig. 1. Phenylacetate (NaPa) and bisphosphonates (BPs) molecules.

from the high concentrations (up to micromolars) that are needed to achieve efficacy in vivo. Since we think that these molecules remain of potential use in cancer because they target specific step involved in both primary tumor growth and metastasis formation, we are developing new strategies that aim to increase their efficacy using drug delivery systems in specific cancer cells localized in specific sites. Herein, we will present all these strategies, first by using polymers for NaPa, and secondly using chemical transformation of the compounds, in particular esterification for the bisphosphonates. Also we will present possible future directions, such as the use of new polymers as well as new delivery systems like nanotechnologies.

2. Glycoaminoglycan polymer strategy

2.1 Carboxybenzylamide dextran (CMDB) and NaPa combination

Carboxymethyl benzylamide dextran derivative (in particular CMDB7) inhibits breast cancer cell proliferation *in vitro* and in nude mice (Bagheri-Yarmand et al, 1992, 1997, 1998a, b, 1999). This *in vitro* effect is associated with a decrease in the S-phase cell population and with an accumulation of cells in G1 phase of cell cycle (Bagheri-Yarmand et al, 1992). CMDB7 disrupts the mitogenic effect of growth factors by preventing their binding to specific receptors as reported for Fibroblast Growth Factor-2 and -4 (FGF2, FGF4, Bagheri-Yarmand et al, 1998a), Platelet-Derived Growth Factor-BB and Transforming Growth Factor-β1 (PDGF-BB, TGFB Bagheri-Yarmand et al, 1998b). *In vivo*, CMDB7 treatment reduces the growth of MCF-7ras (Bagheri-Yarmand et al, 1998b) and FGF4-transfected HBL100 xenografts and decreases the tumor angiogenesis (Bagheri-Yarmand et al, 1998a). Sodium phenylacetate (NaPa), a physiological metabolite of phenylalanine, is normally found in human plasma at micromolar concentrations. At higher concentrations, NaPa is reported to induce the cytostasis and the reversion of malignant phenotype of different cancer cells *in vitro* (Samid et al, 1993, 1994, 1997, 2000; Adam et al, 1995). Furthermore, NaPa is described to modulate the synthesis and/or the release of some growth factors (Ferrandina et al, 1997; Thibout et al, 1998) and to increase, in synergistic manner, the effect of some molecules affecting the growth factor pathways (Prasanna et al, 1996; Samid et al, 1993). For example, NaPa potentiates the antitumor activity of tamoxifen by increasing apoptosis in breast cancer xenografts in nude mice. Finally, NaPa has been used in phase I and II clinical trials on patients with malignant tumors (Chang et al., 1999; Thibault et al, 1994). In basis of this data, we have evaluated *in vitro* and *in vivo* the efficacy of combined treatment with NaPa and an industrial dextran derivative LS4 (Sterilyo Laboratories) whose composition is similar to CMDB7 one, on breast cancer cell growth. We have used the MCF-7ras cell line obtained by transfection of MCF-7 cells, isolated from pleural metastasis of breast adenocarcinoma, with v-Ha-ras oncogene. The MCF-7ras cells secrete high quantities of TGFα, TGFβ, epithelial growth factor (EGF) and insulin growth factor (IGF) (Albini et al, 1986). This cell line represents an oestrogen-independent cellular model corresponding to some malignant breast tumors (Spandidos and Agnantis, 1984) and does no require oestrogen supplementation to induce a high incidence of tumors in nude mice (Sommers et al, 1990). The analysis of CMDBLS4-NaPa combination effect is performed by the isobole method.

NaPa enhances the dextran derivative CMDBLS4 antiproliferative effect on breast cancer MCF-7ras cells both *in vitro* and *in vivo*. Indeed, NaPa or CMDBLS4, delivered alone for 7 weeks, inhibits MCF-7ras tumor growth by 60% and 40%, respectively, while the CMDBLS4-NaPa combination decreases MCF-7ras tumor growth by 83% without any toxicity. The effectiveness of the NaPa and CMDBLS4 combination can be explained by their distinct mechanisms of action. MCF-7ras breast cancer cells secrete an important amount of mitogenic growth factors such as TGFβ and PDGF (Bronzert et al, 1987; Dickson et al, 1987; Knabbe et al, 1987). The mitogenic effects of these growth factors can be reduced by inhibition of their synthesis or/and their action on target cells. Treatment of cells with NaPa decreases the mitogenic activity of MCF-7ras conditioned medium on BALBc/3T3. The possible mechanism is a modulation of the synthesis and the release of growth factors like TGFβ in MCF-7ras breast cancer cells (Thibout et al, 1998). CMDBLS4, when added to conditioned medium, inhibits conditioned medium mitogenic effect on BALBc/3T3 fibroblasts. This finding argues for CMDBLS4 interactions with growth factors contained in CM. Indeed, previous studies have shown that dextran derivatives interact with heparin-binding growth factors like TGFβ, PDGFBB or FGF-2 and inhibit their mitogenic effect (Bagheri-Yarmand et al, 1998a, b). All our and others' observations suggest that NaPa and CMDBLS4 act on distinct targets involved in the tumor development. NaPa alters the mitogenic growth factor production and renders the tumor cells quiescent in the G1 phase while CMDBLS4 interacts with MCF-7ras growth factors and inhibits their mitogenic activities.

aCMDBLS4 (Ac; mM)	NaPa (Bc; mM)	% I	CMDBLS4 (Ae; mM)	NaPa (Be; mM)	D
48 h					
3.7	0.75	33	18.5	17	0.44b
7.4	1.5	45.8	>18.5	30	0.45b
14.8	3	48.1	>18.5	32.1	0.89
18.5	4	50	>18.5	34	1.12
72 h					
3.7	0.75	51.4	>18.5	20.6	0.23b
7.4	1.5	54.8	>18.5	23	0.46b
14.8	3	53.3	>18.5	24	0.93
18.5	4	60.2	>18.5	29	1.13

Table 1. Effects of NaPa and CMDBLS4 combination with a ratio = 5 on MCF-7ras cell proliferation. [a] Ac and Bc, concentrations of agents A and B used in the combination treatment; Ae and Be,concentrations of agents A and B able to produce the same magnitude of effect if used individually. D combination index If D=1 the effect is additive, id D<1, the effect is synergistic.[b] $P < 0.05$. % of inhibition determined by MTT assay:[1-(absorbance of cells in medium containing agents/absorbance of cells in control culture medium)]× 100.(Di Benedetto et al., 2001).

2.2 Carboxybenzylamide –phenylacetate dextran (NaPaC)

NaPa molecule enhances, in a synergistic or additive manner, the inhibitory effect of CMDB on breast cancer cell growth *in vitro* and in nude mice when administrated at a CMDB/NaPa ratio of 4 (Di Benedetto et al., 2001). To obtain a new drug with the same properties but easier to use as a future anti-cancer molecule than the combined treatment, we have performed the esterification of CMDB by NaPa respecting the synergistic CMDB/NaPa ratio. We have then investigated the *in vitro* and *in vivo* effects of this new dextran derivative, phenylacetate carboxymethyl benzylamide dextran, named NaPaC, on breast cancer cell proliferation as well as its apoptotic and anti-angiogenic effects.

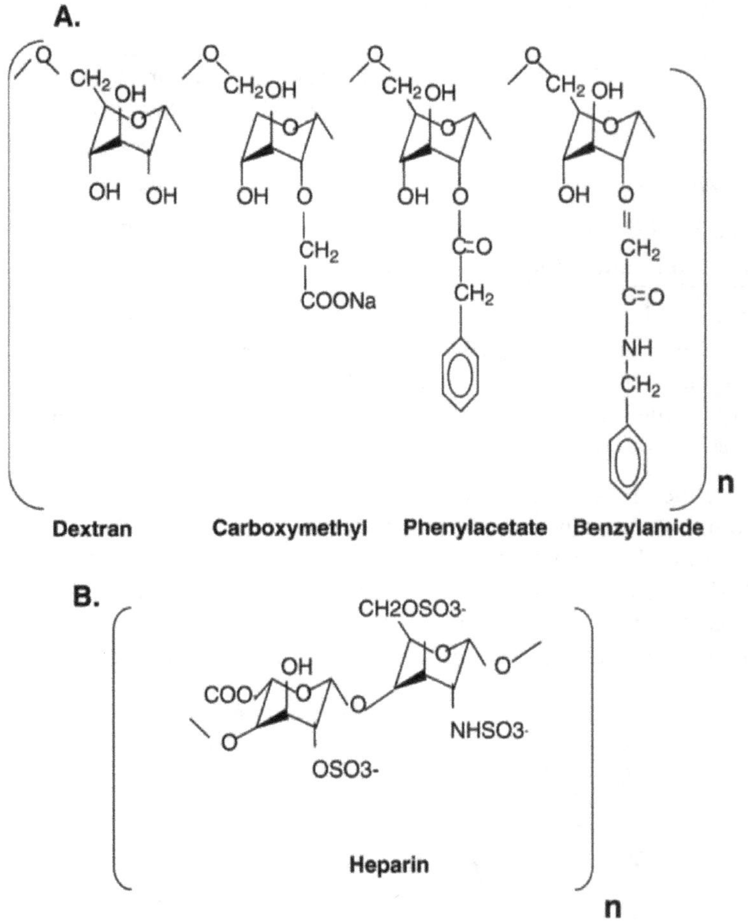

Fig. 2. Carboxymethylbenzylamide-NaPa (NaPac) (A) and heparin (B) molecules (Di Benedetto et al., 2002).

Interestingly, NaPaC inhibits the growth of breast cancer MCF-7ras cells at a concentration lower than CMDB or NaPa. The comparison of IC50 for three drugs supplies the additional evidence for the highly enhanced efficiency of NaPaC as compared to CMDB and NaPa (Table 2). Therefore, the hybrid molecule retains at least the additive effect of its two components observed previously (Di Benedetto et al., 2001). This effect is not only specifc to MCF-7 ras cells as similar results are obtained for other breast cancer cell lines, including MCF-7, MDA-MB-231 and MDA-MB-435. NaPaC inhibited in vivo MCF-7ras tumor growth more efficiently and at lower dose than CMDB or NaPa. This can be explained by the fact that NaPaC gathers the antiproliferative, aponecrotic and anti-angiogenic actions generally admitted to lead *in vivo* to concerted inhibition of tumor growth. The inhibition of the endothelium growth, causing the impaired delivery of nutrients and oxygen to tumor, leads to tumor cell death. Indeed, we observed *in vivo* that the inhibition of MCF-7ras tumor growth by NaPaC is concomitant with a poor microvessel density (as compared to control) at short-time treatment and with multifocal necrotic areas at long-term administration. Therefore, NaPaC is more efficient than CMDB or NaPa and decreases the microvessel density at dose lower than its components.

Treatment	Tumor (volume) at Day 1 (mm^3)	Tumor (volume) at day 5(mm^3)	Tumour growth (%)
Control	221±90	2103±328	-
NaP4 40 m/ kg (0.25 mmol/ kg)	157±30	990±192	57
CMDB 150 mg/kg (1.85 μmol/kg)	199±70	1326±281	33
NaPaC 15 m/kg (0.18 mmol/ kg)	167±40	717±203	66

Table 2. Inhibition of MCF-7ras tumor growth by NaPaC and its components, CMDB and NaPa. MCF-7ras cells were inoculated s.c in nude mice near the fad pad. After tumor uptake, the animals were treated for 7 weeks with NaPa (n=10), CMDB (n=10) and NaPaC (n=10). Tumor volume (+s.e.m.) for different experimental groups were compared to control (Di Benedetto et al., 2002).

Of note, no necrotic areas were detected in tumors treated with CMDB or NaPa alone. In accord with our *in vivo* results on tumor neovascularization, NaPaC *in vitro* inhibits the growth of human endothelial cells more efficiently that CMDB or NaPa. The mechanisms involved in CMDB and NaPa actions on endothelial cell proliferation seem to be distinct. CMDB interacts directly with VEGF165 (Hamma-Kourbali et al., 2001), the most specific angiogenic factor (Plouet et al., 1989) and inhibits the VEGF165-induced HUVE-C-C growth.

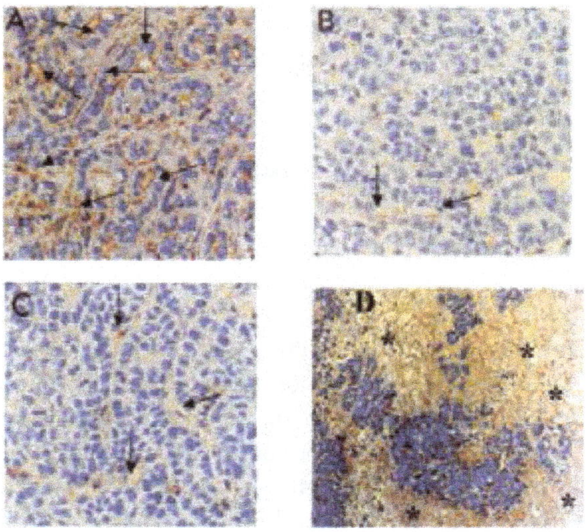

Fig. 3. Inhibition of MCF-7ras tumor angiogenesis by NaPaC, CMDB and NaPa. Microvessel staining of tumors untreated (A) and treated with 150 mg/kg CMDB (B), 40 mg/kg NaPa (C) or 15 mg/kg NaPaC (D), twice a week, for 7 weeks, was performed using GSL-1 lectin. Necrotic areas in panel d are indicated with the asterisks. Magnification X250 was used for panels A,B and C, and magnification X100 was applied for panel D. The representative microvessels in panels A±C are marked with the arrows (Di Benedetto et al., 2002).

In our laboratory, we observe that NaPa do not interact with VEGF 165 molecule, and has no effect on VEGF165-dependent cell growth. Up to date, the mechanism of NaPa action on HUVE-C-C growth is unknown. Concerning NaPaC, it inherits the CMDB ability to interact with angiogenic growth factor and blocks the VEGF165-induced endothelial cell proliferation at lower concentration than CMDB (Fig. 4). However, the involvement of the NaPa mechanism in NaPaC action on HUVE-C-C growth is still unknown.

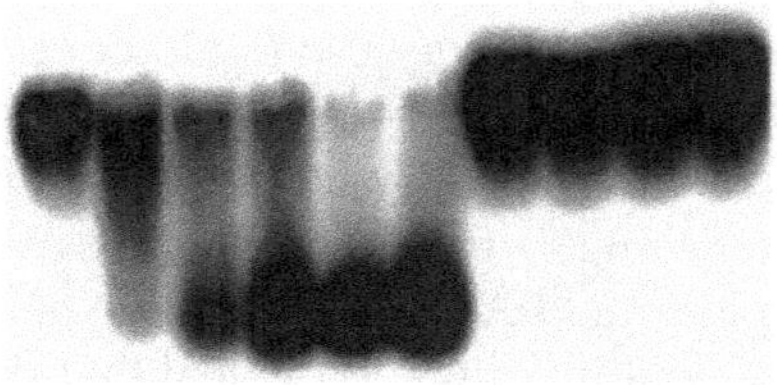

Fig. 4. NaPaC directly interacts with VEGF165. After a 1 h incubation of 125I-VEGF165 (105 c.p.m.=3 ng) with NaPaC or NaPa at 48C, the mixtures (10 ml) were electrophoretically analysed in non denaturant 1% agarose gel at pH 7.0. Lane 1 represents the migration of 125I-VEGF165 alone; lanes 2 ± 6 correspond to 0.6, 1.8, 5.5, 15 or 48 mM NaPaC; lanes 7 ± 10 represent the shifts after addition of 1.0, 5.0, 10 or 20 mM NaPa (Di Benedetto et al., 2003).

Finally, it is noteworthy that NaPa treatments at high concentrations can induce pathological effects (Thibault et al., 1994; Chang et al., 1999). The use of non-toxic new molecule, NaPaC, should limit side effects of NaPa and increase its therapeutic efficacy. In conclusion, NaPaC provides additional interesting clues in developing new anti-cancer drugs with specific triple activity: antiproliferative, aponecrotic and anti-angiogenic. The inhibition of angiogenesis is crucial for blocking tumor progression since tumor-associated high-density neovascularization is responsible for development of metastases.

3. Bisphosphonate esterifications

Bisphosphonates (BPs) have long been used in metabolic bone disease as osteoporosis, tumor-associated hypercalcaemia and metastases-induced osteolysis due to their ability to inhibit bone resorption. BPs are able to bind divalent cations like Ca^{2+} or zinc, constituting the basis of their bone-targeting property and their inhibition of the proteolytic activity of matrix metalloproteinases (MMP), respectively. The nature of their side chains gives rise to a variety of possible structures and stereochemistry determining their different potencies (Clezardin et al., 2005; Cleardin et al., 2003; Caraglia et al., 2006; Green, 2003). Non-nitrogen containing BPs (non N-BPs) act by forming non hydrolysable ATP-analogues and are less effective than nitrogen-containing BPs (N-BPs) in inhibiting bone metastasis (Roger et al., 2003). However, Zoledronate treatment of patients are reported to induce toxic side effect characterised by osteonecrosis of the jaw while non N-BP did not produce this effect (Van den Wingaert, 2006; Diel et al., 2007). N-BPs, such as zoledronate, act on the mevalonate pathway, inhibiting the farnesyl diphosphate synthase (FPP) and thereby depleting the cells of the farnesyl (FPP) or geranylgeranyl (GGPP) diphosphate isoprenoids (Roelofs et al., 2006). Isoprenoids are required for translocation and anchorage of small G proteins like Rho or Ras to the plasma membrane assuring their ultimate involvement in signal transduction during several important normal and tumor cellular pathways. However, *in vivo* efficacy of all BPs on extra-osseous sites or primary tumors is still debated. Only a small number of studies have demonstrated their *in vivo* antiproliferative activity on tumors or metastasis present in soft tissues (Stresing et al., 2007). The reasons are the poor oral bioavaibility (0.3-7% in humans) due to chelation of metal ions by phosphonic acid group inside the digestive lumen, poor membrane permeability due to poor BP lipophilicity as well as strong uptake by bone tissue (Ezra & Colomb, 2000). Previously, new strategy to overcome BP hydrophilicity is masking the phosphonic acid with organic protecting groups and introducing hydrophobic functions in the side chain (Migianu et al., 2005). An esterified BP with methyl group displays antitumor growth and antiangiogenic activities on A431 tumors, being more effective *in vivo* than *in vitro* (Ledoux et al., 2006). In order to further increase the lipophilicity of BPs (and their entering into the cells), we have synthesized new aromatic 1-hydroxymethylene-1,1-bisphosphonic acids containing phenyl or halogen phenyl ring in their side chains. Interestingly, these compounds exhibit potent antiproliferative activities *in vitro* on human epidermoid A431 cells (Guenin et al., 2005). In parallel, recently crystallographic and computational investigation reveal that the presence of phenyl ring in the side chain permitted non N-BPs to interact with farnesyl enzyme (Mao et al., 2006). Based on these data, we have synthesized a class of BPs that contains bromobenzyl in their side chains (BP7033Br, Fig. 5), as well assymmetrically esterified one of each phosphonic acids with aromatic groups (BP7033Br ALK, Fig. 5).

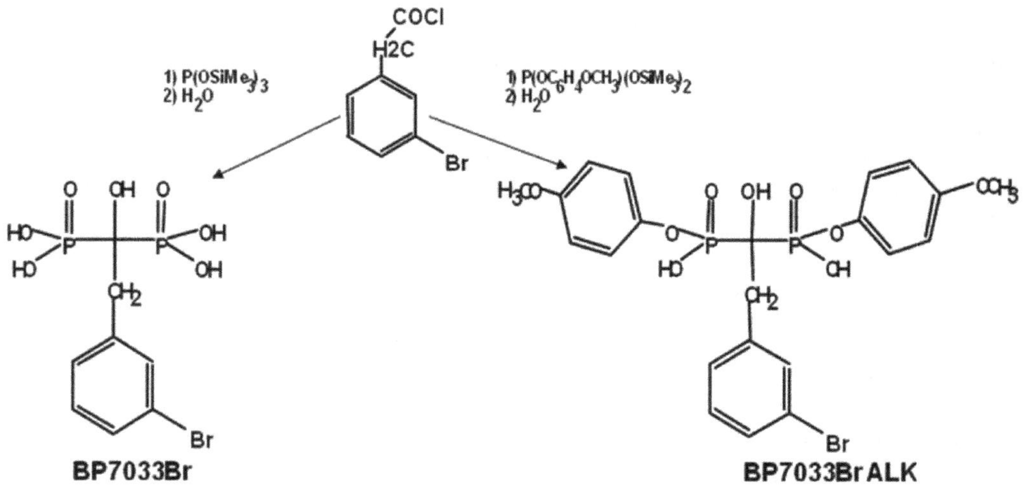

Fig. 5. Chemical structure of BP7033Br and BP7033Br ALK (Abdelkarim et al., 2009).

BPs represents an emerging class of drugs for cancer therapy and new class of non-N-BPs which exhibits higher antiproliferative activities on breast cancer cells compared to previously described non-N-BPs such as clodronate (Journe et al., 2004). Both types of m-bromobenzyl BPs inhibit the viability of several breast cancer cell lines with different estrogen-receptor statuses (Fig. 6). The esterified BP is the more effective on estrogen-responsive cells since the maximal inhibition is reached at 250 μM in contrast to non esterified BP that does not induce maximal inhibition even at 1 mM. In addition, at 250 μM, BP7033Br ALK is effective on cells independently from the estrogen-receptor status. Both types of our BP inhibits viability of estrogen non-responsive cells and particularly that of MDA-MB-231 and D3H2LN cells, the last cell line being the more aggressive ones. Indeed, it is worth to note that dramatic improvement of antiproliferative effect of non-N-BPs on breast cancer cells is reached since clodronate at the same concentration range (200 μM) and the same time-treatment (72h) do not reduce MDA-MB-231 cell viability (Fromigue et al., 2000; Monkkonene et al., 2008; Senaratne et al., 2000). In addition, clodronate demonstrates mitogenic effects via MCF7 estrogenic receptor (Journe et al., 2004) and we never observe this effect with our BPs. Based on our results, it appears also that BP7033Br ALK antiproliferative effect is estrogen-receptor-independent. The occurrence of this new effect of non-N-BPs could result from the addition of aromatic functions in the side chain. Heterocycle in the side chain is implicated in the induction of cell apoptosis by preventing the prenylation of signalling proteins such as Ras or Rho (Luckman et al., 1998). Inhibition of Ras processing using non bromo-containing BP7033 is also reached (Hamma-kourbali et al., 2003). Also, the addition of phenyl function in the side chain of BPs rendered the catalytic pocket of geranyl and/or farnesyl synthase enzymes of the mevalonate pathway more accessible (Mao et al., 2006; Steeg et al., 2006). BP7033Br ALK reduces MDA-MB-231 and D3H2LN cell viabilities about 90% with a concentration 4-fold inferior to that of BP7033Br.

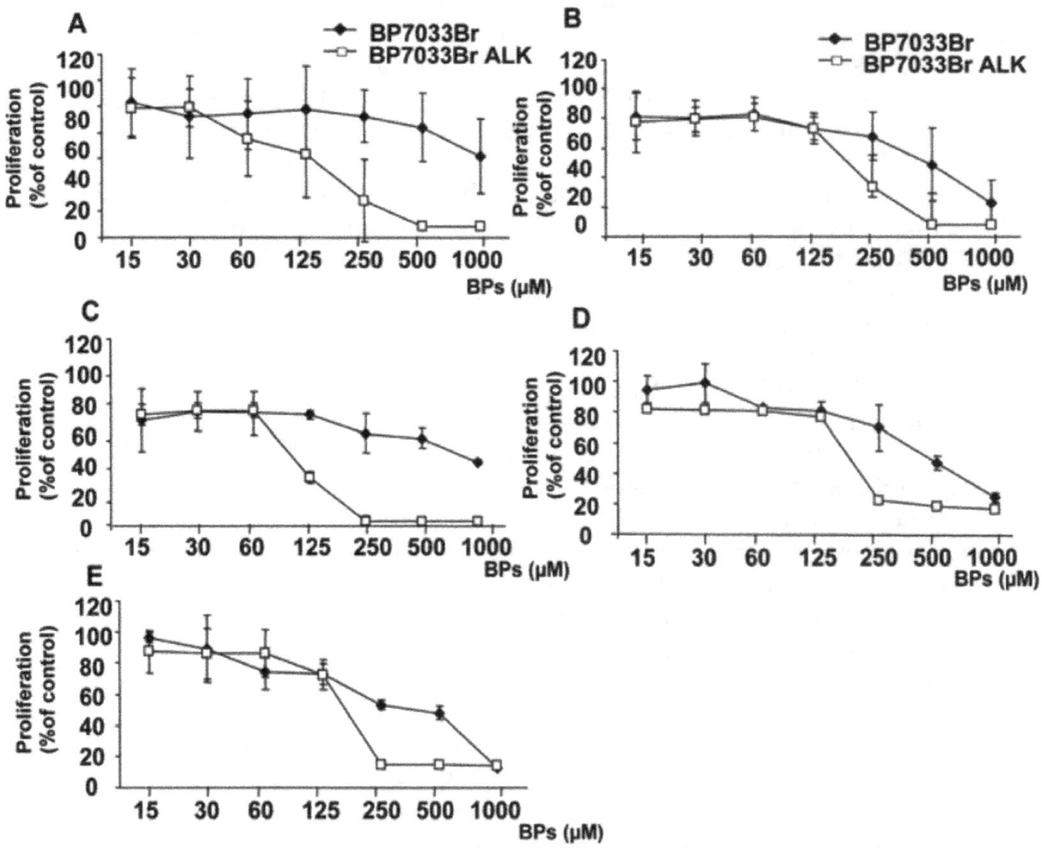

Fig. 6. BP7033Br and BP7033Br ALK inhibited viability of different breast cancer cells. T47D (A), MCF-7 (B), SKBR3 (C), MDA-MB-231 (D) or D3H2LN cells (E) ($1x10^5$) were treated with BP7033Br and BP7033Br ALK at increasing concentrations for 72h. Then, the cells were washed and incubated with 0.1 mL of MTT (2 mg/mL) for 4 h. Optical density was measured at 570 nm using a Labsystems Multiskan MS microplate reader. Data represents the mean value (± SD) of three independent experiments (Abdelkarim et al., 2009).

These data are in agreement with previous results on epidermoid A431 cell proliferation that show a beneficial effect of esterification of the phosphonic groups (Guenin et al., 2005; Ledoux et al., 2006). Our hypothesis is that such esterified compounds rendered BPs more hydrophobic increasing their cell uptake and could therefore act like prodrugs releasing active BP into the cells. In accordance, characterisation of the hydrophilicity demonstrated a shift toward lipophilicity of the BP7033Br ALK compound (Log P values of -0.75 versus -031, respectively). Alternatively, one could also hypothesize that esterified BPs have their own mechanisms since they block the cells into the S phase while non esterified BPs inhibits the G0/G1 cell phase transition. On the other hand, both type of BPs (esterified or not) induce cell death apoptosis of both MDA-MB-231 and D3H2LN cells. These results are interesting since D3H2LN cells have a greater metastatic potential than MDA-MB-231 and consequently could be more resistant to apoptosis, as it is described for metastatic cells (Wang et al., 2002; Winter et al., 2008). Both BPs induce strong D3H2LN metastatic cell apoptosis but the concentration of the esterified analogue used is 2-fold lower. Also, the two BPs inhibits migration of MDA-MB-231 cell lines with a more important effect obtained with BP7033Br ALK. In contrast, BP7033Br ALK is less effective in inhibiting D3H2LN cell lines invasion concomitant with a less important effect on MMP-9 and MMP-2 activities. BP7033Br strongly inhibits MMP-9 and MMP-2, the major form of metalloproteinases present in extracellular matrix. Since MMPs are zinc-dependent endopeptidases, we speculate that the reduction of BP7033Br ALK effect could be due to a reduction of available phosphonic acid groups able to chelate zinc and consequently inhibit MMPs. These results are in agreement with previous studies which show that MMPs inhibition activity by BPs is related to zinc chelation (Clezardin et al., 2003). However, we hypothesise that release of BP7033Br ALK with free phosphonic group could be more important in *in vivo* system because of the presence of phosphodiesterases in serum.

BPs antitumor effects have been mainly observed on D3H2LN xenografts growth and metastasis (Fig. 7). D3H2LN cells have been derived from a MDA-MB-231 subclone isolated from a lymph node metastases and induce an increased xenograft tumor growth as compared to parental cells when injected *in vivo* (Jenkins et al., 2005). Both BP7033Br and BP7033Br ALK inhibit D3H2LN tumor growth after intratumoral injection of about 286 µg BPs per mouse twice a week during 21 days. We establish that this new class of BPs is the most potent among the current non N-BPs since clodronate, even used at 1600 mg twice daily during several weeks (as compared to BP7033 ALK corresponding human dose of 770 mg twice a week during only 2 weeks) fails to reduce primary tumor growth (Winter et al., 2008). Also, BPs are 10-fold more potent than the non halogenated phenyl analogues (Sebbah-Louriki et al., 2002). In addition, BP7033Br ALK better inhibits D3H2LN vessel density than BP7033Br. This point is also supported by the large necrosis area not detected in BP7033Br treated tumors. In addition, we cannot exclude that these large necrosis areas could also be due to a greater amount of esterified BP penetrating into tumor to induce cell death. As compared to N-BPs, it is noteworthy that risedronate or ibandronate failed to inhibit MDA-MB-231 tumor growth in nude mice (Higara et al., 2001, Sasaki et al., 1995). Furthermore, no pre-clinical works demonstrate an antiproliferative effect of zoledronate on primary breast tumor growth in nude mice. The only study demonstrating an inhibition effect of zoledronate on primary tumor growth uses mesothelioma tumors which involves calcification that could uptake the drug (Wakchoure et al., 2006) In addition, the efficacy of zoledronate on bone metastasis seems to be supported by its affinity for osseous tissues rather than its direct antiproliferative effect on tumor cells (Winter et al., 2008).

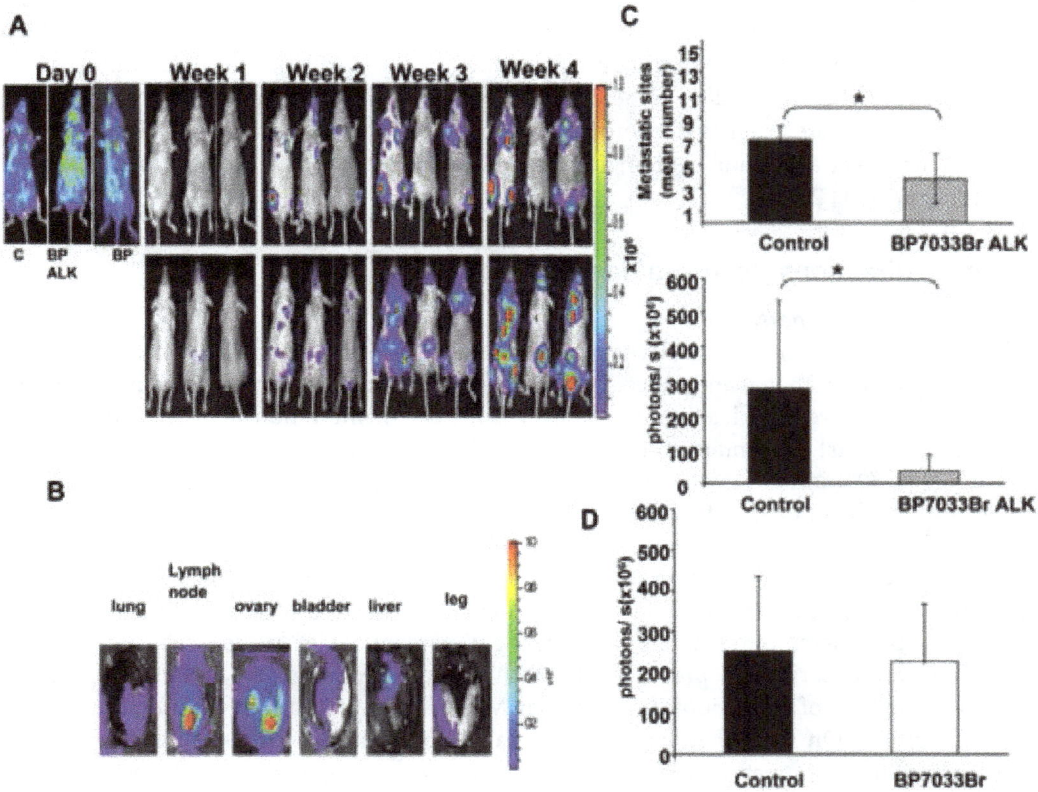

Fig. 7. Only BP7033Br ALK inhibited D3H2LN metastasis. D3H2LN cells were injected into the left ventricle of nude mice (n=7). Day 0 showed the successful intracardiac cells injection. Within 2 weeks, when metastasis were initiated, mice were treated with BP7033Br ALK or BP7033Br (A). At the indicated days, the bioluminescence images were acquired for control (c, left panel) and BPs treated mice (BP7033BrALK and BP7033Br middle and right panel, respectively). *Ex vivo* data confirm soft tissue metastasis from D3H2LN cells injection (B). Quantification of the mean metastatic sites and the photons/s after BP7033Br ALK treatment (C). Quantification the photons/s after BP7033Br treatment (D). Each column represents a mean (±SD) of three independent experiments. $*P_{\text{versus control}} < 0.05$ (Abdelkarim et al., 2009).

Also, zoledronate is a compound rapidly eliminated from plasma, resulting in renal excretion, rapid bone or calcified tissues uptake and accumulation partly due to its phosphonic functions. We have recently showed that the symmetrical esterification of the phosphonic groups may improved BPs soft tissue bioavaibility limiting osseous or calcified tissue uptake (Ref). Also, as their chemical structures are close to the apomine BP, which presents aliphatic ester group, their half-life are expected to be close to that found for this drug (156 h with micromolar plasma concentration, (Alberts et al., 2001). Thus, esterified BP7033Br ALK abrogates angiogenesis, both soft tissue and bone metastasis whereas BP7033Br does not. Noteworthy, in BP7033Br treated mice, luminescence signalling of leg osseous metastasis is not significantly reduced because 2/7 mice do not respond to the treatment in contrast to BP7033Br ALK treatment that induces significant reduction (Ref). Indeed, the esterified functions seem to be important for the BPs distribution within the systemic system and less for local injection (subcutaneous tumors) since the two N-BPs studied both inhibit D3H2LN xenograft growth. Of note, N-BPs induced osteonecrosis of treated patients (Diel et al., 2007) whereas no apparent side effects have been observed with non N-BPs. Therefore, esterified m-bromobenzyl non N-BPs constitute a new class of drugs with potent direct antitumor, antiangiogenic and antimetastatic efficacy on breast tumors (Abdelkarim et al., 2009).

4. Future directions Polynass/nanotechnologies

4.1 PolyNASS polymers

Polymers display antiproliferative, aponecrotic and anti-angiogenic effects without cytotoxicity on endothelial and cancer cells. Indeed, after 4 days of incubation, only 0,6μM of 20MA/80NaSS is required to induce 85% of cell growth inhibition of MDA-MB-231 cell growth. In contrast and interestingly, in HUVECs cells, polymers 50MA/50NaSS is more efficient with 70% inhibition achieved with 0,06μM (Fig. 8). The effect of 20MA/80NaSS on breast tumor cell is not specific only to MDA-MB-231 cells since it also inhibits other breast cancer cell lines MCF-7 (Skhiri *et al.*, 2008).The inhibition achieved with MA/NaSS polymers is comparable to that obtained in non invasive breast carcinoma cell MCF-7 (Skhiri *et al.*, 2008)and the inhibition effect varies in function of percentage of carboxylate and sufonate content in polymers. Interestingly, the strongly percentage of tumor cell proliferation inhibition was observed in presence of 20MA/80NaSS polymer. At 6μM, this polymer induces up to 80% of inhibition of the cellular MDA-MB-231cancer cell proliferation after 4 days of culture. On the other hand, at the same concentration, the polyNaSS effect on cellular proliferation was much lower (60%). Indeed, the presence of two groupings carboxylate and sufonate is necessary and plays an important role in breast cancer anti-proliferation inhibition activity. Also, it seems that similar proportion (50 MA/50 NASS) of functional subunits is rather an interesting chemical composition to obtain the optimal inhibition of endothelial cells proliferation. In addition, it seems that a strong proportion of sulfonate units in polymers is necessary for a high antiproliferative activity in cancer cells while the equal proportion of the functional groups are necessary for the endothelial cells. These results suggest that the mechanism implicated in the inhibition of the two types of cells is different. The effect of these two copolymers on HUVEC and MDA-MB231 cell cycle was also different as a decrease of cells in the S-phase and an accumulation of cells in G0/G1-phase were observed. In conclusion, these new type of polymers could lead to the development of new anti-cancer drugs with specific triple activity: antiproliferative, aponecrotic and anti-angiogenic. Since the development of resistant tumor cell clones can be a serious problem, the inhibition of angiogenesis is crucial for blocking tumour progression since tumor associated high density neovascularization is responsible for development of metastases. Therefore, polymers could be good candidate by selectively inhibiting tumor cells or endothelial cells in basis of their composition.

In addition, these kinds of molecule could be conjugated with specific drugs (copolymers) that will target genes specific to endothelial or tumors cell activities enhancing in this way, the benefit of the therapies. It is to note that in contrast to glycoaminoglycan like polymers, PolyNASS polymer synthesis is better controlled in basis of their chemical composition that is determined by titration of carboxylic groups and ^{1}H NMR.

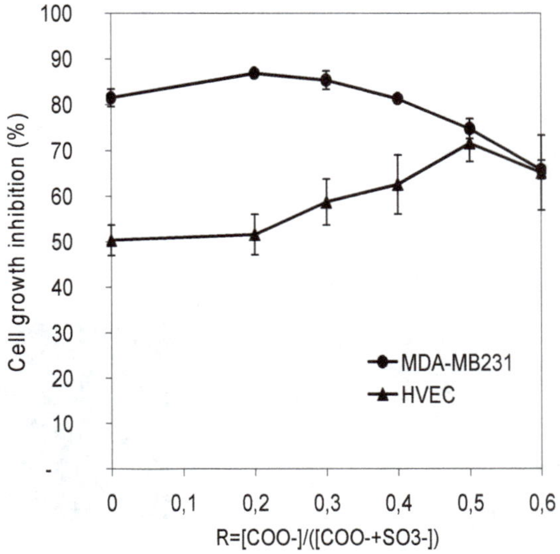

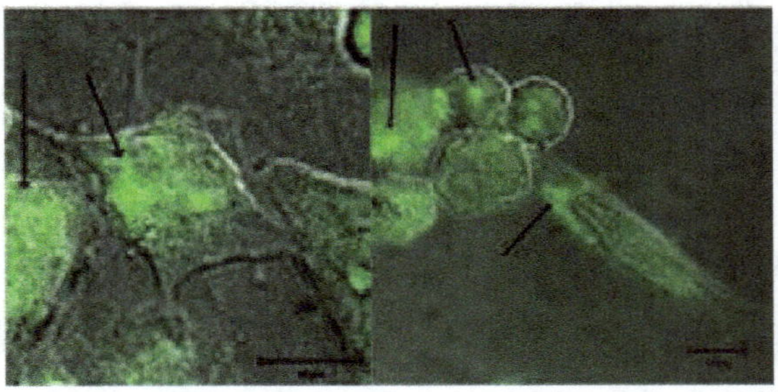

Fig. 8. Stucture-function relationship of PolyNASS copolymers and penetration into MDA-MB-231 tumor (left) and HUVEC endothelial cells (right).

4.2 Nanotechnologies

An innovative multimodal system, which combines magnetic targeting of therapeutic agents with both magnetic resonance and fluorescence imaging into one system has been recently described (Bennayou et al., 2011). This new magnetic nanoplatform consists of superparamagnetic γFe_2O_3 nanoparticles, used clinically as an MRI contrast agent, conjugated to therapeutic molecules of the hydroxylmethylene bisphosphonate family (HMBPs): alendronate with an amine function as the terminal group. *In vitro* tests with breast cancer cells show that the γFe_2O_3@alendronate hybrid nanomaterial reduces cell viability and acts as a drug delivery system. The presence of both γFe_2O_3@alendronate and a magnetic field significantly reduced the development of tumors. The amine functionalities can be used as precursor groups for the covalent coupling of peptides or monoclonal antibodies for specific biological targeting. The feasibility of this process is demonstrated by coupling rhodamine B, a fluorescence marker, to the γFe_2O_3@alendronate nanohybrid. The system shows fluorescent properties and high affinity for cells. Therefore, magnetic and fluorescent nanoparticles are potential candidates for smart drug-delivery systems. Also, the superparamagnetic behaviour of such nanoparticles may be exploited as MRI contrast agents to improve therapeutic diagnostics.

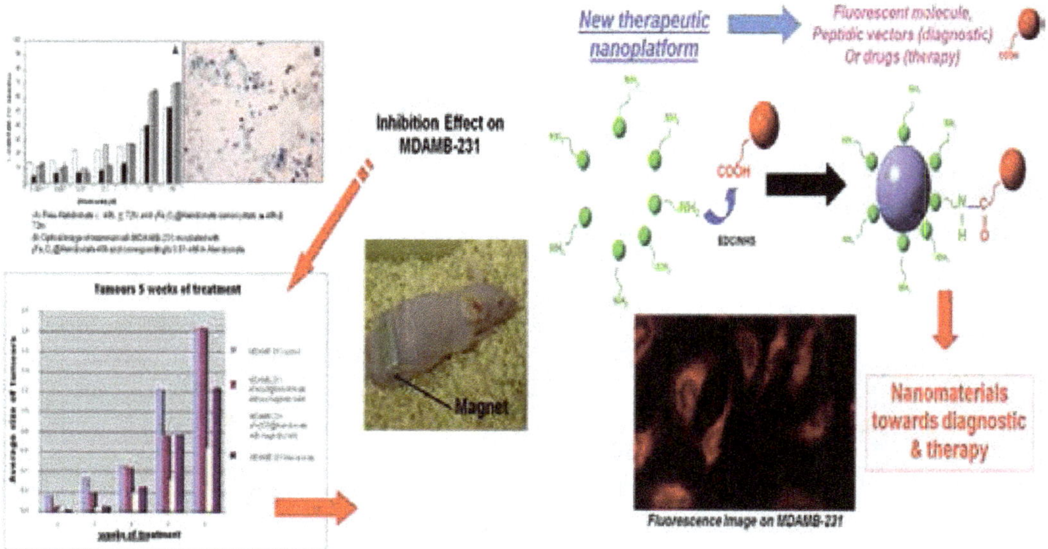

Fig. 9. Nanoplatform showing the possibility to graft BPs on superparamagnetic γFe_2O_3 nanoparticles.

5. References

Abdelkarim M, Guenin E, Sainte-Catherine O, Vintonenko N, Peyri N, Perret GY & Crepin M, Khatib AM, Lecouvey M, Di Benedetto M. (2009) *Plos one.* New symmetrically esterified m-bromobenzyl non- aminobisphosphonates inhibited breast cancer growth and metastases. 4(3):e4685.

Alberts S, Hallum AV, Stratton-Custis M, Garcia D J, Gleason-Guzman M, Salmon SE, Santabarbara P, Niesor EJ, Floret S &Bentzen CL. (2001) *Clin CancerRes.* Phase I pharmacokinetic trial and correlative in vitro phase II tumorkinetic study of apomine (SR-45023A), a novel oral biphosphonate anticancerdrug. 7: 1246–1250.

Anderson JM. (2001) *Annual Rev Mat Res.* Biological responses to materials. 31:81-110.

Bagheri-Yarmand R, Morere JF, Letouneur D, Jozefonvicz J, Israel L & Crepin M (1992) *Anticancer Res.* Inhibitory effect of dextran derivatives in vitro on the growth characteristics of premalignant and malignant human mammary epithelial cell lines. 12: 1641–1646.

Bagheri-Yarmand R, Kourbali Y, Mabilat C, Morere JF, Martin A, Lu LH, Soria C, Jozefonvicz J & Crepin M (1998a). *Br J of Cancer.* The supression of fibroblast growth factor2/fibroblast growth factor 4- dependent tumor angiogenesis and growth by the anti-growth factor activity of dextran derivative (CMDB7).78: 111–118.

Bagheri-Yarmand R, Kourbali Y, Morere JF, Jozefonvicz J & Crepin M (1998b) *Cell Growth Differ* Inhibition of MCF-7ras tumor growth by benzylamide dextran: blockage of the paracrine effect and receptor binding of transforming growth factor β1 and platelet-derived growth factor-BB. 9: 497–504.

Bagheri-Yarmand R, Kourbali Y, Rath AM, Vassy R, Martin A, Jozefonvicz J, Soria C, He L &Crépin M (1999) *Cancer Res.* Carboxymethyl benzylamide dextran blocks angiogenesis of MDA-MB 435 breast carcinoma xenografted in fad pad and its lung metastases in nude mice. 59: 507–510

Bagheri-Yarmand R, Liu JF, Ledoux D, Morere JF &Crépin M (1997) *Biochem Biophys Res Commun* Inhibition of human breast epithelial HBL 100 cell proliferation by a dextran derivative (CMDB7) with FGF2 autocrine loop. 239:424–428.

Benyettou F, Lalatonne Y, Chebbi I, Benedetto MD, Serfaty JM, Lecouvey M & MotteL. (2011) *Phys Chem Chem Phys.* A multimodal magnetic resonance imaging nanoplatform for cancer theranostics. In press

Bronzert K, Pantazis P, Antoniades HN, Kasid A, Davidson N, Dickson RB & Lippman ME (1987) *Proc. Natl. Acad. Sci.* USA.Synthesis and secretion of platelet-derived growth factor by human breast cancer cell lines. 84: 5763–5767.

Caraglia M, Santini D, Marra M, Vincenzi B, Tonini G, & Budillon A. (2006) *Endocr Relat Cancer* Emerging anti-cancer molecular mechanisms of aminobisphosphonates. 13: 7–26.

Chang SM, Kuhn JG, Robin HI, Clifford Schold S, Spence AM, Berger MS, Metha MP, Bozik ME, Pollack I, Schiff D, Gilbert M, Rankin C & Prados MD (1999) *J Clin Oncol* Phase II study of phenylacetate in patients with recurrent malignant glioma: a north American brain tumor concortium. 17: 984–990.

Clezardin P, Fournier P, Boissier S, Peyruchaud O (2003) *Curr Med Chem.* In vitro and in vivo antitumor effects of bisphosphonates. 10: 173–180.

Clezardin P, Ebetino FH, Fournier P (2005) Bisphosphonates and cancer induced bone disease: beyond their antiresorptive activity. Cancer Res 65:4971–4974

Cunha GR, Alarid ET, Turner T, Donjacour AA, Boutin EL, Foster BA (1992). *J Androl.* Normal and abnormal development of the male urogenital tract. Role of androgens, mesenchymal-epithelial interactions, and growth factors. 13(6):465-75.

Di Benedetto M, Kourbali Y, Starzec A, Vassy R, Jozefonvicz J,Perret G, Crepin M & Kraemer M. *Br. J. Cancer.* Sodium phenylacetate enhances the inhibitory effect of dextran derivative on breast cancer cell growth in vitro and in nude mice. 85 (2001) 917–923

Di Benedetto M, Starzec A, Colombo BM, Briane D, Perret GY, Kraemer M & Crépin M. Aponecrotic, antiangiogenic and antiproliferative effects of a novel dextran derivative on breast cancer growth in vitro and in vivo. Br J Pharmacol. 135(2002) 1859-71.

Di Benedetto M, Starzec A, Vassy R, Perret GY, Crépin M & Kraemer M. Inhibition of epidermoid carcinoma A431 cell growth and angiogenesis in nude mice by early and late treatment with a novel dextran derivative. Br J Cancer. 16;88 (2003) 1987-94.

Dickson RB, Kasid A, Huff KK, Bates SE, Knabbe C, Bronzert D, Gelman EP and Lippman ME (1987). *Proc Natl Acad Sci USA* Activation of growth factor secretion in tumorigenic,states of breast cancer induced by 17β estradiol or V-Ha-ras oncogene. 84: 837–841.

Diel IJ, Fogelman I, Al-Nawas B, Hoffmeister B, Migliorati C, et al. Gligorov J, Väänänen K, Pylkkänen L, Pecherstorfer M & Aapro MS. (2007) *Crit Rev Oncol Hematol.* Pathophysiology, risk factors and management of bisphosphonate-associated osteonecrosis of the jaw: Is there a diverse relationship of amino- and nonaminobisphosphonates? 64: 198–207.

Ducan R, Vicent MJ, Greco F, Nicholson RI. (2005) *Endocrine-related Cancer* Polymer-drug conjugates: towards a novel approach for the treatment of endocrine-related cancer. 12:S189-S199.

Ezra A & Golomb G (2000) *Adv Drug Deliv Rev* Administration routes and delivery systems ofbisphosphonates for the treatment of bone resorption. 42:175–195.

Ferrandina G, Melichar B, Loercher A, Verschaegen CF, Kudelka AP, Edwards CL, Scambia G, Kavanagh JJ, Abbruzzese JL & Freedman RS (1997) *Cancer Res.* Growth inhibitory effects of sodium phenylacetate (NSC 3039) on ovarian carcinoma cells in vitro. 57: 4309–4315.

Fromigue O, Lagneaux L & Body JJ (2000) *J Bone Miner Res.* Bisphosphonates induce breast cancer cell death in vitro. 15(11): 2211–2221.

Guenin E, Ledoux D, Oudar O, Lecouvey M & Kraemer M (2005) *Anticancer Res.* Structureactivity relationships of a new class of aromatic bisphosphonates that inhibit tumor cell proliferation in vitro. 25: 1139–1145.

Green JR (2003) *Cancer* Antitumor effects of bisphosphonates. 97: 840–847.

Hamma-Kourbali Y, Di Benedetto M, Ledoux D, Oudar O, Leroux Y, Lecouvey M & Kraemer M.(2003) *Biochem Biophys Res Comm.* A novel non-containing-nitrogen bisphosphonate inhibits both in vitro and in vivo angiogenesis. 310: 816–882.

Hamma-Kourbali Y, Vassy R, , Starzec A, Le Meuth-Metzinger V, Oudar O,Bagheri-Yarmand R, Perret G & Crepin M (2001). *J.Biol.Chem.* VEGF165 activities are inhibited by carboxymethyl benzylamide dextran competing for heparin binding to VEGF165 and VEGF165 : KDR complexes. 276, 39748- 39754.

Haslam SZ &Woodward TL (2001) *Breast Cancer Res.* Reciprocal regulation of extracellular matrix proteins and ovarian steroid activity in the mammary gland. 3(6):365-72.

Hiraga T, Williams PJ, Mundy GR & Yoneda T. (2001) *Cancer Res.* The bisphosphonate ibandronate promotes apoptosis in MDA-MB-231 human breast cancer cells in bone metastases.1;61(11):4418-24.

Jenkins DE, Hornig YS, Oei Y, Dusich J & Purchio T (2005) *Breast Cancer Res* Bioluminescenthuman breast cancer cell lines that permit rapid and sensitive in vivo detection of mammary tumors and multiple metastases in immune deficient mice. 7(4): 444–454.

Journe F, Chaboteaux C, Dumon J-C, Leclercq, Laurent G & Body J-J (2004) *Brit J Cancer.* Steroid-free medium discloses oestrogenic effects of bisphosphonate clodronate on breast cancer cells. 91: 1703–1710.

Knabbe C, Wakefield L, Flanders K, Kasid A, Derynck R, Lippman ME andDickson RB (1987) *Cell* Evidence that TGF β is a hormonally regulated negative growth factor in human breast cancer cell lines. 48: 417–428

Ledoux D, Hamma-Kourbali Y, Di Benedetto M, Foucault-Bertaud A, Oudar O, Sainte-Catherine O, Lecouvey M &Kraemer M. (2006) *Anti-Cancer Drugs.* A new dimethyl ester bisphosphonate inhibits angiogenesis and growth of human epidermoid carcinoma xenograft in nude mice. 17: 479–485.

Luckman SP, Hughes DE, Coxon FP, Russell GG & Rogers MJ (1998) *J Bone MinerRes* Nitrogencontaining biophosphonates inhibit the mevalonate pathway and prevent posttranslational prenylation of GTP- binding proteins, including Ras. 7(4): 581-599.

Mao J, Mukherjee S, Zhang Y, Cao R, Sanders JM, Song Y, Zhang Y, Meints GA, GaoYG, Mukkamala D, Hudock MP & Oldfield E. (2006) *J Am Chem Soc.* Solid-state NMR, crystallographic, and computational investigation of bisphosphonates and farnesyl diphosphate synthase-bisphosphonate complexes. 128:14485–14497.

Matsumura Y & Maeda H. *Cancer Res* A new concept for macromolecular therapeutics in cancer chemotherapy: mechanism of tumoritopic accumulation of proteins and the antitumour agent SMANCS. 6:6387-6392, 1986.

Migianu E, Monteil M, Even P & Lecouvey M (2005) *Nucleosides Nucleotides Nucleic Acids.* Novel approach to nucleoside-59-(1-hydroxymethylene-1, 1-bisphosphonates): synthesis of new AZT analogues. 24: 121–133.

Monkkonen H, Kuokkanen J, Holen I, Evans A, Lefley DV, Jauhiainen M, Auriola S &Mönkkönen J. (2008). *Anticancer Drugs.* Bisphosphonate-induced ATP analog formation and its effect on inhibition of cancer cell growth. 19(4): 391–399.

Noguchi Y, Wu J, Ducan R, Strohalm J, Ulbrich K, Akaike T & Maeda H. (1998) *Japanese J. Cancer Res.* Early phase tumor accumulation of macromolecules: a great difference in clearance rate between tumor and normal tissues. 89: 307-314.

Perret GY & Crepin M (2008) *Fundamental & Clinical Pharmacology.* New pharmacological strategies against metastatic spread. 5: 465-492.

Plouet J, Schilling J, & Gospodarowicz D. (1989). *EMBO J.* Isolation and characterization of a newly identifed endothelial cellmitogen produced by AtT-20 cells. 8, 373 ± 378.

Prasanna P, Thilbault A, Liu L& Samid D (1996) *Clin Cancer Res.* Lipid metabolism as a target for brain cancer therapy: synergistic activity of lovastatin and sodium phenylacetate and phenylbutyrate. 2: 865- 872.

Roelofs AJ, Thompson K, Gordon S & Rogers MJ (2006) *Clin Cancer Res* Molecular mechanisms of action of bisphosphonates: current status. 12: 6222s–6230s.

Rogers MJ (2003) *Curr Pharm Des.* New insights into the molecular mechanisms of action of bisphosphonates. 9(32): 2643–2658.

Samid D, Shack S &Myers CE (1993) *J Clin Invest.* Selective growth arrest and phenotypic reversion of prostate cancer cells in vitro by non toxic pharmalogical concentration of phenylacetate. 91: 2288–2295.

Samid D, Ram Z, Hudgins WR, Shack S, Liu L, Walbindge S, Oldfild EH & Myers CE (1994) *Cancer Res.* Selective activity of phenylacetate against malignant gliomas: ressemblance to fetal brain damage in phenylketonuria. 54: 891–895.

Samid D, Hudgins WR, Shack S, Liu L, Prasanna P & Myers CE (1997) *Adv Exp Med Biol.* Phenylacetate a nd phenylbutyrate as novel, nontoxic differenciation inducers. 400A: 501–505.

Samid D, Wells M, Greene ME, Shen W, Palmer CN & Thibault A (2000). *Clin Cancer Res.* Peroxisome proliferator-activated receptor gamma as a novel target in cancer therapy: binding and activation by an aromatic fatty acid with clinical antitumor activity. 3: 933–941.

Sasaki A, Boyce BF, Story B, Wright KR, Chapman M, Boyce R, Mundy GR 1Yoneda T.(1995) *Cancer res.* Bisphosphonate risedronate reduces metastatic human breast cancer burden in bone. 15;55(16):3551-7.

Sebbah-Louriki M, Colombo BM, el Manouni D, Martin A, Salzmann JL, Leroux Y, Perret GY & Crepin M. (2002) *Anticancer Res.* A new phenylacetate-bisphosphonate inhibits breast cancer cell growth by proapoptotic and antiangiogenic effectsin nude mice.22(6C): 3925–3931.

Senaratne SG, Pirianov G, Mansi JL, Arnett TR & Colston KW (2000) *Br J Cancer.* Bisphosphonates induce apoptosis in human breast cancer cell lines. 82(8): 1459–1468.

Seymour LW, Miyamoto Y, Brereton M, Subr V, Strohalm J & Ducan R. *European J. cancer.* Influence of molecular size of passive tumor-accumulation of soluble macromolecular drug carriers. 5:766-770, 1995.

Shekhar MP, Pauley R & Heppner G (2003) Breast Cancer Res. Host microenvironment in breast cancer development: extracellular matrix-stromal cell contribution to neoplastic phenotype of epithelial cells in the breast. 5(3):130-5.

Skhiri, L, Pavon-Djavid, G, Helary, G, Bartegi, A, & Migonney, V. *Pathologie Biologie.* New antitumor agent: In vitro activity on breast carcinoma cells,, 2008, 57, 3, Pages 9-15.

Sommers CL, Papageorge A, Wilding G & Gelmann EP (1990) *Cancer Res* Growth properties and tumorigenesis of MCF-7 cells transfected with isogenic mutants of rasH. 50: 67–71.

Spandidos DA & Agnantis NJ (1984). *Anticancer Res.* Human malignant tumors of the breast as compared to their respective normal tissue have elevated expression of the Harvey ras oncogene: 4: 269- 272.

Steeg PS (2006). *Nature Med.* Tumor metastasis: mechanistic insights and clinical challenges.12(8): 895- 904.

Stresing V, Daubine F, Benzaid I, Monkkonen H &Clezardin P (2007) *Cancer Lett.* Bisphosphonates in cancer therapy. 257 (1): 16–35.

Thibault A, Cooper MR, Figureg WD, Venzan DJ, Sartor OA, Tompkins AC, Weinberg MS, Headlee DJ, Mc Coll Na, Samid D & Myers CE (1994) *Cancer Res.* A phase I and pharmacokinetic study of intravenous phenylacetate in patients with cancer. 54: 1690–1694

Thibout D, Di Benedetto M, Kraemer M, Sainte-Catherine O, Derbin C & Crepin M (1998) *Anticancer Res* Sodium phenylacetate modulates the synthesis of autocrine and paracrine growth factors secreted by breast cancer cell lines.18: 2657–2662.

Van den Wyngaert T, Huizing MT, Vermoken JB (2006) *Ann Oncol.* Bisphosphonates and osteonecrosis of the jaw: cause and effect of a post hoc fallacy? 17:1197–1204.

Wakchoure S, Merrell MA, Aldrich W, Millender-Swain T, Harris KW, Triozzi P & Selander KS. (2006) *Clin Cancer Res.* Bisphosphonates inhibit the growth of mesothelioma cells in vitro and in vivo. 1;12(9):2862-8.

Wang W, Wyckoff JB, Frohlich VC, Oleynikov Y, Hu¨ttelmaier S, Zavadil J, Cermak L & Bottinger EP, Singer RH, White JG, Segall JE & Condeelis JS. (2002) *Cancer Res.* Single cell behaviour in metastatic primary tumors correlated with gene expression patterns revealed by molecular profiling. 62: 6278–6288.

Winter M, Holen I & Coleman RZ (2008) *Cancer Treat rev.* Exploring the anti-tumor activity of bisphosphonates in early breast cancer. 34(5): 453–75.

2

Ectopic Synthesis of Coagulation Factor VII in Breast Cancer Cells: Mechanisms, Functional Correlates, and Potential for a New Therapeutic Target

Shiro Koizume and Yohei Miyagi
Molecular Pathology & Genetics Division,
Kanagawa Cancer Center Research Institute,
Japan

1. Introduction

Recent advances in the development of therapeutic strategies have enabled the cure of a considerable amount of cases of breast cancer patients. However, breast cancer is a worldwide problem since this disease remains a common cause of cancer death in women throughout the world (Álvarez 2010). Although breast cancer can be regulated by chemotherapy, there are still difficulties with treating recurrence and triple-negative breast cancer without therapeutic molecular targets (HER2 and hormone receptors) (Foulkes et al. 2010). Therefore, it is necessary to increase the knowledge of breast cancer biology and investigate target molecules to facilitate therapeutic strategy toward aggressive breast cancers.

Hypercoagulation is a common complication of cancer patients and also correlates with mortality (Ten Cate & Falanga 2007). In fact, it has been reported that the risk of venous thromboembolism (VTE) is highest for cancers of the ovary, pancreas, liver (Iodice et al., 2008), and breast during chemotherapy (Kirwan et al. 2008).

Blood coagulation factor VII (fVII) is a key enzyme of the extrinsic coagulation cascade that is produced predominantly by hepatocytes (Furie & Furie 1988). Tissue factor (TF) is a 47-kD transmembrane glycoprotein and a cellular receptor of fVII. Blood coagulation factor VII from blood plasma bound to TF is converted to its active form (fVIIa) and activates a downstream extrinsic coagulation cascade, leading to fibrin deposition (Fig. 1).

It has been reported that plasma TF levels are higher in cancer patients including advanced breast cancer (Ueno et al. 2000). Furthermore, breast cancer cells secrete cell membrane-derived microvesicles containing TF antigen under pathological conditions, resulting in coagulation activation (Davila et al. 2008). Therefore, TF-fVIIa formation can be a major cause of thromboembolic disease.

A number of studies have demonstrated that tissue factor-fVIIa complex formation on the cell surface also initiates key pathogenic events including activation of cell motility, invasiveness, cell survival, and angiogenesis (Milsom & Rak 2009). Recently, growing experimental evidence has also suggested that TF contributes to tumor initiation (Milsom & Rak 2009). Given that fVII presents on the invasive edge of various cancer tissues (Fischer et al. 1999;

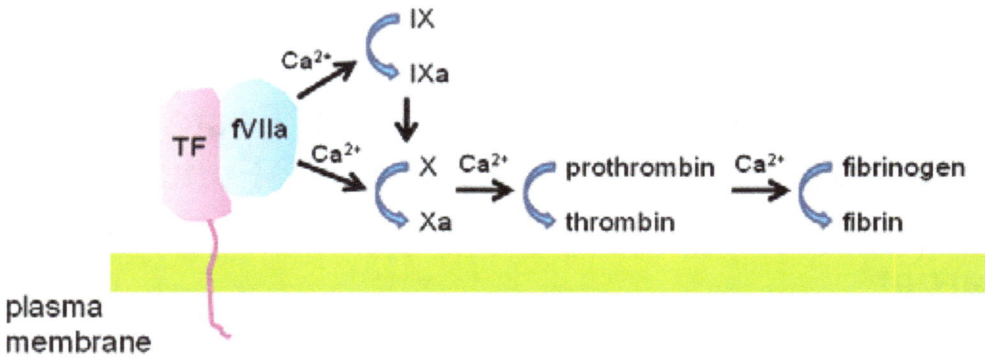

Fig. 1. Extrinsic coagulation cascade initiated by TF-fVIIa complex formation.
TF-fVIIa complex formation on the cell surface triggers an extrinsic coagulation cascade. TF-fVIIa initiates coagulation by activating factor X, resulting in fibrin deposition *via* formation of thrombin. The mechanism of mediation *via* factor IX activation is also possible.

Zacharski et al. 1993), this suggests that TF-fVIIa complex formation may play a critical role in malignant phenotype expression of clinical tumors. Therefore, anti-TF strategy may be applicable to breast cancer although a probable side effect of bleeding should be considered. Blood plasma has been considered to be a predominant source of fVII present on cancer cell surfaces since most plasma proteins including fVII are produced in the liver. Blood coagulation factor VII is believed to penetrate through hyperpermeabilized blood vessels around tumor tissues (McDonald & Baluk 2002), and then associate with the integral membrane protein TF of cancer cells. However, various cancer cells can ectopically synthesize fVII (Koizume et al. 2006). Notably, breast cancer cells were found to constitutively and highly express fVII mRNA by RT-PCR analysis. Further, functional fVII exists as a complex with TF on the cell surface (Koizume et al. 2006). Unsurprisingly, fVII mRNA expression is frequently found in surgical specimens of breast cancer (Koizume et al. 2009), suggesting that fVII is synthesized in cancer tissues of patients and that ectopic fVII synthesis may play an important role in the biology of breast cancer. Therefore, inhibition of ectopic fVII synthesis without affecting fVII secreted from the liver may be a useful therapeutic approach for breast cancer patients. In this chapter, recent progress in breast cancer biology associated with TF-fVIIa signaling and in the biology of ectopic synthesis of fVII in breast cancer cells will be summarized. In addition to descriptions based on previously published data, new data mainly concerning cell growth accelerating characteristics of ectopic fVII in breast cancer cells will be presented. Finally, potential future therapeutic strategies of breast cancer targeting ectopic fVII will be discussed. Recently a target molecule specifically associated with the ectopically active *FVII* gene promoter but not with the *FVII* promoter in hepatocytes (Koizume et al. 2009) was found. Therefore, ectopic fVII synthesis can be selectively blocked without disturbing the normal haemostatic process.

2. Biology of TF-fVIIa signaling in breast cancer cells

Considerable progress has been made towards understanding of how cancer cells depend on TF-fVIIa complex formation to express their malignant phenotypes (Milsom & Rak 2009;

Mackman & Taubman 2009; Schaffner & Ruf 2009). To date, a number of studies concerning TF-fVIIa signaling have been performed using breast cancer cell lines such as MDA-MB-231, MCF-7, and BT549, possibly because they express relatively high levels of TF, and their phenotypes such as motility and invasiveness are TF-dependent (Jiang et al. 2008; Morris et al. 2006). Among these cell lines, MDA-MB-231 synthesizes a considerable amount of TF and is a frequently used cell line as a good TF-dependent breast cancer model. Its characteristics such as motility, invasiveness, and growth are highly TF-dependent in response to fVII *in vitro* (Hjortoe et al. 2004; Jiang et al. 2004; Morris et al. 2006) and *in vivo* (Versteeg et al. 2008a & b).

TF-fVIIa signaling mechanisms potentially resulting in breast cancer phenotypes can be classified into three categories. The first is signaling mediated by TF-fVIIa binary complex formation. Various experimental evidence has suggested that activation of a G protein-coupled receptor, protease activated receptor 2 (PAR2) rather than PAR1 by the TF-fVIIa complex plays a crucial role in phenotypic expression of breast cancer cells through activation of the mitogen-activated protein kinase cascade (Hjortoe et al. 2004; Morris et al. 2006; Versteeg et al. 2008a). Second, TF-fVIIa signaling could involve coagulation factor X (fX) to transmit signals. The TF-fVIIa complex may further interact with fX to produce the TF-fVIIa-fXa ternary complex (Jiang et al. 2004). Breast cancer phenotypes mediated *via* TF-fVIIa-fXa complex formation may not only cause PAR2 signaling but also activate PAR1 to initiate thrombin signaling. This ternary complex may also activate the mTOR pathway in breast cancer cells (Jiang et al. 2008). Third, the G protein–independent pathway of PAR2 signaling is also possible in breast cancer cells (Schaffner et al. 2010). PAR2 recruits a scaffold protein, β-arrestin, to support extracellular signal-regulated kinase signaling to enhance cell motility. In any case, TF-fVIIa signaling may eventually enhance expression of downstream effectors, such as IL-8 (Hjortoe et al. 2004), Cyr61 (Pendurthi et al. 2000), CTGF (Pendurthi et al. 2000), VEGF (Liu & Mueller 2006), CXCL1 (Albrektsen et al. 2007; Versteeg et al. 2008b), Birc3 (Albrektsen et al. 2007), CUX1 (Wilson et al. 2009), and CSF (Albrektsen et al. 2007), which then contribute to malignant phenotype expression of breast cancers.

While phenotypes regulated by TF-fVIIa formation seem dependent on PAR2 signaling, breast cancer cells could augment invasiveness and tumorigenesis by PAR1 signaling (Booden et al. 2004). PAR1 is a thrombin receptor that is highly expressed in invasive breast cancer cells. Treatment of breast cancer cells with thrombin increases cellular invasion in a PAR1-dependent manner. On the other hand, PAR1 can be a receptor of matrix metalloprotease-1 secreted from stromal cells and it enhances invasiveness and tumorigenesis of MDA-MB-231 cells (Boire et al. 2005). Therefore, it is likely that the relative importance of PAR1 and PAR2 signaling in breast cancer progression is dependent on the tumor microenvironment.

Characteristics of breast cancer cells might be influenced by exogenous TF in patients. Recent *in vitro* experiments revealed that growth and metastatic properties of breast cancer cells can also be affected by TF in a paracrine manner (Collier et al. 2008). Treatment with recombinant TF mimicking stroma-derived TF enables breast cancer cells to be more invasive and proliferative *via* activation of β1-integrins and/or PAR2 signaling cascades, followed by down-regulation of estrogen receptor gene expression.

3. Expression of TF in breast cancer tissues

3.1 Expression of TF activity in breast cancer tissues

Immunohistochemical analyses have revealed that breast cancer tissues as well as ovarian and pancreatic cancer tissues highly express TF (Contrino et al. 1996; Ueno et al. 2000).

Although the mechanisms of this overexpression have not been clearly defined, transcriptional up-regulation appears to be a major cause of this aberrant expression. Mechanisms of transcriptional regulation of the TF gene (*F3*) have been well characterized (Mackman 1995). Basal *F3* gene expression is known to be regulated by various transcription factors such as Sp1, AP-1, and NFκB. Given that AP-1 and NFκB are major factors activated in breast cancer (Benz & Yau 2008), it is likely that aberrant activation of these factors is associated with higher TF levels. Indeed, it has been reported that the *F3* gene promoter is highly occupied by these transcription factors in MDA-MB-231 cells, whereas the promoter is weakly bound in TF low-expressing MCF-7 cells (Zhou et al. 1998).

Inducible expression of the *F3* gene is another plausible cause of high TF expression in cancer tissues. Expression of TF is known to be affected by various environmental stimuli such as exposure to cytokines, growth factors, and hypoxia (Milsom & Rak 2009), leading to activation of AP-1 and NFκB. Therefore, expression levels of TF can be varied depending on the tumor microenvironment. Besides environmental factors, expression of TF is also affected by oncogenic events such as activation of ras, p53, PTEN, and EGFR (Milsom & Rak 2009). Expression of the *F3* gene can be up-regulated through signaling cascade downstream of these effectors.

The transcription factor Egr-1 is also known to play a major role in inducible TF expression (Mackman 1995). Briefly, Sp1 mainly contributes to basal up-regulation of *F3* transcription. However, once cells are stimulated with various factors associated with the cellular microenvironment, expression of Egr-1 is induced in cancer cells. Since Egr-1 shares DNA binding sites with Sp1, it could thus substitute Sp1 binding within the promoter region to enhance TF transcription under pathological conditions.

Post transcriptional regulation may also determine TF expression or activity level in breast cancer cells. A major mechanism is inhibition by tissue factor pathway inhibitor (TFPI), directly inhibiting serine protease activity of TF-fVIIa (Milsom & Rak 2009). Indeed, it was recently reported that breast cancer tissues highly express TFPI (Sierko et al. 2010). In addition, TFPI may augment cell adhesion (Fischer et al. 1999) and invasiveness (Sierko et al. 2010) through interaction with the TF-fVIIa complex. Another post-transcriptional mechanism is functional modification by conformational change. Procoagulant activity of TF can be regulated by conformational change called encryption/decryption, possibly mediated *via* multiple mechanisms (Bach 2006). However, recent studies using MDA-MB-231 cell suggested that de-encryption of TF is caused *via* interaction with anionic phospholipids rather than intra-molecular disulfide exchange (Pendurthi et al. 2007). Only decrypted TF can exert its procoagulant activity, while encrypted TF still has the ability to transmit signals. It was recently found that a microRNA (miR-19) could bind to 3′-UTR of the TF transcript to repress translation in breast cancer cells (Zhang et al. 2010). This study showed that miR-19 is abundant in a TF low-expressing breast cancer cell line, MCF-7, suggesting that regulation by this microRNA may be a determinant of TF levels in breast cancer tissues.

In addition to cell surface expression, breast cancer cells can secrete TF as microparticles derived from cell membrane fragments in response to various stimuli *in vitro* and *in vivo* (Tilley et al. 2008; Davila et al. 2008); therefore, this circulating TF may increase the risk of thrombosis in patients. Further, besides expression in tumor parenchyma cells, tumor stroma produces TF to promote breast cancer metastasis (Vrana et al. 1996). Growth factors secreted from breast cancer cells may stimulate stromal cells to produce TF, resulting in breast cancer progression.

3.2 Relationship between TF expression and clinical outcome of breast cancer patients

Activation of platelets (Kirwan et al. 2008) and elevation of plasma TF levels (Davila et al. 2008) are candidate determinants for the development of thrombosis in cancer patients. Indeed, VTE post chemotherapy is relatively frequent for breast cancer patients, and therefore, the relationship between haemostatic markers and thrombosis was investigated (Kirwan et al. 2008). This study showed that plasma TF levels of patients were significantly higher than those of non-cancer controls, but they were not elevated in response to chemotherapy, suggesting that chemotherapy-induced VTE is due to TF-independent mechanisms.

On the other hand, analysis with clinical samples revealed that TF is highly expressed in breast cancer patients. It has been reported that TF is expressed in vascular endothelial cells in invasive breast cancer tissues, suggesting that TF may be a marker for angiogenic phenotypes of breast cancer (Contrino et al. 1996). As well as tissue expression including stromal, vascular endothelial, and monocytic expression, TF levels are elevated in plasma of breast cancer patients. Although it was found that there was no difference in plasma TF levels between normal and benign tumors, primary and recurrent cancer patients showed significantly higher TF levels (Ueno et al. 2000). These expression patterns of TF are correlated with those in tissue samples. These TF levels are associated with tumor grade and can be an independent prognostic indicator. Further, TF levels in urine of breast cancer patients also correlate with disease malignancy (Lwaleed et al. 1999), suggesting that measurement of TF expression has some clinical advantages.

Although molecular mechanisms linking TF levels and cancer phenotypes can be explained by multiple cellular events downstream of TF-fVIIa signaling pathways, recent immunohistochemical analyses have revealed that phosphorylation of the cytoplasmic domain of TF correlates with expression levels of TF and other proteins known to be associated with recurrence and aggressive phenotypes of breast cancers (Rydén et al. 2010). This study showed that TF phosphorylation associated with PAR2 expression correlates with recurrence in breast cancer patients. A recent *in vivo* study by the same group showed that the cytoplasmic domain of TF cooperates with PAR2 to promote breast cancer development through modulating the angiogenic response (Schaffner et al. 2010), providing a rationale for the observed clinical association.

4. Ectopic expression of coagulation factor VII in breast cancer cells

Although the major source of fVII is the liver under normal conditions, various cancer cells could ectopically synthesize fVII (Koizume et al. 2006). Notably, breast cancer cell lines, such as YMB-1, MDA-MB-453, and MCF-7, constitutively and highly express fVII mRNA as shown by RT-PCR analysis (Koizume et al. 2006). Recently, we additionally found by real-time RT-PCR analysis that a breast cancer cell line, T47D, highly expresses fVII, and its mRNA level is comparable with that of YMB-1 (data not shown). Cancer cells that express fVII exhibit fXa-generating activity depending on TF-fVIIa complex formation, suggesting that ectopically synthesized fVII is functional and may play an important role in the progression of breast cancer. As mentioned above, fVII expression is frequent in surgical specimens of breast cancer by RT-PCR and immunohistochemical analyses (Koizume et al. 2009).

4.1 Mechanism of constitutive fVII synthesis in breast cancer cells

Transcript levels of fVII are higher in breast cancer cells, and therefore, it was examined whether the *FVII* gene is activated in breast cancer cells. It is known that binding of a transcription factor, HNF-4 is crucial for *FVII* gene activation in hepatocytes. However, HNF-4 is not responsible for *FVII* expression in breast cancer cells as shown by immunoblotting and chromatin immunoprecipitation (ChIP) analyses (Koizume et al. 2009). Reporter gene analysis showed that the authentic *FVII* promoter region could fully activate reporter activity in breast cancer cells. As expected, deletion of the HNF-4 binding site from the *FVII* promoter construct showed that reporter activity is not significantly impaired, further supporting the idea that HNF-4 is dispensable for ectopic *FVII* expression. Further, analysis with a reporter construct without a Sp1 transcription factor binding site showed a marked decrease in promoter activity in breast cancer cells (Koizume et al. 2009). These results indicate that Sp1 binding to the promoter region is essential for constitutive *FVII* activation in breast cancer cells.

Histone acetylation within the gene promoter region is a crucial step for transcriptional activation, and therefore, epigenetic factors responsible for ectopic *FVII* expression were further explored (Koizume et al. 2009). Histone acetyltransferases (HATs) associated with the *FVII* promoter in breast cancer cells were examined. ChIP analysis revealed that major HATs, p300 and CBP are associated with the *FVII* promoter region in breast cancer cells. On the other hand, other HATs, PCAF and SRC-1, can also interact with the hepatocytic *FVII* promoter. Notably, the *FVII* promoter in HepG2 cells is devoid of p300 and CBP. ChIP analysis showed that histone H4 is hyperacetylated within the active *FVII* promoter in various cells, suggesting that p300 and CBP may be responsible for histone acetylation within the *FVII* promoter region in breast cancer cells, although various HATs can contribute to the acetylation in hepatocytes.

fVII production in hepatocellular carcinoma and breast cancer cells was detected by western blotting and colorimetric analysis (Koizume et al. 2009). Unlike hepatocytes, fVII synthesized in YMB-1 cells is not secreted into culture media, suggesting that ectopically synthesized fVII is involved in TF-fVIIa complex formation on the cell surface in an autocrine manner.

4.2 Induction of fVII expression in breast cancer cells under hypoxic conditions

FVII transcription is inducible under hypoxia and hypoxia mimetic ($CoCl_2$ treatment) conditions depending on the cell type (Koizume et al. 2006). To date, several cell lines have been found to express the fVII transcript in response to hypoxia. As ovarian cancer cells tend to express fVII in response to hypoxia (Koizume et al. 2006; Yokota et al. 2009), it was next tested whether breast cancer cell lines inducibly express fVII mRNA under hypoxic conditions. It was revealed that cell lines with high fVII expression, such as YMB-1 and MDA-MB-453, do not enhance fVII transcript levels in response to hypoxic stimuli (Koizume et al. 2009). However, we recently found that fVII mRNA is inducible in MDA-MB-468 cells under $CoCl_2$ treatment conditions (Fig. 2A), suggesting that induction of fVII in breast cancer cells is cell-type dependent.

Detailed mechanisms of this hypoxic induction have not been defined yet. However, it is likely that a hypoxia inducible factor, HIF-2α, may contribute to the activation. Chromatin immunoprecipitation analysis revealed that although both HIF-1α and HIF-2α are inducible under hypoxia-mimetic conditions (Fig. 2B), HIF-2α predominantly binds to the *FVII* promoter region in MDA-MB-468 cells (Fig. 2C), as in the case of OVSAYO cells (Koizume et al. 2006).

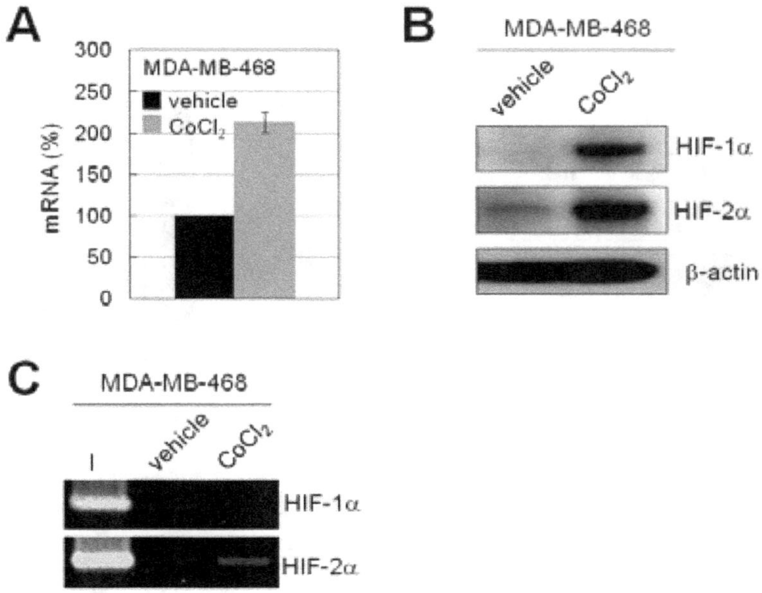

Fig. 2. Induction of the fVII transcript in MDA-MB-468 cells.
(A) *FVII* activation in MDA-MB-468 cells treated with $CoCl_2$. Cells were cultured for 4 hours in the presence or absence of 500 μM $CoCl_2$, and then fVII mRNA levels were analyzed by real-time RT-PCR analysis. *Columns*, mean (n = 2); *bars*, SD. (B) Western blotting analysis of HIF expression in MDA-MB-468 cells cultured with or without 500 μM $CoCl_2$ for 4 hours. (C) Chromatin immunoprecipitation (ChIP) analysis of HIFs binding to the *FVII* promoter in MDA-MB-468 cells. Cells were cultured in the presence or absence of 500 μM $CoCl_2$ for 4 hours, and then subjected to ChIP analysis. I indicates input sonicated DNA fragments without immunoprecipitation.

Notably, unlike typical transcriptional activation mechanisms by HIFs (Majmundar et al. 2010), the promoter region bound by HIF-2α is devoid of the hypoxia responsible element (Koizume et al. 2006), and therefore, novel mechanisms of transcriptional regulation may contribute to *FVII* activation under hypoxia.

5. Ectopically expressed fVII can enhance proliferation of breast cancer cells

As in the case of exogenous fVII treatment of cancer cells, ectopically expressed fVII augments motility and invasiveness of breast cancer cells, MDA-MB-453, as well as ovarian cancer cells, OVSAYO (Koizume et al. 2006). Growth and development of some breast tumors are dependent on TF-fVIIa formation, followed by activation of PAR2 signaling (Versteeg et al. 2008a & b). This is characteristic of *in vivo* conditions since TF expression does not contribute to cell growth in monolayer culture (Yu et al. 2005; Versteeg et al. 2008a). These results may simply be due to the absence of fVII in culture media and/or reflect the importance of host components of the tumor microenvironment (Jessani et al. 2004). Therefore, we tested whether proliferation of breast cancer cells *in vitro* is affected by ectopic fVII synthesis. The cell lines YMB-1 and MDA-MB-453 were selected for this purpose since these cells highly express fVII mRNA (Koizume et al. 2006).

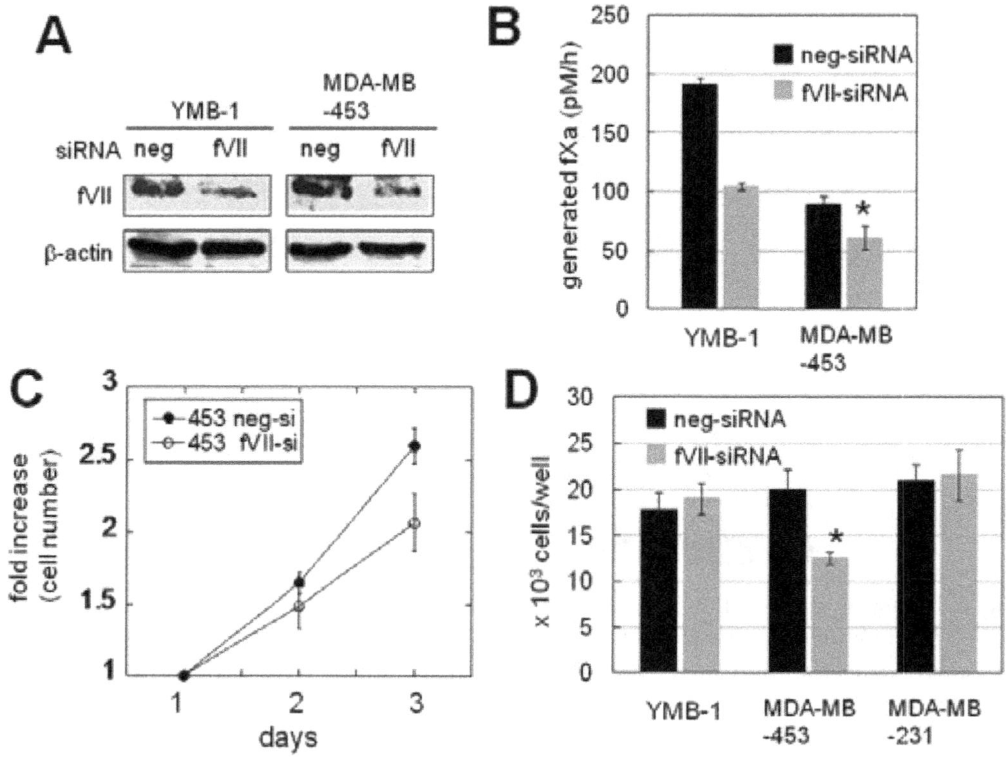

Fig. 3. Blood coagulation factor VII contributes to cell proliferation of MDA-MB-453 cells. (A) Knockdown of fVII expressed in YMB-1 and MDA-MB-453 cells. Cells were transfected with negative control- or fVII-siRNA. After 43 hours of transfection, whole cell lysates were analyzed by immunoblotting. (B) fXa generation analysis of breast cancer cells transfected with siRNA of fVII. Forty-three hours post transfection, cells were examined for fXa generation activity. *Columns*, mean (n = 3); *bars*, SD. *$P < 0.05$ (two-sided Student's t test). (C, D) Cell proliferation analysis of fVII-expressing (YMB-1 and MDA-MB-453) and non-expressing (MDA-MB-231) breast cancer cells after transfection of negative control- or fVII-siRNA. *Columns*, mean (n = 3); *bars*, SD. *$P < 0.05$ (two-sided Student's t test).

Expression of fVII in YMB-1 and MDA-MB-453 cells is suppressed by small interference RNA (siRNA) transfection, resulting in reduction of protein levels (Fig. 3A) and cell surface procoagulant activity (Fig. 3B). After 24 hours post transfection, monitoring of cell growth was obtained by colorimetric assay. Growth of MDA-MB-453 cells was considerably diminished by fVII suppression (Fig. 3C and D). On the other hand, proliferation of YMB-1 cells was not affected after 3 days post transfection (Fig. 3D). As expected, proliferation of MDA-MB-231 cells without fVII expression was not affected by siRNA transfection (Fig. 3D), suggesting that fVII can enhance breast cancer cell proliferation, but the effect is cell-type dependent. Western blotting of hormone receptors (Koizume et al. 2009) and fluorescent *in situ* hybridization analysis of *ERBB2* amplification showed that YMB-1 cells correspond to the "triple negative" molecular subtype, although MDA-MB-453 cells are HER-2 positive (data not shown).

To test whether triple-negative breast cancer cells are unresponsive to ectopically synthesized fVII to activate cell proliferation, we next tested the effect of forced fVII expression on proliferation of other triple-negative breast cancer cells.

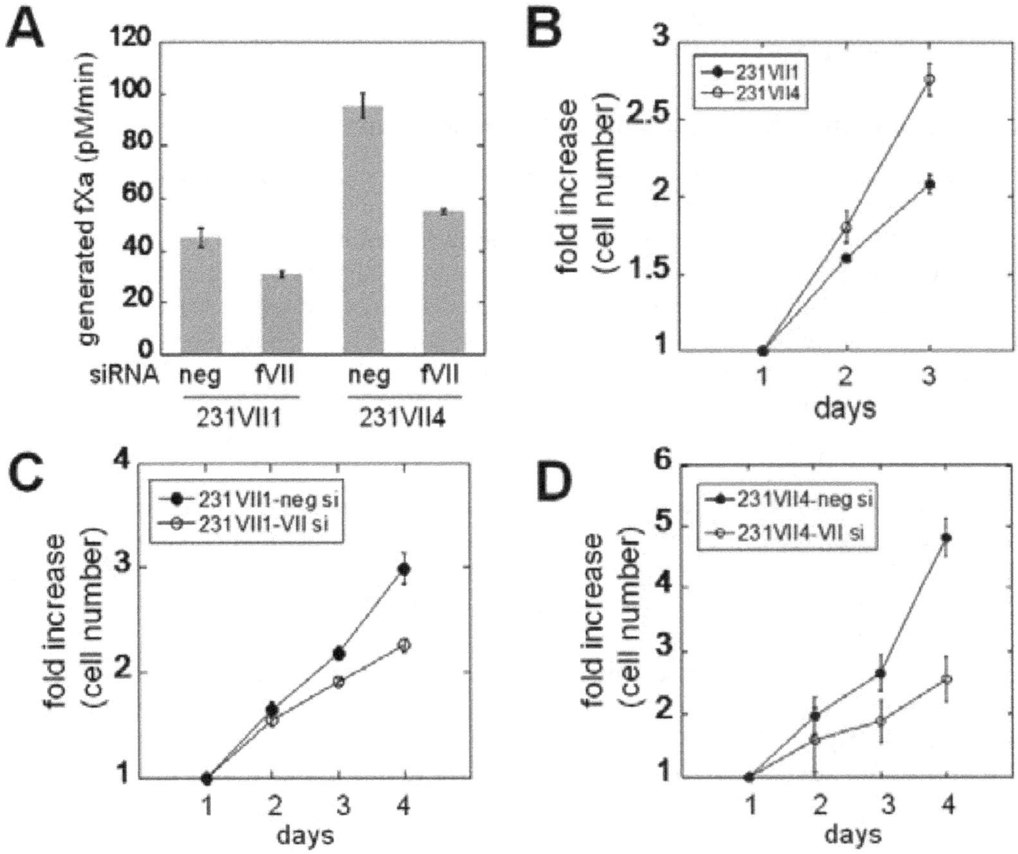

Fig. 4. Effect of fVII overexpression on proliferation of MDA-MB-231 cells.
(A) Procoagulant activity of fVII in MDA-MB-231 cells transfected with fVII. Cloned cells (231VII1 and 231 VII4) constitutively overexpressing fVII were transfected with negative control- or fVII-siRNA and then, examined for fXa generation activity. *Columns*, mean (n = 2); *bars*, SD. (B) Cell proliferation analysis of fVII-expressing cells with different procoagulant activity shown in (A). *Columns*, mean (n = 3); *bars*, SD. (C) Effect of fVII suppression on cell proliferation of 231VII1 cells. After 24 hours of fVII- or negative control-siRNA transfection, cells were examined for proliferation activity. *Columns*, mean (n = 3); *bars*, SD. (D) Effect of fVII suppression on cell proliferation of 231VII4 cells. After 24 hours of fVII- or negative control- siRNA transfection, cells were examined for proliferation activity. *Columns*, mean (n = 3); *bars*, SD.

MDA-MB-231 cell was used for experiments since this cell line without fVII expression highly expresses TF and its growth *in vivo* is dependent on TF-fVIIa signaling (Versteeg et al. 2008a & b). Cell clones stably expressing fVII were prepared and fVII expression levels were analyzed by western blotting (data not shown) and fXa generation assay (Fig. 4A). Two cell clones with variation in fVII expression levels (Fig. 4A) were selected. Cell proliferation assay with these cells showed that the higher fVII is expressed, the faster breast cancer cells proliferate (Fig. 4B). Suppression of fVII synthesis by RNAi restored cell proliferation efficiency (Fig. 4C & D), while it did not affect proliferation of parental MDA-MB-231 cells (Fig. 3D). These results show that ectopically expressed fVII can accelerate proliferation of triple-negative breast cancer cells.

6. Strategy to inhibit ectopic fVII synthesis in breast cancer cells

6.1 Inhibition of ectopic fVII synthesis in breast cancer cells by curcumin

The expression of fVII may contribute to breast cancer metastasis and growth. Therefore, targeting fVII expression may be therapeutically beneficial if ectopic fVII could be specifically inhibited without precluding function of fVII secreted from the liver. We showed that the ectopically activated *FVII* promoter is associated with p300 and CBP, while the *FVII* promoter in hepatocytes can be bound by various HATs, suggesting that targeting p300 and CBP activities may fulfil selective inhibition (Koizume et al. 2009). To date, curcumin, a component of spice turmeric, is the only known compound to selectively block p300/CBP HAT activity. Therefore, the effect of this small compound on ectopic *FVII* expression in breast cancer cells was tested (Koizume et al. 2009). The breast cancer cells YMB-1 and MDA-MB-453 were cultured in the presence of curcumin, and then fVII mRNA levels were analyzed by real-time RT-PCR analysis. It was found that curcumin markedly reduced fVII transcript levels in these cells in a dose-dependent manner, while normal expression of *FVII* in hepatic cells was only weakly impaired (Koizume et al. 2009). Additionally, TF mRNA was not significantly diminished by the same curcumin concentrations in these cells. Furthermore, anacardic acid, another natural small compound inhibitor for p300 and PCAF, did not selectively inhibit ectopic *FVII* expression, suggesting that curcumin targets p300/CBP activity (Koizume et al. 2009). The effect of curcumin on *FVII* expression was further examined at the protein level and it was confirmed that curcumin selectively inhibits ectopic fVII synthesis, consistent with the results of mRNA analysis. However, HAT activity associated with the *FVII* promoter in hepatocytes including p300 and CBP is heterogeneous. Furthermore, we showed selective blockade of ectopic fVII synthesis using a limited number of cell lines; therefore it is possible that hepatocytic fVII synthesis can be considerably impaired by curcumin if p300/CBP is a major coactivator of the *FVII* gene.

We tested whether curcumin treatment inhibits proliferation of fVII-expressing breast cancer cells. YMB-1 and MDA-MB-453 cells were cultured in the presence of curcumin as in the case of transcript analysis, and then cell proliferation was evaluated. As in the case of siRNA experiments, it was found that growth of YMB-1 was not reduced (data not shown) but proliferation of MDA-MB-453 cells was significantly impaired (~50% inhibition after 3 days post curcumin addition). We further tested whether the pro-proliferation effect of ectopic fVII is dependent on TF-fVIIa formation on the cell surface. MDA-MB-453 cells were then cultured with anti-TF (5G9 or 10H10) antibody or negative control IgG. Cell proliferation after antibody addition was analyzed by colorimetric assay. We found that treatment of cells with these antibodies did not affect cell proliferation (Fig. 5A).

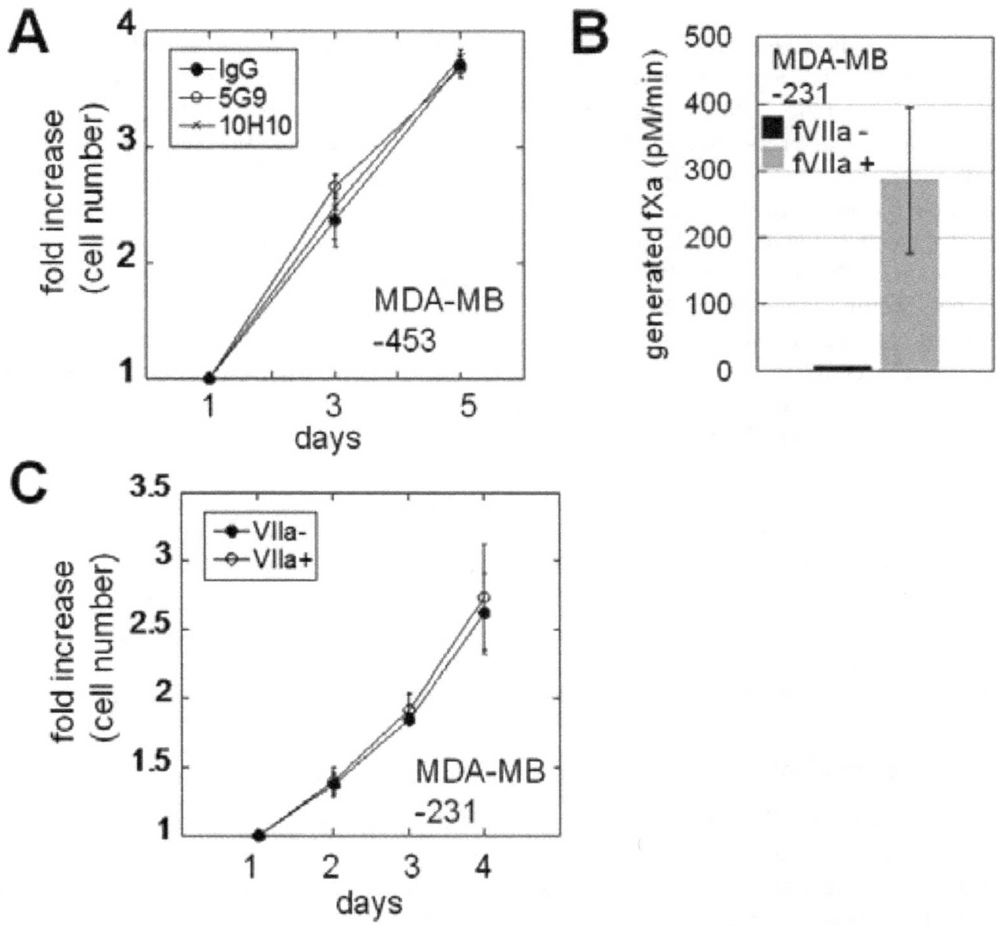

Fig. 5. Effect of TF-fVIIa formation on proliferation of breast cancer cells.
(A) Cell proliferation analysis of MDA-MB-453 cells treated with anti-TF antibodies. Cells had 50 μg/ml of IgG, Mab-5G9, or Mab-10H10 added, and then viable cells were monitored by colorimetric assay. *Columns*, mean (n = 3); *bars*, SD. (B) fXa generation analysis of MDA-MB-231 cells treated with fVIIa. After 1 hour post addition of 10 nM fVIIa, cells were washed twice and then fXa-generating activity due to TF-fVIIa formation on the cell surface was examined by colorimetric assay. *Columns*, mean (n = 2); *bars*, SD. (C) Cells were cultured with or without 20 nM fVIIa. After 2 hours post fVIIa addition, cell proliferation was estimated by colorimetric assay. *Columns*, mean (n = 3); *bars*, SD.

The same results were obtained by cell proliferation experiments (data not shown) with anti-PAR1 and -PAR2 antibodies (Koizume et al. 2006). We further tested the effect of TF-fVIIa protease activity on cell proliferation by adding fVIIa to cell culture media. We confirmed that MDA-MB-231 cells pre-treated with fVIIa strongly generate pro-coagulant activity (Fig. 5B), but cell proliferation was not affected in the presence of fVIIa (Fig. 5C). These data indicate that mechanisms independent of TF-fVIIa formation on the cell surface may be involved in acceleration of cell proliferation driven by ectopic fVII synthesis.

6.2 Other effects of curcumin may augment anti-breast cancer efficacy of ectopic fVII repression

Curcumin has been widely studied because this compound exhibits various anti-cancer effects such as pro-apoptotic, anti-angiogenic, and anti-metastatic activities (Sa & Das 2008). Therefore, anti-ectopic fVII activity in combination with other effects of curcumin may cooperate to suppress malignant phenotype expression of breast cancers. Many investigators have reported that curcumin has pro-apoptotic activity in cancer cells. The molecular mechanism of this effect can be attributed to repression of transcription factors crucial for cell survival. Curcumin can inhibit binding of Egr-1, NFκB, and AP-1 to target genes *in vitro* (Bierhaus et al. 1997; Pendurthi et al. 1997), resulting in down-regulation of proteins essential for tolerance to cell death. Indeed, pro-apoptotic effects of curcumin have also been observed *in vivo* using mouse xenograft breast tumor models (Adams et al. 2004; Shoji et al. 2008). A chemosensitizing effect of curcumin *via* inhibition of the above transcription factors (Goel & Aggarwal 2010) or by targeting proteasomes (Landis-Piwowar et al. 2006; Zhang et al. 2007) has also been reported. Therefore, anti-cancer activity of curcumin can be a result of complex cellular events induced by inhibition of multiple target molecules. In addition, induction of TF expression under cellular stress can be suppressed by curcumin since the *F3* gene is a target of Egr-1, NFκB, and AP-1 for regulation (Bierhaus et al. 1997; Pendruthi et al. 1997). This indicates that curcumin can block a pathologically increased fraction of TF without impairing normal TF expression responsible for extrinsic hemostasis. Since anti-TF strategy may be therapeutically beneficial (Schaffner & Ruf 2009), use of curcumin may be advantageous since this compound could synergistically block malignant phenotypes caused by TF-ectopic fVIIa signaling without causing bleeding.

7. Future directions

Many breast cancer cell lines constitutively and highly express fVII (Fig. 6). Given that TF-fVIIa signaling can be a major mechanism of malignant phenotype expression of breast cancers through enhancement of metastasis, angiogenesis, and anti-apoptotic effects, breast cancer cells possibly synthesize fVII as an optional means to survive in a severe tumor microenvironment unique to mammary tissue. In addition, ectopic fVII can promote cell proliferation. Since transcript and immunohistochemical analyses of clinical samples showed that breast cancer tissues frequently express fVII, anti-breast cancer strategies targeting ectopic fVII should be considered.

It was found that curcumin selectively inhibits ectopic fVII synthesis by precluding p300/CBP binding to the *FVII* promoter region. Since animal studies have shown that curcumin can cure cardiovascular diseases by targeting p300 activity (Morimoto et al. 2008; Li et al. 2008), anti-p300 strategy by curcumin treatment is clinically applicable without significant toxicity. Therefore, for the next step, it will be necessary to examine whether an anti-p300/CBP strategy against fVII-expressing breast cancer is also effective *in vivo*. In addition, an anti-p300/CBP strategy may be compromised since HATs can be targeted to the hepatocytic *FVII* promoter. It is therefore necessary to discover novel molecular targets more specifically associated with ectopic fVII synthesis. Furthermore, although we showed that blockade of ectopic fVII synthesis by RNAi or curcumin treatment could repress cell proliferation, this inhibitory effect is cell-type dependent. Therefore, mechanistic understanding of this difference is also required to predict breast cancer cells responsive to an anti-ectopic fVII strategy.

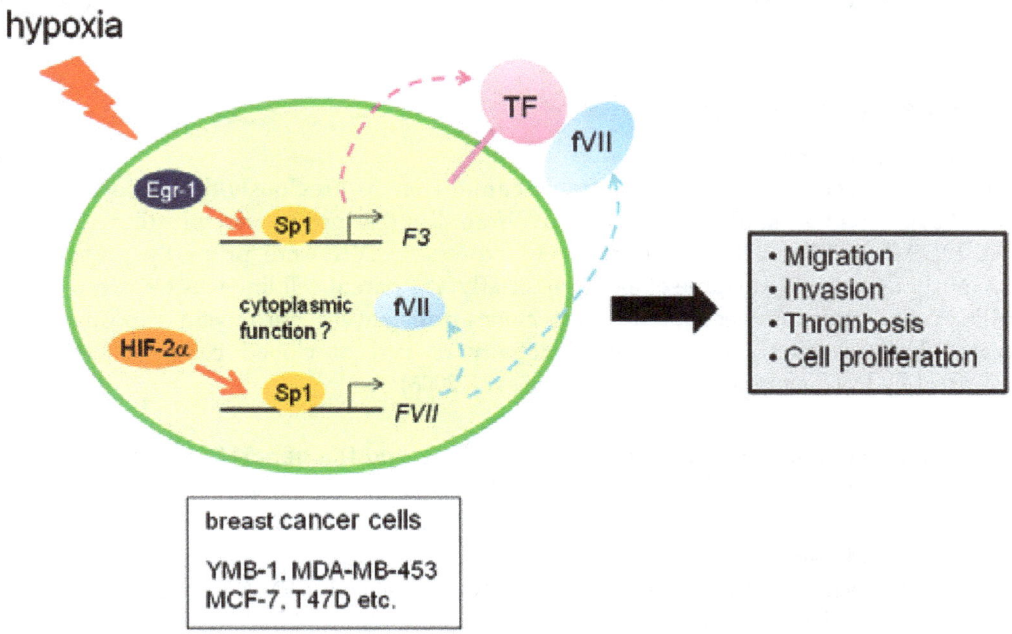

Fig. 6. Breast cancer phenotypes potentially augmented by ectopic fVII expression.
Blood coagulation factor VII can be synthesized *via* transcription from the *FVII* gene constitutively activated by activators such as Sp1 in breast cancer cells. Hypoxic stress may enhance this transcription *via* activation of the *FVII* promoter by binding of the transcription factor HIF-2α. Ectopic fVII activity may be strengthened since expression of its cellular receptor, TF, can also be increased *via F3* gene activation *via* Sp1 substitution by Egr-1 under pathological conditions such as hypoxia. Red symbols are indicative of events expected to occur under hypoxia. Bent arrows are indicative of transcriptional activation. Dotted arrows designate protein expression.

From the clinical point of view, it is essential to reveal relationships between fVII expression and various clinical parameters, such as chemoresistance, relapse, and overall survival to predict patients who may benefit from anti-TF-fVIIa treatment. Notably, breast cancer prognosis is known to closely correlate with pathological complete response after adjuvant chemotherapy (Ross et al. 2008). Therefore, it is worth investigating whether chemoresistant patients express high levels of fVII as a survival factor so that fVII can be targeted to improve prognosis.

Finally, many questions concerning the biology of ectopic fVII synthesis remain unanswered. Why do breast cancer cells tend to synthesize more fVII compared with other cancer cells? How does ectopically expressed fVII associate with TF to express TF-fVIIa complex on the cell surface? It would also be intriguing to investigate whether ectopically expressed fVII has novel functions other than authentic TF-fVIIa signaling. Notably, ectopic fVII might have a cytoplasmic function since we found that ectopic fVII accelerates breast cancer cell proliferation, possibly *via* a cell surface TF-fVIIa-independent mechanism. More specifically, does cytoplasmic fVII exist without complexing with TF to play a biological role? A more detailed understanding of how ectopic fVII expression is regulated and how it can contribute to breast cancer biology will be essential for translating current knowledge to therapeutic strategies.

8. Materials and methods

8.1 Cell lines and reagents

Human cancer cell lines, antibodies, and curcumin were as previously described (Koizume et al. 2009). fVIIa was kindly provided by Wolfram Ruf (Scripps Research Institute, La Jolla, CA). MDA-MB-231 cell lines constitutively expressing fVII were primarily prepared as previously described (Koizume et al. 2006). Briefly, the parent cell line was transfected with pIRES/fVII expression vector, and then clones resistant to puromycin exposure were isolated by passaging. The expression activity of fVII of cloned cells was primarily confirmed by fXa generation assay (Koizume et al. 2006).

8.2 Chromatin immunoprecipitation, real-time PCR, and fXa generation analysis

These experiments were performed as previously described (Koizume et al., 2006).

8.3 RNAi experiments

Small interference RNA (siRNA) for fVII was ON-TARGET plus SMART pool (Dharmacon, Lafayette, CA). Silencer Negative Control 1 RNAi (Ambion, Austin, TX) was used for non-specific siRNA transfection. Transfection of siRNA was performed using the Neon™ transfection system (Invitrogen, Carlsbad, CA).

8.4 Cell proliferation assay

Cell proliferation was analyzed using CellTiter 96 Aqueous One Solution Cell Proliferation Assay (Promega, Madison, WI).

9. Acknowledgments

This work was partly supported by a Grant-in-Aid for the Encouragement of Basic Science and Technology from the Science and Technology Office of the Kanagawa Prefectural Government (S. Koizume), and by a grant from the Japanese Ministry of Education, Culture, Sports, Science and Technology (Y. Miyagi).

10. References

Adams, B. K., Ferstl, E. M., Davis, M. C., Herold, M., Kurtkaya, S., Camalier R. F., Hollingshead, M. G., Kaur, G., Rickles, F. R., Snyder, J. P., Liotta, D. C., Shoji, M. (2004) *Bioorg. Med. Chem.*, 12, 3871-3883.

Albrektsen, T., Sorensen, B. B., Hjortoe, G. M. Fleckner, J., Rao, L. V. M., Petersen, L. C. (2007) *J. Thromb. Haemost.*, 5, 1588-1597.

Álvarez, R. H., (2010) *Breast Cancer Res.*, 12, S1-18.

Bach, R. R. (2006) *Arterioscler. Thromb. Vasc. Biol.*, 26, 456-461.

Benz, C. C. & Yau, C. (2008) *Nat. Rev. Cancer*, 8, 875-879.

Bierhaus, A., Zhang, Y., Quehenberger, P., Luther, T., Haase, M., Muller, M., Mackman, N., Ziegler, R., Nawroth P. P. (1997) *Thromb. Haemost.*, 77, 772-782.

Boire, A., Covic, L., Agarwal, A., Jacques, S., Sherifi, S., Kuliopulos, A. (2005) *Cell*, 120, 303-313.

Booden, M. A., Eckert, L. B., Der, C. J., Trejo, J. (2004) *Mol. Cell. Biol.*, 24, 1990-1999.

Collier, M. E. W., Li Cao, Ettelaie, C. (2008) *Mol. Cancer. Res.*, 6, 1807-1818.

Contrino, J., Hair, G., Kreutzer, D., Rickles, F. R. (1996) *Nature Med.* 2, 209-215.

Davila, M., Amirkhosravi, A., Coll, E., Desai, H., Robles, L., Colon, J., Baker, C. H., Francis, J. L. (2008) *J. Thromb. Haemost.*, 6, 1517-1524.

Fischer, E. G., Riewald, M., Huang, H. Y., Miyagi, Y., Kubota, Y., Mueller, B. M., Ruf, W. (1999) *J. Clin. Invest.*, 104, 1213-1221.

Foulkes, W. D., Smith, I. E., Reis-Filho, J. S., (2010) *N. Engl. J. Med.*, 363, 1938-1948.

Furie, B. & Furie, B. C. (1988) *Cell*, 53, 505-518.

Goel, A. & Aggarwal, B. B., (2010) *Nutr. Cancer*, 62, 919-930.

Hjortoe, G. M. Petersen, L. C., Albrektsen, T., Sorensen, B. B., Norby, P. L., Mandal, S. K., Pendurthi, U. R., Rao, M. V. (2004) *Blood*, 103, 3029-3037.

Iodice, S., Gandini, S., Lohr, M., Lowenfels, A. B., Maisonneuve, P. (2008) *J. Thromb. Haemost.*, 6, 781-788.

Jiang, X.; Bailly, M. A.; Panneti, T. S.; Cappello, M.; Konigsberg, W. H.; Bromberg, M. E. (2004) *J. Thromb. Haemost.*, 2, 93-101.

Jessani, N., Humphrey, M., McDonald, W. H., Niessen, S., Masuda, K., Gangadharan, B., Yates, J. R. III., Mueller, B. M., Cravatt, B. F. (2004) *Proc. Natl. Acad. Sci. USA.* 101, 13756-13761.

Jiang, X.; Zhu, S., Panetti, T. S.; Bromberg, M. E. (2008) *Thromb. Haemost.*, 100, 127-133.

Kirwan, C. C., McDowell, G., McCollum, C. N., Kumar, S., Byrne, G. J., (2008) *Br. J. Cancer.* 99, 1000-1006.

Koizume, S., Jin, M-S., Miyagi, E., Hirahara, F., Nakamura, Y., Piao, J-H., Asai, A., Yoshida, A., Tsuchiya, E., Ruf, W., Miyagi, Y., (2006) *Cancer Res.*, 66, 9453-9460.

Koizume, S., Yokota, Y., Miyagi, E., Hirahara, F., Nakamura, Y., Sakuma, Y., Yoshida, A., Kameda, Y., Tsuchiya, E., Ruf, W., Miyagi, Y. (2009) *Mol. Cancer Res.*, 7, 1928-1936.

Li, H-L., Liu, C., de Couto, G., Ouzounian, M., Sun, M., Wang, A-B., Huang, Y., He, C-W., Shi, Y., Chen, X., Nghiem, M. P., Liu, Y., Chen, M., Dawood, F., Fukuoka, M., Maekawa, Y., Zhang, L., Leask, A., Ghosh, A. K., Kirshenbaum, L. A., Liu, P. P. (2008) *J. Clin. Invest.*, 118, 879-893.

Liu, Y. & Mueller, B. M. (2006) *Biochem. Biophys. Res. Commun.*, 344, 1263-1270.

Landis-Piwowar, K. R., Milacic, V., Chen, D., Yang, H., Zhao, Y., Chan, T. H., Yan, B., Dou, Q. P. (2006) *Drug. Resist. Updat.*, 9, 263-273.

Lwaleed, B. A., Chisholm, M., Francis, J. L., (1999) *J. Pathol.* 187, 291-294.

Mackman, N. (1995) *FASEB J.*, 9, 883-889.

Mackman, N. & Taubman, M. (2009) *Arterioscler. Thromb. Vasc. Biol.*, 29, 1986-1988.

Majmundar, A. J., Wong, W. J., Simon, M. C. (2010) *Mol. Cell*, 40, 294-309.

McDonald, D. M. & Baluk, P., (2002) *Cancer Res.*, 62, 5381-5385.

Milsom, C. & Rak, J. (2009) *Pathol. Haemost. Thromb.*, 36, 160-176.

Morimoto, T., Sunagawa, Y., Kawamura, T., Takaya, T., Wada, H., Nagasawa, A., Komeda, M., Fujita, M., Shimatsu, A., Kita, T., Hasegawa, K. (2008) *J. Clin. Invest.*, 118, 868-878.

Morris, D. R., Ding, Y., Ricks, T. K., Gullapalli, A., Wolfe, B. L., Trejo, J. (2006) *Cancer Res.*, 66, 307-314.

Pendurthi, U. R., Williams, J. T., Rao, L. V. (1997), *Arterioscler Thromb. Vasc. Biol.*, 17, 3406-3413.

Pendurthi, U. R., Allen, K. E., Ezban, M., Rao, V. M. (2000) *J. Biol. Chem.*, 275, 14632-14641.

Pendurthi, U. R., Ghosh, S., Mandal, S. K., Rao, V. M. (2007) *Blood*, 110, 3900-3908.

Ross, J. S., Hatzis, C., Symmans, W. F., Pusztai, L., Hortobagyi, G. N. (2008) *The Oncologist*, 13, 477-493.

Rydén, L., Grabau, D., Schaffner, F., Jönson, P-E., Ruf, W., Belting, M., (2010) *Int. J. Cancer*, 126, 2330-2340.

Sa, G. & Das, T. (2008) *Cell Division*, 3, 1-14.

Schaffner, F. & Ruf. W. (2009) *Arterioscler. Thromb. Vasc. Biol.*, 29, 1999-2004.

Schaffner, F., Versteeg, H. H., Schillert, A., Yokota, N., Petersen. L. C., Mueller, B. M., Ruf, W. (2010) *Blood*, 116, 6106-6113.

Shoji, M., Sun, A., Kisiel, W., Lu, Y. J., Shim, H., McCarey, B. E., Nichols, C., Parker, E. T., Pohl, J., Mosley, C. A., Alizadeh, A. R., Liotta, D. C., Snyder, J. P., (2008) *J. Drug Target*, 16, 185-197.

Sierko, E., Wojtukiewicz, M. Z., Zimnoch, L., Kisiel, W. (2010) *Thromb. Haemost.*, 103, 198-204.

Ten Cate, H. & Falanga, A. (2007) *Pathophysiol Haemost. Thromb.*, 36, 122-130.

Tilley, R. E., Holsher, T., Belani, R., Nieva, J., Mackman, N., (2008) *Thromb. Res.*, 122, 604-609.

Ueno, T., Toi, M., Koike, M., Nakamura, S., Tominaga, T., (2000) *Br. J. Cancer*. 83, 164-170.

Versteeg, H. H., Schaffner, F., Kerver, M., Petersen, H. H., Ahamed, J., Felding-Habermann, Takada, Y., Mueller, B. M., Ruf, W. (2008a) *Blood*, 111, 190-199.

Versteeg, H. H., Schaffner, F., Kerver, M., Ellies, L. G., Andre-Gordon, P., Mueller, B. M., Ruf, W. (2008b) *Cancer Res.*, 68, 7219-7227.

Vrana, J. A., Stang, M. T., Grande, J. P., Getz, M. J., (1996) *Cancer Res.*, 56, 5063-5070.

Wilson, B. J., Harada, R., leDuy, L., Hollenberg, M. D., Nepveu, A. (2009) *J. Biol. Chem.* 284, 36-45.

Yokota, N., Koizume, S., Miyagi, E., Hirahara, F., Nakamura, Y., Kikuchi, K., Ruf, W., Sakuma, Y., Tsuchiya, E., Miyagi, Y. (2009) *Br. J. Cancer*, 101, 2023-2029.

Yu, J. L., May, L., Lhotak, V., Shahrzad, S., Shirasawa, S., Weitz, J. I., Coomber, B. L. Mackman, N., Rak, J. W. (2005) *Blood*, 105, 1734-1741.

Zacharski, L. R., Memoli, V. A., Ornstein, D. L., Rousseau, S. M., Kisiel, W., Kudryk, B. J. (1993) *J. Natl. Cancer Inst.*, 85, 1225-1230.

Zhang, H. G., Kim, H., Liu, C., Wang, J., Grizzle, W. E., Kimberly, R. P., Barnes, S. (2007) *Biochim. Biophys. Acta.*, 1173, 1116-1123.

Zhang, X., Yu, H., Lou, J. R., Zheng, J., Zhu, H., Popescu, N-I., Lupu, F., Lind, S. E., Ding, W-Q. (2010) *J. Biol. Chem.*, 286, 1429-1435.

Zhou, J. N., Ljungdahl, S., Shoshan, M. C., Swedenborg, J., Linder, S. (1998) *Mol. Carcinog.*, 21, 234-243.

3

Roles and Mechanisms of Estrogen and Estrogen Receptors in Breast Cancer Resistant to Chemotherapy

Weimin Fan[1,2] and Meihua Sui[1,3]
[1]*Program of Innovative Cancer Therapeutics, First Affiliated Hospital of Zhejiang University College of Medicine, Hangzhou*
[2]*Department of Pathology and Laboratory Medicine, Medical University of South Carolina, Charleston*
[3]*Center for Bionanoengineering, Department of Chemical and Biological Engineering, Zhejiang University, Hangzhou*
[1,3]*China*
[2]*USA*

1. Introduction

Breast cancer is the most common malignancy of women in many countries including United States and many European countries. Chemotherapy plays a major role in the treatment of advanced breast cancer, either as an adjuvant to primary therapy or as palliation therapy to improve symptoms and prolong survival. The previous 50 years have seen numerous advances in the properties of chemotherapeutic agents. However, a significant proportion of cancers are inherently unaffected by the administration of anticancer drugs. Furthermore, another considerable proportion of patients undergoing chemotherapy display an initial reduction in tumor size and then relapse with a marked insensitivity to a variety of drugs. Both phenomena are brought about by a resistant phenotype, which presents perhaps the single greatest barrier to successful chemotherapy.

Biological mechanisms contributing to drug resistance may be present *de novo* or arise after exposure to anticancer drugs. At present, drug resistance is considered as a multifactorial phenomenon involving several major mechanisms (1, 2). In general, two main groups of factors contribute to the development of drug resistance. The first group includes pharmacological and physiological factors such as drug metabolism and excretion, inadequate access of the drug to the tumor, inadequate infusion rate and inadequate route of delivery. The second group includes cell- or tissue-specific factors. For example, increased repair of DNA damage, reduced apoptotic cell death, altered metabolism of drugs, increased energy-dependent efflux (*e.g.* ATP-binding cassette transporters) of chemotherapeutic drugs and microRNAs are known factors correlated with the development of anticancer drug resistance (1). In recent years, both clinical observations and experimental studies suggested that steroid hormones and their receptors might also affect the therapeutic efficacy of antineoplastic drugs (3-8).

Traditionally, steroid hormones can be grouped into five groups by the receptors to which they bind: glucocorticoids, mineralocorticoids, androgens, estrogens and progestagens (9-11). Previous studies from our laboratory showed that glucocorticoids, such as dexamethasone, could significantly interfere with the antitumor activities of paclitaxel *in vitro* and *in vivo* (3, 4, 12). Further studies suggest that paclitaxel may induce apoptotic cell death through activation of the NF-κB/IκB signaling pathway, whereas glucocorticoids inhibit paclitaxel-induced apoptosis through induction of IκBα synthesis, which antagonizes paclitaxel-mediated activation of NF-κB and subsequently results in inhibition of paclitaxel-induced apoptosis (4, 13, 14). Considering that cancer patients are routinely pretreated with glucocorticoids (such as dexamethasone) before receiving taxanes (*e.g.* paclitaxel, docetaxel) to prevent taxane-related hypersensitivity reactions or other adverse effects, the finding of glucocorticoid-mediated inhibition of paclitaxel-induced apoptosis raises a clinically relevant question as to whether pretreatment of glucocorticoids might actually interfere with the therapeutic efficacy of paclitaxel. We have recently reviewed the influence and impact of glucocorticoids on drug-induced apoptosis (4). The cuurent article is largely focused on the role of estrogen and estrogen receptors on the resistance to chemotherapy and the potential strategies to reverse the resistance or sensitize ER+ breast tumors to chemotherapy.

2. Estrogen and estrogen receptors in the development and treatment of breast cancer

Estrogens, such as 17-β estradiol (E2) in human, are steroidal sex hormones that are synthesized from cholesterol and primarily secreted by the ovaries. They play a major role in the development and maintenance of the reproductive tract as well as in the development of the mammary glands. Estrogens also maintain bone density and reduce cardiovascular system by regulating cholesterol levels and influence some brain structures (15, 16). However, besides their physiological functions, estrogens are also involved in the development and progression of breast and the uterus cancers and can maintain tumor cell proliferation (15, 16).

Estrogen action is primarily mediated by two types of estrogen receptors (ERs), *i.e.* ERα and ERβ. ERs are members of the superfamily of nuclear receptors (17, 18). ERs in the cell nucleus mediate the effects of the ligand E2 by functioning as transcriptional regulators that access various target gene promoters either by directly binding to specific estrogen response elements (EREs) within the promoter or indirectly by interacting with other transcriptional regulators bound to the promoter. Further, several cases of ligand-independent activation of ERα mediated by its phosphorylation by various signaling pathways have been reported (19). In addition, ERα localized in the extra-nuclear compartment (such as the plasma membrane or cytoplasm ER) of target cells, can also mediate several nongenomic effects of estrogen. These non-genomic actions are associated with the activation of a kinase cascade, such as growth factor receptor kinases (*e.g.* epidermal growth factor receptor). By these means, E2 and ERα facilitate pathways involved in the promotion of cell proliferation, inhibition of apoptosis, stimulation of metastasis, and angiogenesis. Although there is growing evidence that the ERβ may inhibit the action of ERα by heterodimerizing with it, the overall role of ERβ in breast cancer remains to be better clarified. A number of reviews have recently been published on the biological roles of estrogens and molecular activities of ERs (15-20). Unless otherwise specified, ER refers to ERα within this review.

Cumulative analysis of tumor biopsies has shown that ERs present in ~65% of human breast tumors (21, 22). This is consistent with the crucial role of the ERα subtype in breast cancer etiology and progression, and with the role played by estrogens as tumor promoters. It has long been known that breast tumors that express the ERα protein (ER+) behave in a fundamentally different fashion than ER-negative (ER-) tumors with regard to their response to hormonal therapies, given that outcomes are often favorable in ER-positive breast tumors treated by adjuvant endocrine therapy alone (23, 24). Neoadjuvant chemotherapy has a well-established role in the management of early-stage, operable breast cancer, and remains the gold standard downstaging systemic therapy in many centers, regardless of ER status. However, the data from other clinical trials or retrospective analyses suggest that ER status might also affect the efficacy of chemotherapy (5-8). Specifically, it has been observed that some chemotherapeutic agents may be less effective in patients with ER+ tumors than those with ER- tumors.

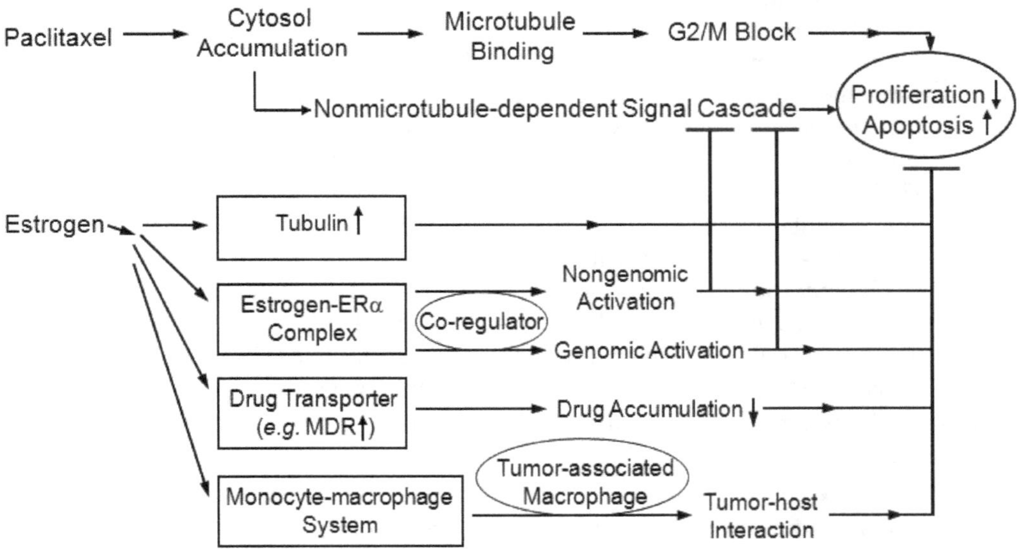

Fig. 1. Hypothesized pathways of estrogen/ER-mediated chemoresistance using paclitaxel as an example. ⊤ and ⋮ represent inhibitory or antagonistic action. MDR, multidrug resistance. There are possible cross-talks between indicated pathways.

3. Current understnding of ER-mediated chemoresistance

More than one decade ago, Lippman ME *et al* first determined the relation between ER and the response rate to cytotoxic chemotherapy in 70 breast cancer patients (6). They found that 34 of 45 patients with low or absent ER values (<10 fmol/mg of cytoplasmic protein) had objective responses to chemotherapy, whereas only 3 of 25 patients with higher ER values (>10 fmol/mg of cytoplasmic protein) responded ($p<0.0001$). There were no statistically significant differences between the two groups in age, menopausal status, disease-free interval, Karnofsky index or prior therapy. Moreover, differences in sites of involvement or type of combination chemotherapy did not account for the increased response rate in ER- patients. This is the first report suggesting that ER status might be an important predictor of response to cytotoxic chemotherapy in breast tumors. Since then, evidence from clinical trials or retrospective analyses is accumulating that improvements in chemotherapy disproportionately benefit breast cancer patients with ER- tumors, in which multiple chemotherapeutic regimens have been tested in these studies (6, 25-33), such as taxanes-, anthracycline- and navelbine-containing regimens. More recently, in a retrospective clinical study conducted by us and our collaborators, we found that primary breast cancer patienhts with ER+ tumors achieved significant lower pathologic response than those with ER- breast tumors when treated with preoperative chemotherapeutic regimens including DEC (docetaxel+epirubicin+cyclophosphamide), VFC (vinorelbine/vincristine+5-fluorouracil+ cyclophosphamide) and EFC (epirubicin+5-fluorouracil+cyclophosphamide) (34).

The involvement of ER in chemoresistance has also been confirmed in a number of *in vitro* studies (5, 7, 8, 35-40). For example, ER- breast cancer tissue was found chemosensitive *in vitro* compared with ER+ tissue against six antitumor drugs including carboquone, adriamycin, mitomycin C, aclacinomycin A, cisplatin and 5-fluorouracil (5). When subjected ER+ human breast cancer MCF-7 and ZR-75–1 cells to paclitaxel or to UV irradiation, marked increases in cell apoptosis were induced. However, these responses were significantly reversed by incubation with E2, which was probably mediated through the plasma membrane estrogen receptor (40). Recently, we established several isogenic ER+ cell lines by stable transfection of ERα expression vectors into ER- breast cancer BCap37 cells to investigate the possible influence of ER on the therapeutic efficacy of paclitaxel and *vinca* alkaloids (7, 8). We found that 17-β estradiol significantly reduced the overall cytotoxicity of these antimicrotubule drugs in ERα-expressing BCap37 but had no influence on the ER-parental cells or ER- MDA-MB-468 cells. Further analyses indicate that expression of ERα in BCap37 cells mainly interferes with the apoptotic cell death but not mitotic arrest induced by these drugs. Moreover, we found that the addition of ICI 182,780 (fulvestrant), a selective ER down-regulator, could completely reverse the above resistance observed in ER+ BCap37 cells, and sensitize MCF-7 and T47D cell lines to the treatment of the above drugs (see Fig. 2). These findings further confirmed the correlation between ERα and drug resistance in ER+ tumor cells.

4. Possible mechanisms of ER-mediaed chemoresistance

Estrogens and ERs are well-known for their critical roles in the development and progression of breast tumors, through genomic or non-genomic pathways as described above. Plentiful data also indicate that estrogens and ER are involved in or interact with a number of apoptosis- or proliferation-related signal pathways existed in tumor cells. Therefore, it is believed that through interaction with and/or regulation on specific or various co-regulators or downstream molecules, estrogen/ER induce chemoresistance in tumor cells by promoting tumor growth and/or inhibiting the antitumor effect of chemotherapeutic drugs. Several mechanisms that may contribute to ER-mediated drug resistance are discussed below. It appears that the underlying mechanisms of ER-mediated chemoresistance are quite complicated and specifically related with the tumor models and chemotherapeutic drugs studied.

4.1 Role of apoptosis-related molecules in ER-mediated chemoresistance

Reduced apoptotic cell death or enhanced tumor cell proliferation are major factors involved in drug resistance. Whereas it is not completely understood how estrogen and ER regulate

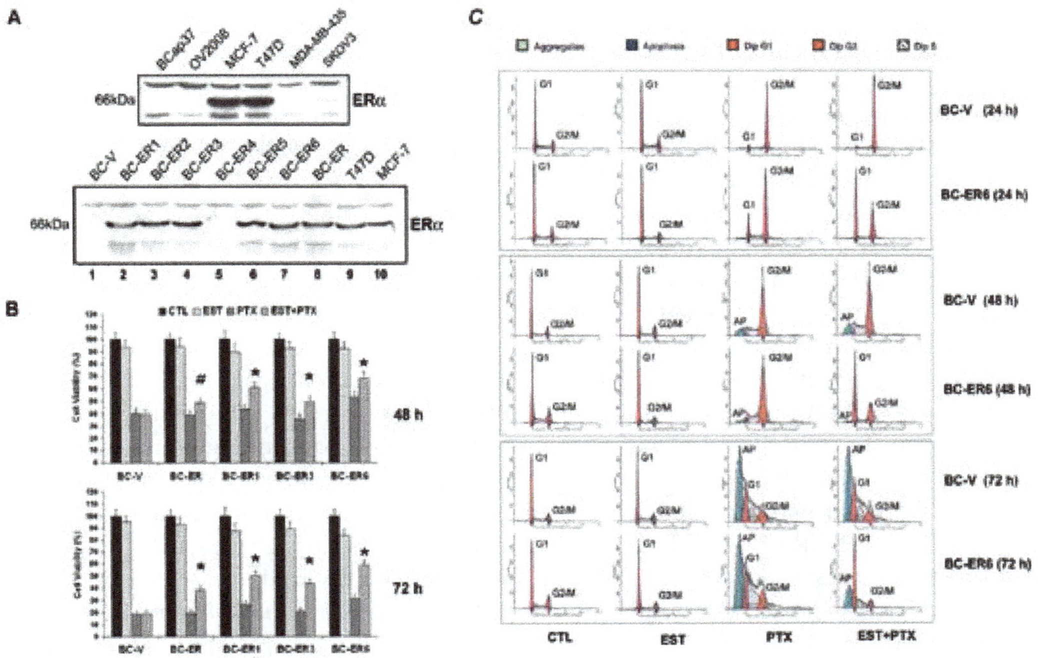

Fig. 2. ERα expression attenuates the anticancer activity of paclitaxel (7). A, protein extracts of BCap37 cells transfected with empty vector (BC-V) or ERα were analyzed by Western blot. T47D and MCF-7 cells were used as positive controls of ERα expression. *B*, cells were treated with 1 nmol/L 17-β estradiol, 50 nmol/L paclitaxel, or the combination treatment in which cells were preincubated with 17- β estradiol for 12 h before paclitaxel treatment. Cell viability was evaluated by MTT assays after both 48 and 72 h of paclitaxel treatment. BC-ER, pooled transfectants of BCap37 transfected with ERα, BC-ER1–7, single clones 1 to 7 of BCap37 transfected with ERα; CTL, control; EST, 17-β estradiol; PTX, paclitaxel. #, $P < 0.05$, when compared with the group treated with paclitaxel alone in the same cell line; *, $P < 0.001$, when compared with the group treated with paclitaxel alone in the same cell line. *C*, cells treated with 1 nmol/L 17-β estradiol, 50 nmol/L paclitaxel, or their combination for indicated time points were harvested, and DNA content stained with propidium iodide for flow cytometric analysis. Peaks corresponding to G1, G2-M, and S phases of the cell cycle and apoptotic cells (AP).

the growth of tumor cells, it is known that hormonal induction of growth factors/receptors such as transforming growth factor α, epidermal growth factor, Her-2 contributes to the proliferative actions of E2 (41-44). Recent studies indicate that several apoptosis-related moleculars or signal pathways, such as bcl-2 and p53, might be involved in E2/ER-mediated resistance to chemotherapy.

Expression of the bcl-2 protein prevents apoptotic cell death induced by a variety of stimuli including most chemotherapeutic agents (45-47). Teixeira C *et al* demonstrated that depletion of estrogen from the medium results in loss of expression of the bcl-2 in MCF-7 cells, whereas reexposure to estrogen markedly induces the bcl-2 expression (48). Moreover, estrogen depletion, the simultaneous treatment of ICI 164,384, or the transfection of bcl-2 antisense significantly sensitized MCF-7 cells to adriamycin, consistent with a decrease in

the bcl-2 levels. Their data suggest that estrogen can promote resistance of ER+ breast cancer cells to chemotherapeutic drugs through a mechanism that involves regulation of the bcl-2, which supports the recent report that bcl-2 expression usually occurs in ER+ breast tumors, whereas ER- breast cancer biopsies tend to lack this protein (48). Another study conducted by Razandi M *et al* showed that in ER+ human breast cancer cells, the apoptosis, activation of c-JNK, phosphorylation of Bcl-2 and Bcl-xl, activation of caspase induced by paclitaxel or UV radiation were significantly reversed by incubation with E2. E2 also independently activated extracellular signal-regulated protein kinase activity, which contributed to the antiapoptotic effects. In addition, our recent studies also demonstrated that E2 significantly inhibited paclitaxel or *vinca a*lkaloids-induced phosphorylations of bcl-2 and c-raf-1, as well as the degradation of IκBα in BCap37 cells transfected with ERα, which was accompanied with decreased sensitivity of BC-ER cells to the above anticancer drugs (7, 8).
In response to various extracellular and intracellular signals, p53 mediates cellular processes, such as apoptosis, cell cycle arrest, and senescence, depending on the signal and the cellular context (49-51). A body of accumulating evidence suggests the possibility of a cross-talk between pathways mediated by ERα and p53. Das GM *et al* demonstrated the direct binding of ERα to p53 both *in vitro* and *in vivo* to endogenous p53 target gene promoters, which subsequently resulted in inhibition of transcriptional activation by p53 (52). They further showed that ERα bound to p53 on endogenous *Survivin* and *MDR1* gene promoters, leading to inhibition of p53-mediated transcriptional repression of these genes. Further, alleviating p53-mediated transcriptional repression of *Survivin* contributes to the ability of ERα to inhibit apoptosis in human breast cancer cells. RNA interference-mediated knockdown of ER resulted in reduced survivin expression and enhanced the propensity of MCF-7 cells to undergo apoptosis in response to staurosporine treatment. These data indicate that countering p53-mediated transcriptional repression of *Survivin* is at least one of the important mechanisms underlying the antiapoptotic function of ERα (53).

4.2 Involvement of tumor growth rate in ER-mediated chemoresistance

Evidence has shown that ER- tumors have a higher growth rate as indicated by a higher labeling index and mitotic index (6). Since many agents used in chemotherapy for breast cancer have some degree of cell-cycle specificity, there might be a correlation between higher growth rate and chemotherapy response (6). Dougherty MK *et al* used three *in vitro* models (MCF-7, T47D and ZR-75) to examine and compare growth rates as well as paclitaxel-induced apoptosis in ER+ and ER- clones with the same originate (54). They found that in T47D and ZR-75 cell lines, loss of ER was associated with a decrease in doubling time and an increase in paclitaxel sensitivity. However, when cell culture conditions were altered to achieve equivalent cell proliferation rates, no difference in paclitaxel sensitivity was observed. Similarly, an ER- clone of MCF-7 cells that did not exhibit an enhanced growth rate compared to its ER+ counterpart also did not show increased paclitaxel sensitivity. In these *in vitro* models, the decreased sensitivity to paclitaxel appears to be correlated closely with the decreased growth rate observed in ER+ breast tumors (54).

4.3 ABC transportors and ER-mediated chemoresistance

The most widely studied phenomenon of drug resistance is multidrug resistance (MDR) that has been linked to overexpression of a membrane associated P-glycoprotein (1, 2), a member of ATP-binding cassette (ABC) transporter family that functions as an efflux pump for various structurally unrelated anticancer agents, such as the *vinca* alkaloids, anthracyclines and taxanes (1, 2). Several studies have suggested that ABC transporters might be involved in E2/ER-induced drug resistance. For example, E2 increased the cytoplasmic concentration of P-gp in ER+ breast cancer cells that were resistant to doxorubicin treatment (55). In addition, ABCC11 (MRP8) expression is high in high-expressing ER breast cancers, supporting the notion that expression of ABCC11 in ER+ breast cancers may contribute to decreased sensitivity to chemotherapy combinations (56). Interestingly, Sugimoto Y *et al* recently reported that both estrogens (57) and antiestrogens (58) inhibit breast cancer resistance protein (BCRP)-mediated drug resistance. They also found that the physiological levels of E2 down-regulate both endogenous and exogenous BCRP expression in ER+ cells by post-transcriptional mechanisms (59). Moreover, they showed that estrogen decreases P-gp expression in MDR1-transduced, ER+ human breast cancer cells, and this E2-mediated P-gp down-regulation sensitizes tumor cells to vincristine. However, it is possible that the effects of estrogen on P-gp expression may differ in ER+ human breast cancer cells expressing endogenous and exogenous P-gp, which needs to be further assessed in appropriate models (60).

4.4 Enhanced β3-tubulin expression by E2/ER

It has been suggested that certain changes in cytoskeletons, such as tubulin mutations and isoforms, alterations in microtubule-bindings proteins (*e.g.* stathmin, tau), as well as enhanced β3-tubulin expression might be correlated with reduced response to antimicrotubule agent-based chemotherapy or worse outcome in a variety of tumor settings. In *in vitro* studies or in clinical investigations, enhanced expression of β3-tubulin has shown to play a crucial role in the development of chemoresistance to antimicrotubule agents in a variety of tumors such as lung, breast, prostate or orarian cancers (61-66), and has be considered as a predictive marker of paclitaxel resistance (25, 67-70). Nevertheless, the mechanism underlying β3-tubulin expression still remains unclear. In *Drosophila,* β3-tubulin expression is enhanced by an exposure to ecdysone, a steroid hormone, through a transcriptional mechanism (71). Recently, Saussede-Aim J *et al* found that exposure of ER+ MCF-7 cells to estradiol induced β3-tubulin expression in both mRNA and protein levels, while estradiol had no effect on the expression of β3-tubulin in ER- MDA-MB-231 cells (72). They further showed that co-administration of antiestrogens including tamoxifen or fulvestrant, completely abolished the increase of β3-tubulin mRNA levels due to estradiol in MCF-7 cells, implying that estradiol regulates β3-tubulin expression, and thereby induces resistance of ER+ breast tumors to antimicrotubule drugs through an ER-dependent pathway.

4.5 Tumor-host interaction in ER-mediated chemoresistance

Estrogen regulates differentiation, maturation and function of many cell types in monocyte-macrophage system directly or indirectly *via* other cells by autocrine/paracrine mechanisms (73). Estrogen effects on this system are primarily repressive, and mainly mediated by repression of expression of genes for cytokines or modulation of other inflammatory mediators by the ER-dependent or nongenomic pathways. The ER-dependent mechanisms mostly involve modulation of the NF-kappaB pathway for transcriptional regulation of cytokine or other mediator genes. In the context of hormone-regulated cancer, estrogen can influence production of cytokines or other inflammatory mediators by both tumor cells and tumor-invading macrophages (73). The interactions of breast cancer cells with tumor-associated macrophages, regulation of the monocyte-macrophage system by estrogen and cross-talk between the ER and cytokine-mediated pathways, may play an important role in tumor progression as well as the development of resistance to anticancer treatment (73-75).

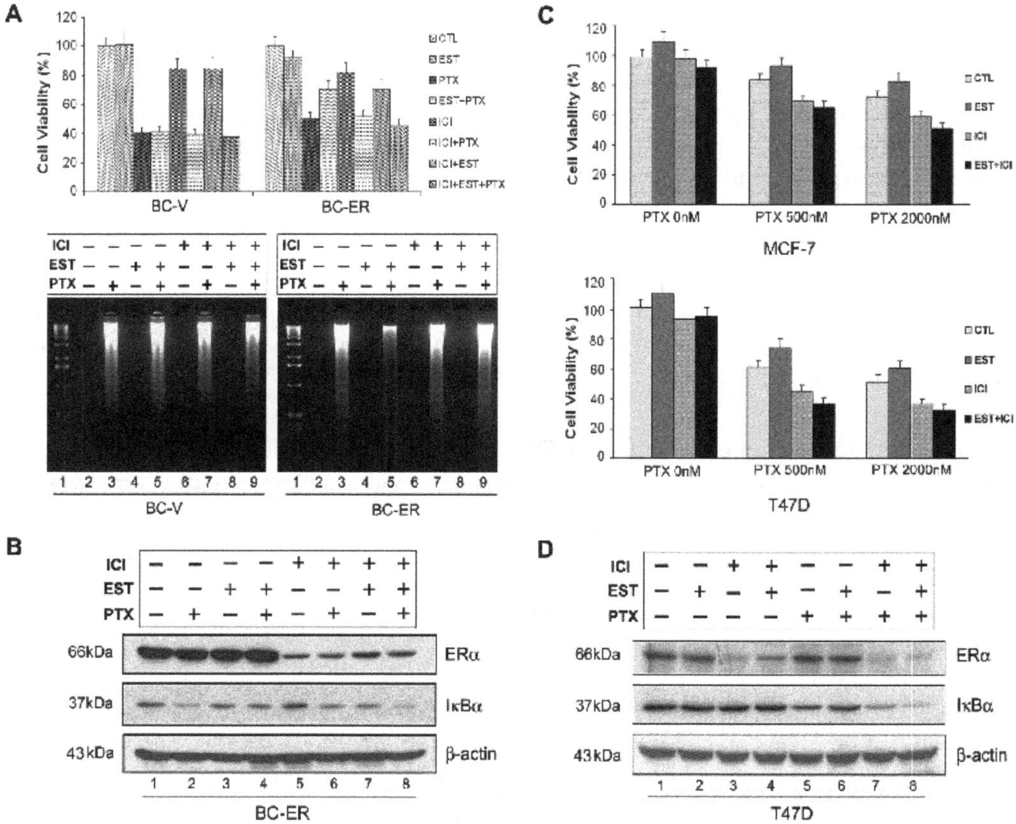

Fig. 3. ICI 182, 780 abrogates the resistance of ERα positive breast tumor cells to paclitaxel (7). BCap37 cells were treated with 1 nmol/L 17-β estradiol, 50 nmol/L paclitaxel, 100 nmol/L ICI 182, 780 or their various combinations. MCF-7 and T47D cells were treated with 100 nmol/L 17-β estradiol, 500 or 2000 nmol/L paclitaxel, 1 μmol/L ICI 182, 780 or their various combinations. *A*, determination of cell viability by MTT assays and apoptosis by DNA fragmentation assays after BC-V and BC-ER cells were exposed to paclitaxel for 48 h. *B*, effect of 17-β estradiol, paclitaxel, ICI 182, 780 and their combinations on the expression of ERα and IκBα in BC-ER cells. *C*, cell viability of MCF-7 and T47D cells after 72 h of paclitaxel treatment with MTT assays. *D*, effect of 17-β estradiol, paclitaxel, ICI 182, 780 and their combinations on the expression of ERα and IκBα in T47D cells. Proteins were extracted from cells after 24 h of paclitaxel treatment.

5. Stratagies to sensitize ER+ breast tumors to chemotherapy

Considering that ERs are expressed in ~65% of human breast cancer, the ER-mediated resistance to chemotherapy has become a big challenge for clinical treatment of breast tumors. Unfortunately, despite the fact that the involvement of ER in drug resistance to chemotherapy has been observed for more than a decade, very few studies have investigated the potential strategies to reverse the ER-mediated chemoresistance or sensitize ER+ breast tumors to chemotherapy. Because the resistance of ER+ breast tumors to chemotherapy is mainly mediated by activation of estrogen/ER signal pathway, it is logical that agents targeting or inhibiting the ER signal pathway may have the potential to reverse the ER-mediated chemoresistance. Indeed, as described below, a number of studies have shown that antiestrogenic agents in combination with chemotherapeutic drugs are of significant therapeutic benefit in ER+ breast cancer over chemotherapy alone. Moreover, recent investigations indicate that the ER-derived peptide, MicroRNAs specifically targeting ER, as well as agents targeting estrogen-related receptors (ERRs) may hold great promise to sensitize ER+ breast tumors to chemotherapy.

5.1 Sensitization of ER+ breast tumors to chemotherapy by SERMs

Selective estrogen receptor modulators (or SERMs) bind ERs but have a mixed agonist/antagonist profile. Tamoxifen and raloxifene are well-known first and second generations of SERMs, respectively (76-78). New SERMs in clinical development include idoxifene, droloxifene, arzoxifene, acolbifene/EM-800, lasofoxifene, TAT-59, ERA-923, toremifene, GW5638/GW7604, *etc* (76-78). Kurebayashi J *et al* found that concurrent treatment of 5-FU and 4-hydroxytamoxifen (4OHT) additively inhibited the growth of ER+ ML-20 and KPL-1 breast cancer cells but not ER- MDA-MB-231 cells (79). They further demonstrated that 4OHT significantly decreased thymidilate synthase activity, which might increase the antitumor activity of 5-FU (79). However, conflicting observations on the interaction between tamoxifen and chemotherapeutic agents including 5-FU and doxorubicin in terms of antitumor activity have been reported by different laboratories (79-83). In addition, Wu L *et al* showed that arzoxifene and 4OHT can inhibit specifically the repopulation of ER+ MCF-7 and T47D breast cancer cells between courses of weekly treatment with 5-FU or methotrexate (84). Most recently, they further confirmed that combined treatment with arzoxifene given between cycles of 5-FU or paclitaxel can inhibit repopulation of MCF-7 breast cancer xenografts (85). They proposed that scheduling of short-acting antiestrogenic agents between courses of adjuvant chemotherapy for human breast cancer has potential to improve the outcome of treatment. Additionally, the increased etoposide cytotoxicity by tamoxifen as compared to cells treated with either drug alone was observed in brain tumor HTB-14 cells expressing ER, which was accompanied with enhanced inhibition of protein kinase C (PKC) and insulin-like growth factor II (IGF-II) (86).

5.2 Sensitization of ER+ breast tumors to chemotherapy by aromatase inhibitors

One strategy to inhibit the activation of estrogen/ER pathway is to block the conversion of estrogen precursors into estrogen by aromatase inhibitors (AIs) (87). Currently, third-generation aromatase inhibitors, such as the non-steroidal agents anastrozole, letrozole and the steroidal agent exemestane, have been introduced into the market as endocrine therapy in postmenopausal patients, either alone or as part of multiple hormonal therapies (88). In addition to the above AIs, cyclooxygenase (COX) inhibitors also decrease aromatase mRNA expression and enzymatic activity (89). A recent study by Chen D *et al* showed that the combination of paclitaxel with exemestane produced additive antitumor effect in cultured human breast cancer cell lines. Interestingly, this additive effect was independent of ERα expression, but dependent on the presence of androstenedione (90). The effects of AIs on sensitivity of ER+ breast tumors to chemotherapy remains unclear and need to be further investigated.

5.3 Sensitization of ER+ breast tumors to chemotherapy by SERDs

The pure antiestrogens, also called selective estrogen receptor downregulators (or SERDs), including fulvestrant (ICI 182, 780), ZK-703, ZK-253, RU58668 and TAS-108, act by decreasing the level of ERs through their ubiquitinylation and subsequent targeting to the proteasome (87). Unlike tamoxifen, fulvestrant is a pure antagonist of estrogen-regulated gene expression that could down-regulat ER expression without any concomitant rise in other growth signal pathways, *e.g.*, EGFR or TGF-α (8, 87). Recently, our laboratory demonstrated that pretreatment with fulvestrant significantly prevented E2-induced resistance to paclitaxel and *vinca* alkaloids in human breast cancer BCap37 cells transfected with ER-expressing vector (BC-ER) while down-regulates the protein levels of ERα in BC-ER cells (7, 8). Similar sensitizing effect of fulvestrant was observed in MCF-7 and T47D breast cancer cells expressing endogenous ERα (7, 8). These results provided additional evidence for the correlation between ERα and the resistance of breast tumors to chemotherapeutic drugs such as paclitaxel and *vinca* alkaloids. More recently, through implanted ER- and ER+ BCap37 cells into athymic nude mice, we established isogenic ER- and ER+ xenograft breast tumor models. Subsequently, we demonstrated that co-treatment of fulvestrant could significantly sensitize ER+ breast tumors to paclitaxel (unpublished data). Because fulvestrant has been successfully used in the treatment of ER+ advanced breast tumors, our experimental results may also suggest the clinical strategy to combine fulvestrant with certain chemotherapeutic drugs for the treatment of ER+ breast tumors.

5.4 Other strategies potentially useful for sensitizing ER+ breast tumors to chemotherapy

In addition to the well-known antiestrogens including the SERMs, AIs and SEDMs, studies have been conducted to explore new agents that may interfere the biological responses medicated by E2/ER. One example is the synthesis of ER-derived peptide. Two ER-derived peptides specifically targeting estradiol/ER action, pY-peptide (Ac-Leu-pTyr-Asp-Leu-Leu-Leu-NH2) and Tat-peptide (Ac-EFVCLKSIILLNS-AAA-RKKRRQRRR-NH2) have shown activity to inhibit the growth of ER+ breast tumors *in vitro* and *in vivo* (91, 92). Moreover, accumulating evidence is revealing an important role of MicroRNAs in anticancer drug resistance (93). Adams *et al* reported that MicroRNA (miR)-206 could decrease endogenous ERα in MCF-7 cells *via* two specific target sites within the 3′-untranslated region of the human ER transcript (22, 94). They further found that miR-206 expression was markedly decreased in ER+ human breast cancer tissues, and that the introduction of miR-206 into estrogen-dependent MCF-7 cells led to the suppression of ERα expression and growth inhibition. These data suggest that miR-206 is a key factor for the regulation of ERα expression in breast cancer, which could be a novel candidate for targeting ER (22, 94).

Nuclear receptor estrogen-related receptor (ERR) family, comprising ERRα, ERRβ and ERRγ, are the closest relatives to ERα after ERβ (95) . The ERRs share several biochemical activities with ERs, bind and regulate transcription *via* estrogen response elements (EREs) and extended ERE half-sites termed ERR response elements (ERREs), but do not bind endogenous estrogens. The ERRs act in an analogous fashion as ERα, but the effect of ERRα binding to an ERE or ERRE can be either negative or positive. ERRα likely plays a role in modulating estrogen responsiveness both by modulating levels of estrogens themselves and expression of estrogen-regulated genes in estrogen target-tissues such as breast cancer. The search for ligands of the ERRs is an active area of research. Targeting ERRs holds great promise and may open new opportunities for the management of breast cancers (95).

As described above, the mechanisms underlying ER-mediated chemoresistance involve ER-coregulatory proteins and cross-talk between plasma membrane-localized ER, nuclear-localized ER and other growth-factor signaling networks, such as EGFR, IGFR, VEGFR and HER2. As a consequence, targeting the ER-coregulators or "cross-talk" pathways may provide opportunities to overcome the ER-mediated chemoresistance, either alone or in combination with agents inhibiting E2/ER activation. However, the mechanisms of ER-mediated chemoresistance need to be further clarified so that effective strategies could be developed to sensitize ER+ breast tumors to chemotherapy.

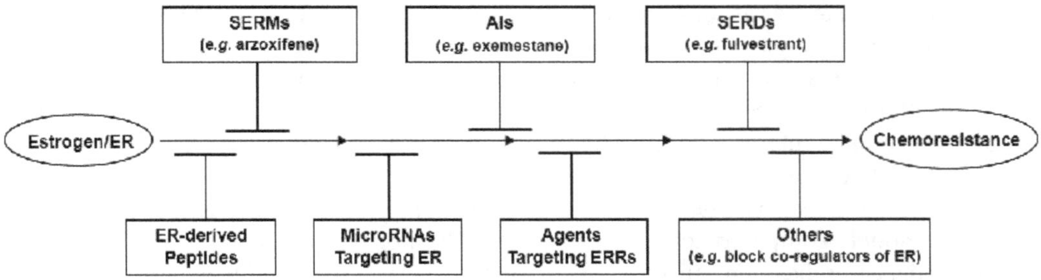

Fig. 4. Possible strategies to reverse ER-mediated chemoresistance or sensitize ER positive tumors to chemotherapy. SERMs, selective estrogen receptor modulators; AIs, aromatase inhibitors; SERDs, selective estrogen receptor down-regulators; ERRs, estrogen-related receptors.

6. Future perspectives

Cumulative data from *in vitro* experiments and clinical investigations have demonstrated the association between ERα expression and the resistance to chemotherapy in breast tumors. However, most of *in vitro* data were based on comparative studies between the tumor cell lines derived from different individuals. Although some paired cell lines were derived under the selective pressure of a low/no estrogen environments, these tumor cells are still not likely to be isogenic because many features, including their proliferative capacity, might have changed due to genetic alterations (54). Thus, it is difficult to elucidate the cellular and molecular mechanisms. The pairs of isogenic breast cell lines generated by stable transfection of ERα or empty vector in our laboratory have provided a valuable model system to investigate the mechanism underlying ERα-mediated breast tumor cell resistance to chemotherapeutic agents. Interestingly, we found that estrogen had marginal effect on microtubule dynamics in breast tumor cells expressing ER (BC-ER) treated with paclitaxel and *vinca* alkaloids, but may decrease the G2-M population through the increase of cells at the G1 phase. This phenomenon is similar to the finding previously reported by Zajchowski *et al.* (96, 97). However, the question still remains whether G1 arrest and decreased G2-M population by estrogen may affect the above drug-induced apoptosis. Further studies are required to elucidate this issue, and it is important to integrate data obtained from breast tumors expressing endogenous ER with those expressing exogenous ER.

Some previous reports about the association between ER status and response to chemotherapy can be confused by the use of chemo-endocrine therapy, where the ER+ population may have responded to the hormonal part of the treatment (98, 99). Moreover, there are heterogeneous in design, in determination of marker and response evaluation, which could be partly responsible for conflicting results about the predictive and prognostic value of these markers (98-103). Therefore, some cautions are required when interpret these results, considering that there are many factors need to be taken into account, such as differences in patient selection, whether the patients were previously untreated with chemotherapy or endocrine therapy, type of chemotherapy, size of the study, follow-up time, different evaluation methods, different cut-off value of ER or other related markers, interactions between combined chemotherapeutic drugs, *etc.*

Compared to the available *in vitro* and clinical reports, very few animal studies have been conducted to determine the role and underlying mechanisms of estrogen and ER in development of chemoresistance, as well as to explorer the potential strategies to reverse the ER-mediated drug resistance. However, appropriate animal models may provide us with easily controlled ways to further evaluate various signal pathways/molecules *in vivo*, to determine the differences between *in vitro* and *in vivo* models, to test chemotherapeutic drugs that we have interests, to investigate agents that may hold promise to sensitize ER+ breast tumors to chemotherapy, either alone or in desirable combinations/sequences. There are less variables need to be taken into account when interpret or analyze the data obtained in animal models compared to clinical patients. The hope to overcome the ER-mediated chemoresistance relies on further clarification of specific pathways or molecules contributing most significantly to the resistance. More exhaustive and systematic attempts to provide this information are essential to reach deeper understandings on ER-mediated chemoresistance in breast tumors. Moreover, it is known that breast cancer patients show a wide range of ER expression levels, and the levels of ER expression in individual patients change during disease progression and/or in response to systemic therapies. Thus, the treatment plan for breast cancer patients might need to be optimized based on the most up-to-date molecular characteristics and responses to therapy in individuals.

7. Acknowledgements

This work was supported in part by Grants NNSF-81071880, NNSF-30973456, ZJ-DST-2008C14079 and NIH CA92880 (to Fan W).

8. References

Raguz, S.;Yagüe, E. Resistance to chemotherapy: new treatments and novel insights into an old problem. *Br. J. Cancer*, 2008, 99(3), 387-391.

Luqmani, Y.A. Mechanisms of drug resistance in cancer chemotherapy. *Med. Princ. Pract.*, 2005, 14 Suppl 1, 35-48

Sui, M.; Chen, F.; Chen, Z.; Fan, W. Glucocorticoids interfere with therapeutic efficacy of paclitaxel against human breast and ovarian xenograft tumors. *Int. J. Cancer.*, 2006, 119, 712–717.

Fan, W.; Sui, M.; Huang, Y. Glucocorticoids selectively inhibit paclitaxel-induced apoptosis: mechanisms and its clinical impact. *Curr. Med. Chem.*, 2004, 403–411.

Maehara, Y.; Emi ,Y.; Sakaguchi, Y.; Kusumoto ,T.; Kakeji, Y.; Kohnoe, S.; Sugimachi,

K. Estrogen receptor-negative breast cancer tissue is chemosensitive in vitro compared with estrogen-receptor-positive tissue. *Eur. Surg. Res.*, 1990, 50–55.

Lippman, M.E.; Allegra, J.C.; Thompson, E.B.; Simon, R.; Barlock, A.; Green, L.; Huff, K.K.; Do, H.M.; Aitken, S.C.; Warren, R. The relation between estrogen receptors and response rate to cytotoxic chemotherapy in metastatic breast cancer. *N. Engl. J .Med.*, 1978, 298, 1223–1228.

Sui, M.; Huang, Y.; Park, B.H.; Davidson, N.E.; Fan,W. Estrogen receptor alpha mediates breast cancer cell resistance to paclitaxel through inhibition of apoptotic cell death. *Cancer Res.*, 2007, 67(11), 5337-5344.

Sui, M.; Jiang, D.; Hinsch, C.; Fan, W. Fulvestrant (ICI 182,780) sensitizes breast cancer cells expressing estrogen receptor alpha to vinblastine and vinorelbine. *Breast Cancer Res. Treat.*, 2010, 121(2), 335-345.

McEwen, B.S. Steroid hormones: effect on brain development and function. *Horm. Res.*, 1992, 37, 1-10.

Simons, S.S. What goes on behind closed doors: physiological versus pharmacological steroid hormone actions. *Bioessays*, 2008, 30(8), 744-756.

Dowsett, M.; Folkerd, E.; Doody, D.; Haynes, B. The biology of steroid hormones and endocrine treatment of breast cancer. *Breast*, 2005, 452-457.

Fan, W.; Cheng, L.; Norris, J.S.; Willingham, M.C. Glucocorticoids selectively inhibit taxol-induced apoptosis in a human breast cancer cell line. *Cell Pharmacol.*, 1996, 3, 435–440.

Huang, Y.; Fang, Y.; Wu, J.; Dziadyk, J.M.; Zhu, X.; Sui, M.; Fan,W. Regulation of vinca alkaloid-induced apoptosis by NF-κB/IκB pathway in human tumor cells. *Mol. Cancer Ther.*, 2004, 3, 271–277.

Huang,Y.; Johnson, K.R.; Norris, J.S.; Fan, W. Nuclear factorkappaB/IkappaB signaling pathway may contribute to the mediation of paclitaxel-induced apoptosis in solid tumor cells. *Cancer Res.*, 2000, 60, 4426–4432.

O'Lone, R.; Frith, M.C.; Karlsson, E.K.; Hansen, U. Genomic targets of nuclear estrogen receptors. *Mol. Endocrinol.*, 2004, 18(8), 1859-1875.

Simpson, E.R.; Misso, M.; Hewitt, K.N.; Hill, R.A.; Boon, W.C.; Jones, M.E.; Kovacic, A.; Zhou, J.; Clyne, C.D. Estrogen-the good, the bad, and the unexpected. *Endocr. Rev.*, 2005, 26(3), 322-330.

Cordera, F.; Jordan, V.C. Steroid receptors and their role in the biology and control of breast cancer growth. *Semin. Oncol.*, 2006, 33, 631–641.

Conzen, S.D. Nuclear receptors and breast cancer. *Mol. Endocrinol.*, 2008, 22(10), 2215-2228.

Weigel, N.L.; Zhang, Y. Ligand-independent activation of steroid hormone receptors. *J. Mol. Med.*, 1998, 76, 469–479.

Hanstein, B.; Djahansouzi, S.; Dall, P.; Beckmann, M.W.; Bender, H.G. Insights into the molecular biology of the estrogen receptor define novel therapeutic targets for breast cancer. *Eur. J. Endocrinol.*, 2004, 150(3), 243-255.

Dickson, R.B.; Lippman, M.E. Control of human breast cancer by estrogen, growth factors, and oncogenes. *Cancer Treat. Res.*, 1988, 40, 119-165.

Yamashita, H. Current research topics in endocrine therapy for breast cancer. *Int. J. Clin. Oncol.*, 2008, 13(5), 380-383.

Murphy, L.; Cherlet, T.; Lewis, A.; Banu, Y.; Watson, P. New insights into estrogen receptor function in human breast cancer. *Ann. Med.*, 2003, 35, 614–631.

Ariazi, E.A.; Ariazi, J.L.; Cordera, F.; Jordan, V.C. Estrogen receptors as therapeutic targets in breast cancer. *Curr. Top. Med. Chem.*, 2006, 6(3), 181-202.

Pusztai, L. Markers predicting clinical benefit in breast cancer from microtubule-targeting agents. *Ann. Oncol.*, 2007, 18 suppl 12: xii15-20.

Cocquyt, V.F.; Schelfhout, V.R.; Blondeel, P.N.; Depypere, H.T.; Daems, K.K.; Serreyn, R.F.; Praet, M.M.; Van, Belle, S.J. The role of biological markers as predictors of response to preoperative chemotherapy in large primary breast cancer. *Med. Oncol.*, 2003, 20(3), 221-231.

Faneyte, I.F.; Schrama, J.G.; Peterse, J.L.; Remijnse, P.L.; Rodenhuis, S.; van de Vijver, M.J. Breast cancer response to neoadjuvant chemotherapy: predictive markers and relation with outcome. *Br. J. Cancer*, 2003, 88(3), 406-412.

International Breast Cancer Study Group (IBCSG). Endocrine responsiveness and tailoring adjuvant therapy for postmenopausal lymph node-negative breast cancer: a randomized trial. *J. Natl. Cancer. Inst.*, 2002, 94(14), 1054-1065.

Berry, D.A.; Cirrincione, C.; Henderson, I.C.; Citron, M.L.; Budman, D.R.; Goldstein, L.J.; Martino, S.; Perez, E.A.; Muss, H.B.; Norton, L.; Hudis, C.; Winer, E.P. Estrogen-receptor status and outcomes of modern chemotherapy for patients with node-positive breast cancer. *JAMA*, 2006, 295(14), 1658-1667.

Gianni, L.; Zambetti, M.; Clark, K.; Baker, J. Cronin, M.; Wu, J.; Mariani, G.; Rodriguez, J.; Carcangiu, M.; Watson, D.; Valagussa, P.; Rouzier, R.; Symmans, W.F.; Ross, J.S.; Hortobagyi, G.N.; Pusztai, L.; Shak, S. Gene expression profiles in paraffin-embedded core biopsy tissue predict response to chemotherapy in women with locally advanced breast cancer. *J. Clin. Oncol.*, 2005, 23(29), 7265-7277.

Colleoni, M.; Minchella, I.; Mazzarol, G.; Nolè, F.; Peruzzotti, G.; Rocca, A.; Viale, G.; Orlando, L.; Ferretti, G.; Curigliano, G.; Veronesi, P.; Intra, M.; Goldhirsch, A. Response to primary chemotherapy in breast cancer patients with tumors not expressing estrogen and progesterone receptors. *Ann. Oncol.*, 2000, 11, 1057-1059.

MacGrogan, G.; Mauriac, L.; Durand, M.; Bonichon, F.;Trojani, M.; de Mascarel, I.; Coindre, J.M. Primary chemotherapy in breast invasive carcinoma: predictive value of the immunohistochemical detection of hormonal receptors, p53, c-erbB-2, MiB1, pS2 and GST pi. *Br. J .Cancer.*, 1996, 74, 1458-1465.

Stearns, V.; Singh, B.; Tsangaris, T.; Crawford, J.G.; Novielli, A.; Ellis, M.J.; Isaacs, C.; Pennanen, M.; Tibery, C.; Farhad, A.; Slack, R.; Hayes, D.F. A prospective randomized pilot study to evaluate predictors of response in serial core biopsies to single agent neoadjuvant doxorubicin or paclitaxel for patients with locally advanced breast cancer. *Clin. Cancer Res.*, 2003, 9(1), 124-133.

Wang, L.; Jiang, Z.; Sui, M.; Shen, J.; Xu, C.; Fan, W. The potential biomarkers in predicting pathologic response of breast cancer to three different chemotherapy regimens: a case control study. *BMC Cancer*, 2009, 9, 226.

Dittrich, C.; Jakesz, R.; Wrba, F.; Havelec, L.; Haas, O.; Spona, J.; Holzner, H.; Kolb, R.; Moser, K. The human tumour cloning assay in the management of breast cancer patients. *Br. J. Cancer*, 1985, 52(2), 197-203.

Aho, A.J.; Mäenpää, J.U.; Kangas, L.; Söderström, K.O.; Auranen, A.A.; Linna, M. Subrenal capsule assay in human breast cancer. Response to cytostatic drug combinations and correlation with receptor status. *Eur. J. Cancer Clin. Oncol.*, 1985, 21(10), 1133-1140.

Kaufmann, M.; Klinga, K.; Runnebaum, B.; Kubli, F. Hormone receptors in breast cancer and response to chemotherapy. *N. Engl. J .Med*, 1979, 300(18), 1052.

Maehara, Y.; Anai, H.; Kusumoto, H.; Sugimachi, K. Poorly differentiated human gastric carcinoma is more sensitive to antitumor drugs than is well differentiated carcinoma. *Eur. J. Surg. Oncol.*, 1987, 13(3), 203-206.

Allegra, J.C.; Lippman, M.E.; Thompson, E.B.; Simon, R. An association between steroid hormone receptors and response to cytotoxic chemotherapy in patients with metastatic breast cancer. *Cancer Res.*, 1978, 38(11 Pt 2), 4299-4304.

Razandi, M.; Pedram, A.; Levin, E.R. Plasma membrane estrogen receptors signal to antiapoptosis in breast cancer. *Mol. Endocrinol.*, 2000, 14(9), 1434-1447.

Lee, A.V.; Cui, X.; Oesterreich, S. Cross-talk among estrogen receptor, epidermal growth factor, and insulin-like growth factor signaling in breast cancer. *Clin. Cancer. Res.*, 2001, 7(12 Suppl), 4429s-4435s discussion 4411s-4412s.

Chalbos, D.; Philips, A.; Rochefort, H. Genomic cross-talk between the estrogen receptor and growth factor regulatory pathways in estrogen target tissues. *Semin. Cancer. Biol*, 1994, 5(5), 361-368.

Kato, S. Estrogen receptor-mediated cross-talk with growth factor signaling pathways. *Breast Cancer*, 2001, 8(1), 3-9.

Levin, E.R. Bidirectional signaling between the estrogen receptor and the epidermal growth factor receptor. *Mol. Endocrinol.*, 2003, 17(3), 309-317.

Levine, B.; Sinha, S.; Kroemer, G. Bcl-2 family members: dual regulators of apoptosis and autophagy. *Autophagy*, 2008, 4(5), 600-606.

Adams, J.M.; Cory, S. Bcl-2-regulated apoptosis: mechanism and therapeutic potential. *Curr. Opin. Immunol.*, 2007, 19(5), 488-496.

van Delft, M.F.; Huang, D.C. How the Bcl-2 family of proteins interact to regulate apoptosis. *Cell Res.*, 2006, 16(2), 203-213.

Teixeira, C.; Reed, J.C.; Pratt, M.A. Estrogen promotes chemotherapeutic drug resistance by a mechanism involving Bcl-2 proto-oncogene expression in human breast cancer cells. *Cancer Res.*, 1995, 55(17), 3902-3907.

Vousden, K.H.; Lu, X. Live or let die: the cell's response to p53. *Nat. Rev. Cancer*, 2002, 2, 594–604.

Vogelstein, B.; Lane, D.; Levine, A.J. Surfing the p53 network. *Nature*, 2000, 408, 307–310. Hofseth, L.J.; Hussain, S.P.; Harris, C.C. p53: 25 years after its discovery. *Trends Pharmacol. Sci.*, 2004, 25, 177–181.

Liu, W.; Konduri, S.D.; Bansal, S.; Nayak, B.K.; Rajasekaran, S.A.; Karuppayil, S.M.; Rajasekaran, A.K.; Das, G.M. Estrogen receptor α binds p53 tumor suppressor protein directly and represses its function. *J. Biol. Chem.*, 2006, 281, 9837–9840.

Sayeed, A.; Konduri, S.D.; Liu, W.; Bansal, S.; Li, F.; Das, G.M. Estrogen receptor alpha inhibits p53-mediated transcriptional repression: implications for the regulation of apoptosis. *Cancer Res.*, 2007, 67(16), 7746-7755.

Dougherty, M.K.; Schumaker, L.M.; Jordan; V.C.; Welshons W.V.; Curran, E.M.; Ellis, M.J.; El-Ashry, D. Estrogen receptor expression and sensitivity to paclitaxel in breast cancer. *Cancer Biol. Ther.*, 2004, 3(5), 460-467.

Zampieri, L.; Bianchi, P.; Ruff ,P.; Arbuthnot, P. Differential modulation by estradiol of P-glycoprotein drug resistance protein expression in cultured MCF7 and T47D breast cancer cells. *Anticancer Res.*, 2002, 22(4), 2253-2259.

Honorat, M.; Mesnier, A.; Vendrell, J.; Guitton, J.; Bieche, I.; Lidereau, R.; Kruh ,G.D.; Dumontet, C.; Cohen, P.; Payen, L. ABCC11 expression is regulated by estrogen in MCF7 cells, correlated with estrogen receptor alpha expression in postmenopausal breast tumors and overexpressed in tamoxifen-resistant breast cancer cells. *Endocr. Relat. Cancer.*, 2008, 15(1), 125-138.

Imai, Y.; Tsukahara, S.; Ishikawa, E.; Tsuruo, T.; Sugimoto, Y. Estrone and 17-estradiol reverse breast cancer resistance protein-mediated multidrug resistance. *Jpn. J. Cancer Res.*, 2002, 93, 231–235.

Sugimoto, Y.; Tsukahara, S.; Imai, Y.; Sugimoto, Y.; Ueda, K.;Tsuruo, T. Reversal of breast cancer resistance protein-mediated drug resistance by estrogen antagonists and agonists. *Mol. Cancer Ther.*, 2003, 2, 105–112.

Imai, Y.; Ishikawa, E.; Asada, S.; Sugimoto, Y. Estrogen-mediated post transcriptional down-regulation of breast cancer resistance protein/ABCG2. *Cancer Res.*, 2005, 65, 596–604.

utoh, K.; Tsukahara, S.; Mitsuhashi, J.; Katayama, K.; Sugimoto, Y. Estrogen-mediated post transcriptional down-regulation of P-glycoprotein in MDR1-transduced human breast cancer cells. *Cancer Sci.*, 2006, 97(11), 1198-1204.

Rosell, R.; Scagliotti, G.; Danenberg, K.D.; Lord, R.V.; Bepler, G.; Novello, S.; Cooc, J.; Crino, L.; Sanchez, J.J.; Taron, M.; Boni, C.; Da Marinis, F.; Tonato, M.; Marangolo, M.; Gozzelino, F.; Di Constanzo, F.; Rinaldi, M.; Solanga, D.; Stephens, C. Transcripts in pretreatment biopsies from a three-arm randomized trial in metastatic nonsmall-cell lung cancer. *Oncogene*, 22(23), 3548–3553.

Seve, P.; Mackey, J.; Isaac, S.; Tredan, O.; Souquet, P.J.; Perol M, Lai, R.; Voloch, A.; Dumontet, C. Class III beta-tubulin expression in tumor cells predicts response and outcome in patients with non-small cell lung cancer receiving paclitaxel. *Mol. Cancer Ther.*, 2005b, 4(12), 2001–2007.

Shalli, K.; Brown, I.; Heys, S.D.; Schofield, A.C. Alterations of beta-tubulin isotypes in breast cancer cells resistant to docetaxel. *FASEB J.*, 2005, 19(10), 1299–1301.

Ranganathan, S.; Benetatos, C.A.; Colarusso, P.J.; Dexter, D.W.; Hudes, G.R. Altered beta-tubulin isotype expression in paclitaxel-resistant human prostate carcinoma cells. *Br. J. Cancer.*, 1998, 77(4), 562–566.

Kavallaris, M.; Kuo, D.Y.; Burkhart, C.A.; Regl, D.L.; Norris, M.D.; Haber, M.; Horwitz, S.B. Taxol-resistant epithelial ovarian tumors are associated with altered expression of specific beta-tubulin isotypes. *J. Clin. Invest.*, 1997, 100(5), 1282–1293.

Gan, P.P.; Pasquier, E.;Kavallaris, M. Class III beta-tubulin mediates sensitivity to chemotherapeutic drugs in non small cell lung cancer. *Cancer Res.*, 2007, 67(19), 9356–9363.

Tommasi, S.; Mangia, A.; Lacalamita, R.; Bellizzi ,A.; Fedele, V.; Chiriatti, A.; Thomssen, C.; Kendzierski, N.; Latorre, A.; Lorusso, V.; Schittulli, F.; Zito, F.;Kavallaris ,M.; Paradiso, A. Cytoskeleton and paclitaxel sensitivity in breast cancer: the role of beta-tubulins. *Int. J. Cancer*, 2007, 120(10), 2078–2085.

Seve, P.; Dumontet, C. Is class III beta-tubulin a predictive factor in patients receiving tubulin-binding agents? *Lancet Oncol.*, 2008, 9(2), 168–175.

Ferrandina, G.; Zannoni ,G.F.; Martinelli ,E.; Paglia, A.; Gallotta, V.; Mozzetti,S.; Scambia, G.; Ferlini, C. Class III beta-tubulin overexpression is a marker of poor clinical outcome in advanced ovarian cancer patients. *Clin. Cancer Res.*, 2006, 12(9), 2774–2779.

Sève, P., Isaac, S., Trédan, O., Souquet, P.J., Pachéco, Y., Pérol, M., Lafanéchère, L., Penet, A., Peiller, E.L., Dumontet, C. Expression of class III {beta}-tubulin is predictive of patient outcome in patients with non-small cell lung cancer receiving vinorelbine-based chemotherapy. *Clin. Cancer Res.*, 2005, 11(15):5481-5486.

Bruhat, A.; Dreau, D.; Drake, M.E.; Tourmente, S.; Chapel, S.; Couderc, J.L.; Dastugue, B. Intronic and 50 flanking sequences of the Drosophila beta 3 tubulin gene are essential to confer ecdysone responsiveness. *Mol. Cell. Endocrinol.*, 1993, 94(1), 61–71.

Saussede-Aim, J.; Matera, E.L.; Ferlini, C.; Dumontet, C. Beta3-tubulin is induced by estradiol in human breast carcinoma cells through an estrogen-receptor dependent pathway. *Cell Motil. Cytoskeleton*, 2009, 66(7), 378-388.

Härkönen, P.L.; Väänänen, H.K. Monocyte-macrophage system as a target for estrogen and selective estrogen receptor modulators. *Ann. N. Y. Acad. Sci.*, 2006, 1089, 218- 227.

Seeger, H., Wallwiener, D., Mueck, A.O. Effects of estradiol and progestogens on tumor-necrosis factor-alpha-induced changes of biochemical markers for breast cancer growth and metastasis. *Gynecol. Endocrinol.*, 2008, 24(10), 576-579.

Kramer, P.R., Kramer, S.F., Guan, G. 17 beta-estradiol regulates cytokine release through modulation of CD16 expression in monocytes and monocyte-derived macrophages. *Arthritis Rheum.*, 2004, 50(6), 1967-1975.

Johnston, S.R. Endocrinology and hormone therapy in breast cancer: selective oestrogen receptor modulators and downregulators for breast cancer - have they lost their way? *Breast Cancer Res.*, 2005, 7(3), 119-130.

Osborne, C.K., Zhao, H., Fuqua, S.A. Selective estrogen receptor modulators: structure, function, and clinical use. *J. Clin. Oncol.*, 2000, 18(17), 72-16.

Howell, S.J., Johnston, S.R., Howell, A. The use of selective estrogen receptor modulators and selective estrogen receptor down-regulators in breast cancer. *Best Pract. Res. Clin. Endocrinol. Metab.*, 2004, 18(1), 47-66.

Kurebayashi, J.; Nukatsuka, M.; Nagase, H.; Nomura, T.; Hirono, M.; Yamamoto, Y,; Sugimoto, Y.; Oka, T.; Sonoo, H. Additive antitumor effect of concurrent treatment of 4-hydroxy tamoxifen with 5-fluorouracil but not with doxorubicin in estrogen receptor-positive breast cancer cells. *Cancer Chemother. Pharmacol.*, 2007, 59(4), 515- 525.

Benz, C.; Cadman, E.; Gwin, J.; Wu, T.; Amara, J.; Eisenfeld, A.; Dannies, P. Tamoxifen and 5-fluorouracil in breast cancer: cytotoxic synergism in vitro. *Cancer Res.*, 1983, 43, 5298–5303.

Leonessa, F.; Jacobson, M.; Boyle, B.; Lippman, J.; McGarvey, M.; Clarke, R. Effect of tamoxifen on the multidrug-resistant phenotype in human breast cancer cells: isobologram, drug accumulation, and M(r) 170,000 glycoprotein (gp170) binding studies. *Cancer Res.*, 1994, 54, 441–447.

Osborne, C.K.; Kitten, L.; Arteaga, C.L. Antagonism of chemotherapy-induced cytotoxicity for human breast cancer cells by antiestrogens. *J. Clin. Oncol.*, 1989, 7, 710–717.

Woods, K.E.; Randolph, J.K.; Gewirtz, D.A. Antagonism between tamoxifen and doxorubicin in the MCF-7 human breast tumor cell line. *Biochem. Pharmacol.*, 1994, 47, 1449–1452.

Licun, W.; Tannock, I.F. Selective estrogen receptor modulators as inhibitors of repopulation of human breast cancer cell lines after chemotherapy. *Clin. Cancer Res.*, 2003, 9(12), 4614-4618.

Wu, L.; Tannock, I.F. Effect of the selective estrogen receptor modulator arzoxifene on repopulation of hormone-responsive breast cancer xenografts between courses of chemotherapy. *Clin. Cancer Res.*, 2005, 11(22), 8195-8200.

Ramachandran, C.; Khatib, Z.; Petkarou, A.; Fort ,J.; Fonseca, H.B.; Melnick, S.J.; Escalon, E. Tamoxifen modulation of etoposide cytotoxicity involves inhibition of protein kinase C activity and insulin-like growth factor II expression in brain tumor cells. *J. Neurooncol.*, 2004, 67(1-2), 19-28.

Sola, B.; Renoir, J.M. Antiestrogenic therapies in solid cancers and multiple myeloma. *Curr. Mol. Med.*, 2006, 6(4), 359-368.

Gao, X.P.; Liu, F. New agents in development for breast cancer. *Curr. Opin. Obstet. Gynecol.*, 2007, 19(1), 68-74.

Díaz-Cruz, E.S., Shapiro, C.L., Brueggemeier, R.W. Cyclooxygenase inhibitors suppress aromatase expression and activity in breast cancer cells. *J. Clin. Endocrinol. Metab.*, 2005, 90(5), 2563-2570.

Chen, D.; Hackl ,W.; Ortmann, O.; Treeck, O. Effects of a combination of exemestane and paclitaxel on human tumor cells in vitro. *Anticancer Drugs*, 2004, 15(1), 55-61.

Varricchio, L., Migliaccio, A., Castoria, G., Yamaguchi, H., de Falco, A., Di Domenico, M., Giovannelli, P., Farrar, W., Appella, E., Auricchio, F. Inhibition of estradiol receptor/Src association and cell growth by an estradiol receptor alpha tyrosine- phosphorylated peptide. Mol. Cancer Res., 2007, 5(11):1213-1221.

Castoria, G.; Migliaccio, A.; Giovannelli, P.; Auricchio, F. Cell proliferation regulated by estradiol receptor: therapeutic implications. *Steroids*, 2010, 75(8-9):524-527.

Zheng, T.; Wang, J.; Chen, X.; Liu, L. Role of microRNA in anticancer drug resistance. *Int. J. Cancer*, 2010, 126(1), 2-10.

Adams, B.D.; Furneaux, H.; White, B.A. The micro-ribonucleic acid (miRNA) miR-206 targets the human estrogen receptor-alpha (ERalpha) and represses ERalpha messenger RNA and protein expression in breast cancer cell lines. *Mol. Endocrinol.*, 2007, 21, 1132–1147.

Ariazi, E.A.; Jordan, V.C. Estrogen-related receptors as emerging targets in cancer and metabolic disorders. *Curr. Top. Med. Chem.*, 2006, 6(3), 203-215.

Zajchowski , D.A.; Sager, R.; Webster, L. Estrogen inhibits the growth of estrogen receptor-negative, but not estrogen receptor-positive, human mammary epithelial cells expressing a recombinant estrogen receptor. *Cancer Res.*, 1993, 53, 5004–5011.

Jiang, S.Y.; Jordan, V.C. Growth regulation of estrogen receptor-negative breast cancer cells transfected with complementary DNAs for estrogen receptor. *J. Natl. Cancer Inst.*, 1992, 84(8), 580-591.

DiMarco, B.; Aguggini, S.; Bolsi, G.; Cirillo, F.; Filippini, L.; Betri, E.; Bertoli, G.; Alquati, P.; Dogliotti, L. p53 but not bcl-2 immunostaining is predictive of poor clinical complete response to primary chemotherapy in breast cancer patients. *Clin. Cancer Res.*, 2000, 6, 2751-2758.

Makris, A.; Powles, T.J.; Dowsett ,M.; Osborne, C.K.; Trott, P.A.; Fernando, I.N.; Ashley, S.E.; Ormerod, M.G.; Titley, J.C.; Gregory, R.K.; Allred, D.C. Prediction of response to neoadjuvant chemoendocrine therapy in primary breast carcinomas. *Clin. Cancer Res.*, 1997, 3, 593-600.

Gapinski, P.V.; Donegan, W.L. Estrogen receptors and breast cancer: prognostic and therapeutic implications. *Surgery*, 1980, 88, 386-393.

Hilf, R.; Feldstein, M.L.; Gibson, S.L.; Savlov, E.D. The relative importance of estrogen receptor analysis as a prognostic factor for recurrence or response to chemotherapy in women with breast cancer. *Cancer*, 1980, 45, 1993-2000.

Hilf, R.; Feldstein, M.L.; Savlov, E.D.; Gibson, S.L.; Seneca, B. The lack of relationship between estrogen receptor status and response to chemotherapy. *Cancer*, 1980, 46(12 Suppl), 2797-2800.

Minisini, A.M.; Di Loreto, C.; Mansutti, M.; Artico, D.; Pizzolitto, S.; Piga, A.; Puglisi,

F. Topoisomerase IIalpha and APE/ref-1 are associated with pathologic response to primary anthracycline-based chemotherapy for breast cancer. *Cancer Lett.*, 2005, 224(1), 133-139.

4

Targeting Cas Family Proteins as a Novel Treatment for Breast Cancer

Joerg Kumbrink and Kathrin H. Kirsch
Department of Biochemistry, Boston University School of Medicine, Boston, MA USA

1. Introduction

Frequently, breast cancer is treated before and after surgery with chemotherapy, hormone, and radiation therapies. However, breast cancers can evolve and stop responding to chemotherapeutic drugs, including adriamycin (doxorubicin), and hormone therapy with tamoxifen. A new generation of targeted biological agents demonstrates a high effectiveness at lower toxicity. Treatment with these specific drugs is limited to subsets of breast cancers that depend on their targets, and eventually patients develop resistance to these drugs as well. This strongly indicates the need to develop novel approaches to fight breast tumor cells and to prevent or reduce drug-resistance. The Cas family of proteins play significant roles in development, proliferation, cell cycle control, cell survival, migration, and invasion. Some of its members, in particular p130^{Cas}/*BCAR1*, has been implicated with tamoxifen as well as adriamycin resistance in mammary tumors. Here we review the role of the Cas family of proteins in breast cancer and summarize the potential development of anti-cancer therapeutics targeting this important family of adapter-type proteins.

1.1 Cas family

Proteins of the Cas (Crk-associated substrate) family function as scaffolds for large multi-protein complexes that integrate the response to numerous stimuli including growth factors, integrin engagement, and hormone release (Tikhmyanova *et al.* 2010; Bouton *et al.* 2001). Cas family members comprise p130^{Cas}/*BCAR1* (Sakai *et al.* 1994a; Brinkman *et al.* 2000), HEF1 (also known as *NEDD9*, CASS2, Cas-L) (Law *et al.* 1996; Minegishi *et al.* 1996), Efs/Sin (CASS3) (Alexandropoulos & Baltimore 1996; Ishino *et al.* 1995), and CASS4 (HEPL) (Singh *et al.* 2008). p130^{Cas} is the founding member and was first identified as a major tyrosine-phosphorylated 130 kDa protein in cells transformed by the v-crk and v-src oncogenes (Sakai *et al.* 1994a). HEF1 (human enhancer of filamentation)/*NEDD9* (neural precursor cell expressed, developmentally downregulated 9) was isolated in a screen for human proteins that confer morphoregulatory changes leading to filamentous budding in yeast *Saccharomyces cerevisiae* (Law *et al.* 1996). In addition, HEF1 was independently isolated based on its homology to p130^{Cas} (Minegishi *et al.* 1996).

Efs/Sin (embryonal Fyn-associated substrate/Src-interacting protein) was identified as a protein binding to the Src-homology (SH) 3 domain of Fyn (Alexandropoulos & Baltimore 1996; Ishino *et al.* 1995). Most recently, the fourth member CASS4 (Cas scaffolding protein family member 4)/HEPL (HEF1-Efs-p130^{Cas}-Like) was identified using reiterative BLAST analysis for protein and mRNA sequences of Cas family members (Singh *et al.* 2008). The expression patterns of Cas family members are distinct. p130[Cas] is ubiquitously expressed in adult tissues, suggesting that it plays an essential role in normal cell physiology (Defilippi *et al.* 2006; Sakai *et al.* 1994a). HEF1 is found primarily in lymphocytes and in lung and breast epithelium (Law *et al.* 1996; Law *et al.* 1998; Minegishi *et al.* 1996). Highest levels of Efs/Sin and CASS4 expression are found in the placenta and brain (Ishino *et al.* 1995), and lung and spleen (Singh *et al.* 2008), respectively.

By facilitating the interaction of Src family kinases (SFKs), focal adhesion kinase (FAK), and recruiting the adaptor proteins Crk and Nck, members of the Cas family play significant roles in signaling networks involved in cell survival (Cabodi *et al.* 2006; Kim *et al.* 2004), cell cycle regulation (Law *et al.* 1998; Ma *et al.* 2007; Yamakita *et al.* 1999), proliferation, and invasion (Huang *et al.* 2002; Klemke *et al.* 1998) (as depicted in Figure 1). These cellular programs are frequently deregulated in different cancer types (Cabodi *et al.* 2010a; Henderson & Feigelson 2000; Marcotte & Muller 2008; Hanahan & Weinberg 2011) and concordantly members of the Cas family have been extensively associated with the development and progression of different tumors in particular mammary carcinomas as reviewed in Section 2.

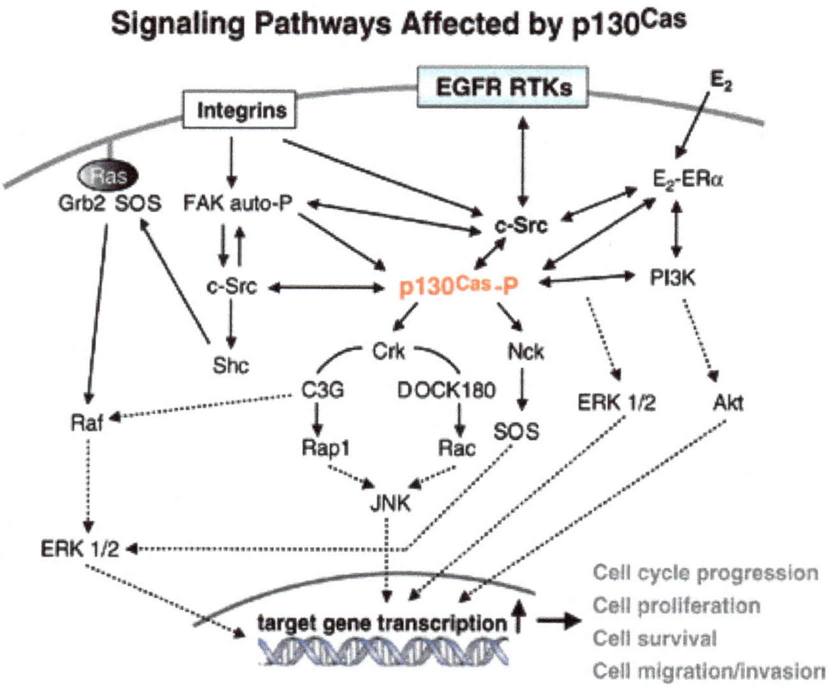

Fig. 1. Major signaling pathways affected by p130[Cas]. Integrin engagement, growth factor-mediated activation of receptor tyrosine kinases (RTKs), and estrogen (E_2)-induced non-genomic estrogen receptor (ER) alpha signaling results in tyrosine phosphorylation of p130[Cas]. The phosphorylated/activated p130[Cas] recruits various effector proteins, thereby generating a signaling node, that activates downstream pathways leading to the induction of transcriptional programs promoting cell cycle progression, proliferation, survival, and migration/invasion. Solid lines depict direct interactions; dashed lines show pathways that have additional steps in between.

1.2 The domain structure of Cas family proteins

Cas proteins exhibit a highly conserved modular domain structure and vary from 561 to 870 amino acids (Tikhmyanova *et al.* 2010). To date no evidence has been found for intrinsic enzymatic activity of the Cas family members. The members are characterized by multiple protein-protein interaction domains including an amino-terminal SH3 domain, a central substrate domain (SD) containing multiple tyrosine phosphorylation sites, a serine-rich region (SER), and a carboxy-terminal domain (CTD) containing a bi-partite Src-binding motif (SBM) (Figure 2). Cas proteins have numerous binding partners for each domain which are summarized in Table 1.

Domain	Interacting partners	Reference
SH3 domain	C3G	(Kirsch *et al.* 1998)
	CMS/CD2AP	(Kirsch *et al.* 1999)
	CIZ	(Nakamoto *et al.* 2000)
	FAK	(Polte & Hanks 1995; Law *et al.* 1996; Singh *et al.* 2008)
	FRANK	(Harte *et al.* 1996)
	PR-39	(Chan & Gallo 1998)
	PTP-1B	(Liu *et al.* 1996)
	PTP-PEST	(Garton *et al.* 1997)
	Pyk2	(Astier *et al.* 1997; Lakkakorpi *et al.* 1999)
Substrate Domain	<u>Crk family:</u> CrkI, CrkII, CrkL	(Burnham *et al.* 1996; Ishino *et al.* 1995; Petruzzelli *et al.* 1996; Sakai *et al.* 1994a; Salgia *et al.* 1996)
	Nck	(Schlaepfer *et al.* 1997)
	SHP-2	(Prasad *et al.* 2001; Yo *et al.* 2009)
	c-Src	(Shin *et al.* 2004)
Serine-rich Domain	14-3-3	(Briknarova *et al.* 2005)
Carboxy-terminal domain	AIP4	(Feng *et al.* 2004)
	APC/C, CDH1	(Nourry *et al.* 2004)
	Bmx/Etk	(Abassi *et al.* 2003)
	<u>NSP family:</u> BCAR3/NSP2, NSP1, CHAT	(Gotoh *et al.* 2000; Lu *et al.* 1999; Sakakibara & Hattori 2000)
	Nephrocystin	(Donaldson *et al.* 2000)
	p130^{Cas}, HEF1, Id2	(Law *et al.* 1999)
	p140Cap	(Di Stefano *et al.* 2004)
	PI3K	(Li *et al.* 2000)
	<u>Src family:</u> c-SRC, LCK, LYN, HCK, FYN, YES	(Alexandropoulos & Baltimore 1996; Ishino *et al.* 1995; Kanda *et al.* 1999; Nakamoto *et al.* 1996; Nasertorabi *et al.* 2006; Nishio & Suzuki 2002; Pellicena & Miller 2001; Singh *et al.* 2008)
Not mapped/ indirect	DDR	(Shintani *et al.* 2008)
	ER alpha	(Cabodi *et al.* 2004)
	Grb2	(Wang *et al.* 2000)
	Smad3	(Liu *et al.* 2000)

Table 1. Interacting partners of Cas family proteins.

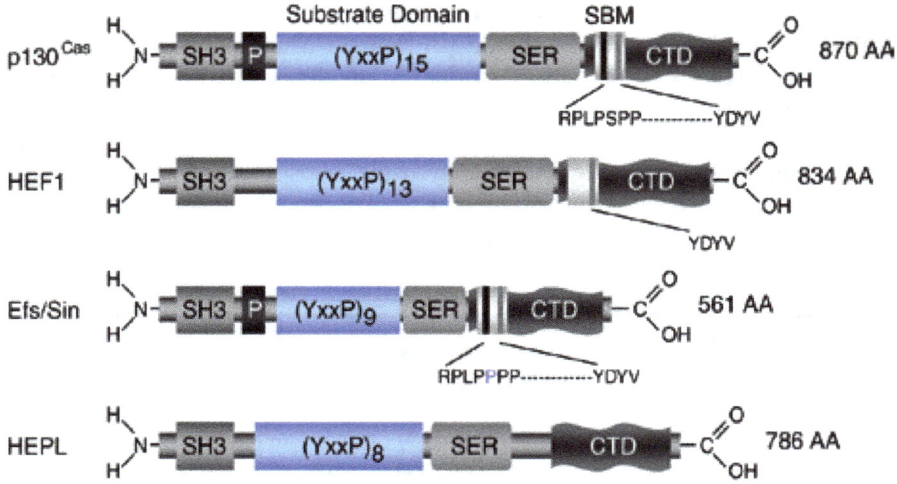

Fig. 2. Domain structure of the Cas family members. SH3, Src homology 3 domain. P, proline-rich region. SER, serine-rich domain. SBM, bi-partite Src-binding motif. CTD, carboxy-terminal domain. The number of YxxP motifs, representing SH2 domain binding sites when phosphorylated, are indicated.

1.2.1 The SH3 domain

The amino-terminal SH3 domain is an interaction module that associates with proteins containing proline-rich motifs with the core consensus sequence PxxP (Ren *et al.* 1993). The SH3 domain of p130Cas selects binding sites sharing the consensus motif *XX*Pp+Pp*X* (where + and *X* represent positively charges and non-conserved residues, respectively; lower case positions contain residues that tend to be proline) (Kirsch *et al.* 1998). The specificity of the p130Cas SH3 domain is strongly dependent on the positively charged amino acid in the position P_2 (see nomenclature in Yu *et al.* 1994). The functional relevance of the interaction of Cas family members with FAK via the Cas SH3 domain has been extensively studied (Polte & Hanks 1995; Parsons *et al.* 2000; Law *et al.* 1996; Singh *et al.* 2008; Provenzano & Keely 2009; Tikhmyanova *et al.* 2010). Utilizing p130Cas SH3 domain deletion mutants, studies indicated that this domain and its interaction with FAK are necessary for phosphorylation and the localization of p130Cas to focal adhesions (FAs) (Nakamoto *et al.* 1997). More recent studies, further explored the temporal and spatial involvement of p130Cas in FA dynamics and showed the influence of p130Cas in FA turnover and controlling the migratory response (Donato *et al.* 2010; Meenderink *et al.* 2010). The p130Cas SH3 domain was shown to be necessary for tyrosine phosphorylation of the SD and the promotion of cell migration (Donato *et al.* 2010), in conditional FAK-deficient mammary tumor cells a reduction in the phosphorylation of Y249 within the p130Cas SD was observed (Provenzano *et al.* 2008). These studies uncovered the significance of the Cas SH3 domain in the spatial regulation of Cas protein function and in particular its role for the phosphorylation of the SD of the Cas proteins (as described in the next section).

1.2.2 The substrate domain (SD)

The SD region of the Cas family members is situated adjacent to the SH3 domain and contains clusters of YxxP tyrosine phosphorylation sites (Figure 2). The SD of p130Cas and

HEF1 contain 15 and 13 YxxP motifs, whereas only eight and nine of these motifs are present in Efs/Sin and HEPL, respectively (Alexandropoulos & Baltimore 1996; Ishino *et al.* 1995; Law *et al.* 1996; Sakai *et al.* 1994a), which upon phosphorylation by Src family members recruit small adaptor proteins such as Crk, CRKII, CrkL, and Nck via their respective SH2 domains (Burnham *et al.* 1996; Harte *et al.* 1996; Minegishi *et al.* 1996).

The SFKs, in particular c-Src, play significant roles in the activation of Cas proteins by phosphorylation of tyrosine residues within the SD, resulting in coupling to downstream effector molecules (Sakai *et al.* 1997; Schlaepfer *et al.* 1997). Correspondingly, c-Src-deficient cells show reduced Cas phosphorylation levels. Furthermore, *in vitro* kinase assays show that c-Src, in comparison to FAK, has a stronger ability to phosphorylate the SD of $p130^{Cas}$ (Ruest *et al.* 2001).

In order to prevent permanent activation of Cas-related pathways, the protein tyrosine phosphatases (PTPs) PTP-1B (Liu *et al.* 1996), PTP-PEST (Garton *et al.* 1997; Cote *et al.* 1998), and leukocyte antigen related (LAR)-PTP (Hoon *et al.* 2003) can be recruited to Cas family members to dephosphorylate Cas proteins and other associated molecules. This results, for instance, in the subsequent cleavage and degradation of the $p130^{Cas}$ protein (Hoon *et al.* 2003; Weng *et al.* 1999) and/or the disassembly of signaling complexes in FAs (Angers-Loustau *et al.* 1999).

The tyrosine phosphorylation/activation status of Cas family members is altered by diverse stimuli, including environmental influences such as growth factors, integrin, and estrogen signaling as well as intrinsic signals, thereby modulating multiple signal transduction networks as depicted in Figure 1 (reviewed in Bouton *et al.* 2001; Cabodi *et al.* 2010a; Tikhmyanova *et al.* 2010). SD phosphorylation correlates with transformation and the effector signaling pathways relevant in breast cancer development and progression involving the Cas family proteins are reviewed in Section 2.

1.2.3 The serine-rich domain (SER)

This domain is situated between the SD and the CTD and is enriched in serines and threonines (Alexandropoulos & Baltimore 1996; Law *et al.* 1996; Sakai *et al.* 1994a; Sakai *et al.* 1994b; Singh *et al.* 2008). Although the SER was initially thought to separate and orient the SD and SBM, several studies identified important properties. During mitosis an increase in the phosphorylation of serine and threonine residues of $p130^{Cas}$ has been observed (Yamakita *et al.* 1999). Notably, adhesion-dependent serine phosphorylation of $p130^{Cas}$ is associated with an invasive phenotype in breast cancer cells (Makkinje *et al.* 2009). The solution structure of the SER of $p130^{Cas}$ was determined by nuclear magnetic resonance spectroscopy revealing that it folds as a four-helix bundle. Site-directed mutagenesis and binding assays characterized this domain as an interaction site for 14-3-3 proteins (Briknarova *et al.* 2005). Proteins of the 14-3-3 family act as chaperones or scaffolds and are involved in signaling, cell cycle control, and apoptosis (reviewed in Bridges & Moorhead 2004).

1.2.4 The carboxy-terminal domain (CTD)

Although the CTD, which folds as a helix-loop-helix (HLH) structure, is the most conserved region among Cas family members, one of the striking differences regarding this domain is the presence or absence of the bi-partite SBM. The SBM consists of a proline-rich motif (RPLP S/P PP) that interacts with the SH3 domain of SFKs and a YDYVHL motif that, when

phosphorylated, interacts with the SH2 domain of SFKs. This region is present in $p130^{Cas}$ and Efs/Sin but absent in CASS4 (Alexandropoulos & Baltimore 1996; Nakamoto *et al.* 1996; Singh *et al.* 2008; Nasertorabi *et al.* 2006). HEF1 contains the SH2 binding motif but lacks the SH3 binding motif (Law *et al.* 1996). This may influence the ability of HEF1 to bind SFKs and to become phosphorylated, since amino acid substitutions in the RPLP S/P PP sequence reduces/abolishes binding to Src (Burnham *et al.* 1999; Burnham *et al.* 2000; Nakamoto *et al.* 1996). However, TGF-β-mediated tyrosine phosphorylation of HEF1 (Zheng & McKeown-Longo 2002) and attachment-induced tyrosine phosphorylation of CASS4 (Singh *et al.* 2008), are both dependent on Src kinase activity. It has been suggested that additonal mechanisms may regulate this modification such as FAK-dependent recruitment of c-Src to $p130^{Cas}$ (Ruest *et al.* 2001). The differences in the SBM of Cas proteins likely indicate distinct functions among the Cas proteins, which are highly dependent on the phosphorylation of the SD by SFKs and represents an important event in different cellular programs (see 1.2.2).
The CTD along with the SH3 domain target $p130^{Cas}$ to FAs, as deletion of the CTD prevents the localization of $p130^{Cas}$ to FAs (Harte *et al.* 2000). In addition, the CTD mediates the homo- and heterodimerization of $p130^{Cas}$ and HEF1 (Law *et al.* 1999) thereby potentially generating additional regulatory mechanisms.

2. Involvement of Cas family members in mammary carcinomas

Over the last decade *in vivo* studies in different organisms and *in vitro* studies in cells in culture accumulated evidence that individual Cas family members play central roles in the development and progression of mammary carcinomas. The $p130^{Cas}$ and HEF1 proteins are the best studied in this context. Primary breast tumors contain elevated $p130^{Cas}$ levels, which correlate with increased rate of relapse and with poor response to tamoxifen treatment (van der Flier *et al.* 2000). Increased $p130^{Cas}$ expression was also found in tumor cells isolated from pleural effusions of breast cancer patients in comparison to primary tumors (Konstantinovsky *et al.* 2010). In feline and canine breast cancers the levels of $p130^{Cas}$ positively correlate with advanced breast disease as well (Scibelli *et al.* 2003). Furthermore, our *in vitro* studies have shown increased $p130^{Cas}$ levels in the tamoxifen resistant breast cancer cells TAM-R (Soni *et al.* 2009), which were derived from tamoxifen sensitive MCF-7 cells (Knowlden *et al.* 2003).
In 2000, Brinkman and colleagues identified the gene of $p130^{Cas}$, in a retroviral insertion screen as a factor that mediates resistance to tamoxifen in breast cancer cell lines (Brinkman *et al.* 2000; Dorssers *et al.* 1993). Subsequently, the gene located on chromosome 16q23.1 was named *BCAR1* (breast cancer anti-estrogen resistance 1). Although HEF1 has a similar domain structure it was unable to support long-term anti-estrogen resistant cell proliferation (Brinkman *et al.* 2009). Chimeric $p130^{Cas}$/HEF1 proteins generated by exchange of defined domains, identified the SD of $p130^{Cas}$ as the region contributing to anti-estrogen resistance in breast cancer cells (Brinkman *et al.* 2009). Accordingly, disruption of the $p130^{Cas}$ signaling node by ectopic expression of an isolated constitutively tyrosine phosphorylated SD of $p130^{Cas}$ in the cytoplasm (as described in detail in Section 3) led to reduced proliferation and re-sensitization of tamoxifen resistant breast cancer cells to tamoxifen (Kirsch *et al.* 2002; Soni *et al.* 2009).
The mechanisms by which Cas proteins may promote mammary carcinomas and acquired tamoxifen resistance are manifold and under extensive investigation. It has been shown that estrogen treatment triggers the rapid and transient association of $p130^{Cas}$ with the estrogen

receptor (ER) alpha in the cytoplasm, thus mediating non-genomic ER signaling in human breast cancer cells (Cabodi *et al.* 2004). This is dependent on c-Src activation and results in the formation of a multi-molecular complex containing p130^{Cas}, c-Src, and the p85 subunit of phosphatidylinositol 3-kinase (PI3K) and subsequent activation of extracellular-signal regulated kinase (ERK) 1/2. Importantly, overexpression of p130^{Cas} as well as short-interfering (si) RNA-mediated reduction of p130^{Cas} experiments in T47D breast cancer cells indicated that p130^{Cas} enhances the estrogen-dependent Src and Erk1/2 activities (and accelerates the kinetics in response to stimulation) (Cabodi *et al.* 2004). Long-term treatment of estrogen-dependent mammary carcinoma cells with the estrogen antagonist tamoxifen led to increased phosphorylation levels of p130^{Cas} (Cowell *et al.* 2006; Soni *et al.* 2009), suggesting that anti-estrogens modulate intrinsic mechanisms to deregulate Cas protein function.

Resistance to the anti-estrogens tamoxifen and fulvestrant, is associated with enhanced growth factor signaling involving the upregulation of epidermal growth factor receptor (EGFR) family and alteration of the AKT signaling pathway (Knowlden *et al.* 2003; Soni *et al.* 2009; Zhang *et al.* 2009; Frogne *et al.* 2009). Consistently, interference with p130^{Cas} signaling results in the attenuation of the ERK and PI3K/Akt survival pathways in breast cancer cells (Soni *et al.* 2009). Moreover, overexpression of p130^{Cas} mediates resistance to the chemotherapeutic drug adriamycin in mammary tumor cells by activating c-Src, Akt, and ERK1/2 growth and survival pathways (Ta *et al.* 2008).

More recent *in vivo* studies in transgenic mice overexpressing p130^{Cas} in mammary epithelial cells, showed substantial mammary epithelial cell hyperplasia during development and pregnancy, and delayed involution (Cabodi *et al.* 2006). Activation of Src, ERK1/2, mitogen-activated protein kinase (MAPK), and Akt pathways contribute to these phenotypes by inducing proliferation and inhibiting apoptosis.

Importantly, accelerated mammary tumor formation has been observed in double transgenic mice that overexpress both p130^{Cas} and the activated form of HER2/neu (human epidermal growth factor receptor 2) compared to the HER2/neu single transgenic mice without p130^{Cas} (Cabodi *et al.* 2006). Delivery of p130^{Cas}/*BCAR1*-specific siRNAs into the mammary gland of transgenic BALB-HER2/neu mice carrying the activated *HER2/neu* oncogene was sufficient to inhibit HER2/neu signaling and decreased the growth of spontaneous tumors *in vivo* (Cabodi *et al.* 2010b).

The balance between canonical and noncanonical transforming growth factor (TGF)-β signaling in mammary carcinomas is also regulated by p130^{Cas} (Wendt *et al.* 2009). Maintaining this balance is critical as TGF-β acts as both a tumor-suppressor or tumor-promoter depending on the tumor microenvironment and tumor stage (as reviewed in Ikushima & Miyazono 2010; Meulmeester & Ten Dijke 2011). Forced expression of either full length p130^{Cas} or the CTD of p130^{Cas} in mammary epithelial cells (MECs) shifted TGF-β signaling from Smad2/3 to p38 MAPK activation resulting in resistance of TGF-β-induced growth arrest and increased invasion and metastasis of MECs *in vivo* utilizing an orthotopic mouse model (Wendt *et al.* 2009).

In addition to p130^{Cas}, HEF1, also mediates TGF-β tumor promoting activities. TGF-β signaling upregulates HEF1 thereby enhancing mammary carcinoma cell scattering and the transition from collective cell motility to single cell motility (Giampieri *et al.* 2009). Similar to the TGF-β study, HEF1 overexpression in MCF-7 breast cancer cells increases the migration and invasion *in vitro* (Fashena *et al.* 2002). In MMTV-polyoma virus middle T antigen

(PyMT) mice crossed with the HEF1-deficient (HEF$^{-/-}$) mice delayed mammary tumor formation and reduced tumor incidence was observed (Izumchenko *et al.* 2009). Most of the mammary tumors excised from PyMT/HEF1$^{-/-}$ mice showed reduced activation of AKT, FAK, Src, and ERK1/2 compared to HEF1 wildtype animals. In contrast, an siRNA screening approach to identify genes that regulate migration in non-transformed mammary epithelial MCF-10A cells demonstrated an inhibitory function of HEF1 on migration (Simpson *et al.* 2008). Furthermore, HEF1 is part of a lung metastasis signature for primary breast cancers (Minn *et al.* 2005). In this study, an orthotopic MDA-MB-231 breast cancer mouse model was used and HEF1 was found to be down-regulated in highly lung metastatic mammary cancer cells. These results may suggest, that high levels of HEF1 contribute to early stages of breast cancer and a loss of expression during tumor progression may promote later stages leading to metastases formation of tumor cells.

In summary, the studies reviewed here indicate the extensive involvement of Cas family members, specifically p130^{Cas} and HEF1, in the transformation of mammary epithelium as well as acquired resistance of breast cancers to several therapeutic agents. The effects of the Cas proteins might be further amplified by simultaneous and synergistic activation of multiple signaling effector pathways, in particular down-stream of the SD of p130^{Cas} and HEF1.

2.1 Role of Cas SD effector protein signaling in mammary carcinomas

As described above, phosphorylaion of the Cas SD and subsequent coupling to effector molecules has been implicated in the transformation of cells, breast cancer progression, and acquired tamoxifen resistance (reviewed in Tikhmyanova *et al.* 2010). To better understand how the SD of the Cas proteins may contribute to these malignant processes the involvement of SD-interacting proteins in breast cancer is reviewed in this section.

2.1.1 The Crk family

Members of the Crk (chicken tumor virus no. 10 regulator of kinase) family, consisting of CRKI, CRKII, generated by alternative splicing of transcripts of the *CRK* gene, and CRKL (CRK-like protein) are SH2 and SH3 domain containing adaptor proteins (Matsuda *et al.* 1992; ten Hoeve *et al.* 1993; Feller & Lewitzky 2006). The Crk family SH2 domains bind to p130^{Cas} upon phosphorylation of the SD and recruit additional downstream effectors via their SH3 domains. The amino-terminal SH3 domain of Crk binds to guanine nucleotide exchange factors (GEFs), including C3G, Sos (Son of sevenless) (Feller *et al.* 1995; Okada & Pessin 1996), and DOCK1 (dedicator of cytokinesis 1, also known as DOCK180) (Hasegawa *et al.* 1996). This complex leads to the activation of the small GTPases Rap1 (Gotoh *et al.* 1995) and Rac (Dolfi *et al.* 1998), and subsequently JNK (c-Jun N-terminal kinase) signaling (shown in part in Figure 1) (Dolfi *et al.* 1998).

Crk proteins have been associated with several different tumor types and especially with the promotion of an invasive phenotype and cell migration (Cabodi *et al.* 2010a; Tikhmyanova *et al.* 2010). Interestingly, Klemke's group was the first to reveal that p130^{Cas}-crk coupling is involved in HER2/neu -mediated cell migration (Spencer *et al.* 2000). Subsequently, Park's group found elevated CrkI and CrkII protein levels in human mammary tumors and showed that siRNA-mediated CrkI/II knockdown results in a significant decrease in migration and invasion of breast cancer cells (Rodrigues *et al.* 2005). More recently, the same group observed in post-pubertal MMTV-CrkII transgenic mice premature ductal branching that was associated with increased proliferation (Fathers *et al.* 2010). The mammary tumor incidence in MMTV-CrkII mice was 17.6% compared to 4% in female control mice with a similar latency of approximately 15 months. While Crk has been shown to induce cell migration, no metastatic lesions were found in any of the MMTV-CrkII animals. This suggests that CrkII plays a more important role at the early stages of breast carcinomas *in vivo*.

2.1.2 The Src-family tyrosine kinases (SFKs)

The SFKs are comprised of ten members of which c-Src, Lck, Lyn, Hck, Fyn, and Yes phosphorylate the SD of the Cas proteins (Alexandropoulos & Baltimore 1996; Ishino *et al.* 1995; Kanda *et al.* 1999; Nakamoto *et al.* 1996; Nasertorabi *et al.* 2006; Nishio & Suzuki 2002; Pellicena & Miller 2001; Singh *et al.* 2008). In addition to phosphorylating the $p130^{Cas}$ SD, c-Src binds to phosphorylated tyrosine residues within SD *in vitro* (Shin *et al.* 2004).

SFKs have a conserved structure containing SH1 (kinase), SH2, SH3, and SH4 (membrane targeting) domains and transactivate interacting partners by phosphorylation resulting in the activation of multiple signaling pathways as presented in part in Figure 1 (reviewed in Mayer & Krop 2010; Wheeler *et al.* 2009). The kinase activity is tightly regulated by tyrosine-phosphorylation on the carboxyl terminus by CSK (c-src tyrosine kinase) resulting in intramolecular binding and an inactive closed conformation (Superti-Furga *et al.* 1993). The precise cellular regulation of c-Src is of major relevance and $p130^{Cas}$ has been postulated to activate c-Src by disrupting the intramolecular inactive conformation (Nasertorabi *et al.* 2006; Burnham *et al.* 2000).

SFKs are central players in multiple cellular programs that are often dysregulated during tumorigenesis and progression and several of the members have been associated with malignant transformation. The founding member c-Src was the first proto-oncogene to be sequenced in the early 1980s (Czernilofsky *et al.* 1980; Schwartz *et al.* 1983; Takeya & Hanafusa 1982) and over the past 30 years several therapeutic agents to inhibit Src kinase activity have been developed and clinical trials are ongoing (summarized in Aleshin & Finn 2010; Mayer & Krop 2010).

Several studies have demonstrated the relevance of Src in breast cancer as enhanced expression and activity of c-Src was observed in human mammary carcinoma cell lines and tumor tissues (Biscardi *et al.* 1998; Jacobs & Rubsamen 1983; Ottenhoff-Kalff *et al.* 1992; Verbeek *et al.* 1996). Studies by Muller's group unequivocally showed that expression of an activated c-Src protein in the mammary gland of mice induces tumor formation, though with long latency (Webster *et al.* 1995). Importantly, tumor formation in transgenic mice expressing the PyMT oncogene under the control of the MMTV promoter is c-Src dependent as PyMT-Src-deficient mice rarely developed mammary tumors, whereas a more rapid tumor progression was found in the MMTV-PyMT control mice (Guy *et al.* 1994). Furthermore, aberrated c-Src expression and activity has been associated with Her2/neu transformation *in vivo* (Muthuswamy & Muller 1995). Several SFK specific inhibitors have been developed which suppress migration and invasion of human breast cancer cells (Vultur *et al.* 2008). These compounds also reduce the incidence of metastasis formation after intracardiac injection of human breast cancer cells in nude mice (Rucci *et al.* 2006).

2.1.3 SHP-2 (Src homology 2 domain-containing protein tyrosine phosphatase)

Through its interactions with numerous proteins via its two SH2 domains, the protein tyrosine phosphatase SHP-2 regulates oncogenic transformation (as reviewed in Matozaki *et al.* 2009). Conflicting results have been reported for a role of SHP-2 in mammary adenocarcinomas in regard to the effect on migration. Upon tyrosine phosphorylation of HEF1, SHP-2 associates with the HEF1 SD and dephosphorylates it thereby inhibiting HEF1-mediated cell migration (Yo *et al.* 2009). Conversely, SHP-2 acts as a positive regulator of migration of MCF7 breast cancer cells *in vitro* and promotes metastasis of MCF7 cells, when injected into the abdominal cavity of nude mice *in vivo* (Wang *et al.* 2005).

2.1.4 The Nck family

Similar to the Crk proteins, the two Nck family members are SH2/SH3 domain-containing adapters which regulate tyrosine kinase signaling (reviewed in Buday *et al.* 2002). Nck was first identified in a screen of a human melanoma cDNA library using antibodies against the melanoma cell adhesion molecule (MCAM) (Lehmann *et al.* 1990). In MCF-7 breast cancer cells, Nck is required for fibroblast growth factor (FGF)-2-induced DNA synthesis (Liu et al. 1999). Furthermore, Nck facilitates invadopodia formation and extracellular matrix (ECM) degradation in various tumor cell lines including breast cancer cells (Stylli et al. 2009).

These studies summarized here emphasize the importance of Cas effector proteins in the promotion of breast cancer *in vitro* and *in vivo*. They highlight the potential importance of targeting the $p130^{Cas}$ signaling node in human breast cancers, as Cas family members might contribute to this malignancy through their association with these SD interacting molecules.

3. Novel strategies to develop therapeutic agents for targeting Cas signaling in mammary carcinomas

Though many studies have suggested that $p130^{Cas}$ and HEF1 are critical for phenotypic changes that drive breast cancer progression and metastasis (see Section 2), no therapeutic agents (drugs) have been developed that target these important proteins. It might be feasible to inactivate cancer promoting adaptor proteins by several mechanisms among them (a) downregulating their expression or (b) by interfering with specific protein-protein interaction modules. Defillipi's group used an RNAi-based approach to mediate downregulation of $p130^{Cas}$ by intranipple injection of siRNA resulting in a reduction of tumor growth in BALB-HER2/neu mice (Cabodi *et al.* 2010b). These results are very promising and may warrant further exploration.

Current research has now revealed a clearer picture regarding the functions of the different domains in $p130^{Cas}$ signaling and tumor formation (see Sections 1 and 2). Therefore, inhibitors targeting individual domains, such as the SD, SH3, and/or CTD domain, might confer additional specificity and maintain the functional properties of the other domains thereby reducing potential adverse effects. As an alternative approach, the Src*/CasSD decoy molecule (Kirsch et al., 2002 and summarized in Section 3.1) could be used as a starting point to develop inhibitors that target only certain Cas functions.

3.1 Blocking $p130^{Cas}$ SD signaling by utilization of a phosphorylated $p130^{Cas}$ SD

As discussed above, the important role for $p130^{Cas}$ in breast cancer has been demonstrated by several groups, with a critical function for the SD emerging in cell transformation. Kirsch and colleagues previously investigated the role of the Cas SD in transformation by functionally separating Cas from upstream signals (Kirsch *et al.* 2002). The $p130^{Cas}$ SD was fused to the Src kinase domain with attenuated activity [activating tyrosine 416 replaced with phenylalanine (Y416F); designated as Src*/CasSD] (Figure 3) (Kmiecik & Shalloway 1987; Piwnica-Worms *et al.* 1987). As controls, a Src kinase inactive mutant (K295M) (Jove *et al.* 1987) fused to the p130^{Cas} SD (Src^{KM}/CasSD) and the isolated Src* were employed (Kirsch *et al.* 2002). The initial hypothesis, that this constitutively phosphorylated chimera would act as dominant active molecule by circumventing upstream signaling had to be revised as the results obtained in transient and stably expressing cell systems revealed a dominant negative effect on downstream signaling. It was subsequently found that the Src*/CasSD chimera attenuated cellular transformation. Expression of Src*/CasSD resulted in a significant reduction of colony formation of v-crk transformed NIH3T3 cells in soft agar assays. Further experiments, suggested that the isolated tyrosine phosphorylated CasSD acts as a decoy for v- and c-Crk thereby blocking the ability of v-crk to transform these cells involving a reduction in JNK activation (Kirsch *et al.* 2002).

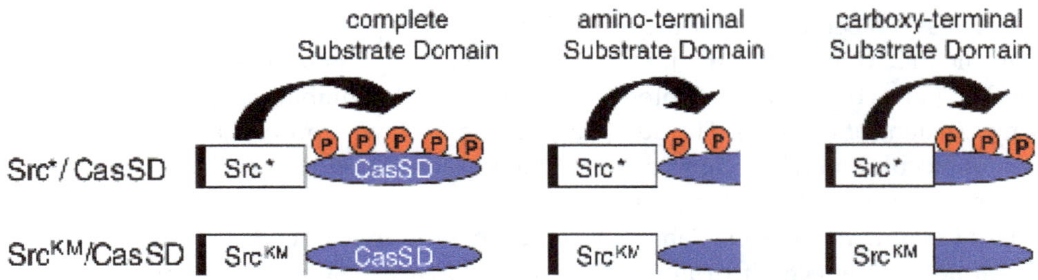

Fig. 3. Representation of the dominant negative p130^{Cas} (Src*/CasSD) and control (Src^{KM}/CasSD) fusion constructs generated by Kirsch and colleagues, 2002. Src*, attenuated Src kinase domain. Src^{KM}, inactive Src kinase domain. CasSD, substrate domain of p130^{Cas}. P, phosphorylation.

Additional studies utilizing this approach in different cellular contexts revealed proof of principle of the Src*/CasSD decoy approach. In BxPC3 pancreatic adenocarcinoma cells the Src*/CasSD expression prevented collagen I-mediated upregulation of N-cadherin and cell scattering (Shintani *et al.* 2008). In tamoxifen resistant breast cancer cells TAM-R, expression of the chimeric molecule attenuated several signaling pathways involved in breast carcinoma progression and acquired tamoxifen resistance (see below) (Soni *et al.* 2009).

TAM-R cells were established by long-term exposure of estrogen-dependent MCF-7 cells to tamoxifen (Hiscox *et al.* 2004). Importantly, similar to anti-estrogen resistant breast cancers, endogenous p130^{Cas} levels are increased and highly phosphorylated in these cells (Soni *et al.* 2009), a further indication that p130^{Cas} contributes to tamoxifen resistance. A major finding of our study investigating the effects of the inhibition of p130^{Cas} by the Src*/CasSD chimera on breast cancer cells was the re-sensitization of TAM-R cells to tamoxifen resulting in increased apoptosis (Soni *et al.* 2009). Of note, the Src*/CasSD induced apoptosis was specific for TAM-R cells and not detected in the parental MCF-7 cells expressing lower p130^{Cas} levels. Moreover, expression of Src*/CasSD resulted in reduced cell numbers of MCF-7 and TAM-R cells and in a reversion to a more epithelial-like phenotype in TAM-R cells. In TAM-R cells, these observations were accompanied by elevated levels of ERα, E-cadherin stabilization at cell-cell boundaries, and reduced migration and consistently, enhanced cell clustering. Furthermore, employment of the Src*/CasSD approach in TAM-R cells led to the reduction of growth factor signaling as seen by an attenuated PI3K/AKT pro-survival pathway, and a reduced activation of the MAPK/ERK pathway (Soni *et al.* 2009).

Taken together, these studies suggest, that blocking endogenous p130Cas function by ectopic expression of a constitutively phosphorylated p130Cas SD may represent an important tool not only for further elucidating the mechanisms by which Cas proteins contribute to breast cancer and other malignancies but also to develop potential therapeutic agents targeting this domain as discussed below.

3.2 The Src*/CasSD decoy approach - a starting point to develop potential therapeutics for breast cancer

The Src*/CasSD approach implies at least two different strategies to inhibit downstream signaling of Cas family proteins: **1.** Develop therapeutic agents reflecting the structure of important parts of the phosphorylated SD (mimetic), which act as a decoy for SD interacting molecules, thereby competing with endogenous Cas proteins for binding partners; **2.** Design compounds that bind to functionally relevant tyrosine motifs in the SD of the endogenous Cas proteins to block the recruitment of SD binding adapter proteins. **3.** Design drugs that bind to the SH2 domains of the interacting proteins as it has been elegantly demonstrated for Grb2 (Growth factor receptor-bound protein 2) inhibitors (Atabey *et al.* 2001; Dharmawardana *et al.* 2006). The advantage of the first two approaches lies in the fact that several molecules may be targeted simultaneously. On the other hand, this can be a disadvantage as well, due to the possibility of a greater degree of unwanted effects.

One requirement for specific inhibition of protein-protein interaction (PPI) and to limit potential adverse effects of drugs is to narrow down the targeting region. This will also increase alternative options for the choice of an application such as the utilization of peptide inhibitors or small-inhibitory molecules (discussed below).

Not all of the YxxP motifs in the Cas SD are phosphorylated by Src, or important for Crk, Src, and/or Nck binding (Kirsch *et al.* 2002; Shin *et al.* 2004) (summarized in Fig. 4), potentially suggesting that smaller fragments of the SD might be sufficient to mediate the inhibition of breast carcinoma progression. Importantly, the initial study describing the Src*/CasSD approach showed that the carboxy-terminal YxxP motifs six to fifteen of the p130Cas SD were necessary for decoying/interacting with Crk (Kirsch *et al.* 2002). This correlated with the identified Crk-SH2 consensus sequence of YDxP (Birge *et al.* 1993; Songyang *et al.* 1993). In addition, the carboxy-terminal part of the p130Cas SD is essential for p130Cas-mediated cell migration (Shin *et al.* 2004). Furthermore, the majority of the 15 and 13 tyrosine motifs

within the p130Cas and HEF1 SD, respectively, belong to two groups of sequences: YQxP and YDxP (Fig. 4B). PhosphoSitePlus™ (Hornbeck *et al.* 2004), a comprehensive resource of known phosphorylation sites, indicated that in both family members the amino-terminal motifs (primarily of the YQxP sequence) in the SD are rarely phosporylated, whereas the carboxy-terminal sites (primarily of the YDxP sequence) are significantly more often phosphorylated as measured by high-throughput mass spectometry screenings (Fig. 4B). In addition, these studies support the hypothesis that a drug based on the Src*/CasSD approach may block signaling mediated by both p130Cas and HEF1 proteins. However, to date no studies addressing the influence of the Src*/CasSD chimera on HEF1 activity, and the importance of the carboxy-terminal part of the Cas SD for mediating the inhibition have been performed.

To test this hypothesis, experiments are currently ongoing in our laboratory using the Src*/CasSD approach to identify and define the smallest region of the SD that retains its inhibitory function in breast cancer *in vitro* and *in vivo*. Subsequently, the structure of this constitutively phosphorylated peptide could be resolved by crystallization and *in silico* protein structure modeling, which may provide a starting point to design therapeutic agents for future testing.

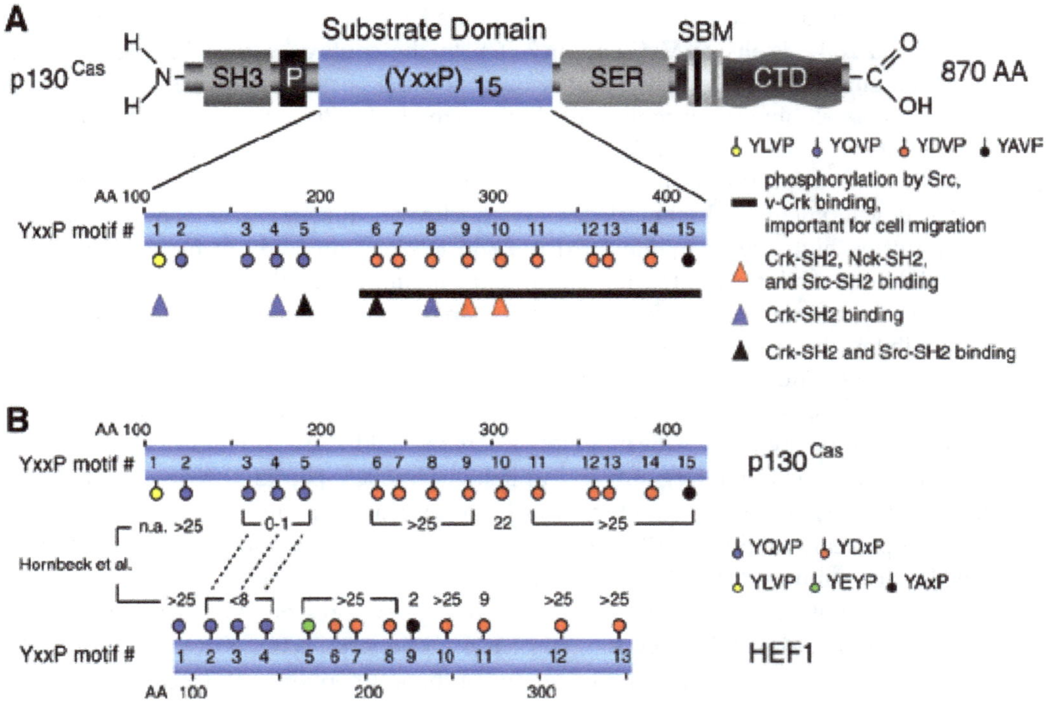

Fig. 4. Representation of the YxxP motifs in the p130^{Cas} and HEF1 substrate domains. A, Interaction partners for p130^{Cas} and a region important for cell migration are indicated. SH3, Src homology 3 domain. P, proline-rich region. SER, serine-rich domain. SBM, bi-partite Src-binding motif. CTD, carboxy-terminal domain. B, Comparison of the YxxP motifs in the SD of p130^{Cas} and HEF1. The number of studies showing phosphorylation of certain motifs by high-throughput mass spectometry screening as curated at PhosphoSitePlus™ (Hornbeck *et al.* 2004) are indicated. n.a., not available.

4. Overview of potential approaches for targeting cytoplasmic adapter proteins

Over the past 15 years progress has been made in drug development and different novel approaches have become avaible to diversify the options of drug design and functional screening. For instance, humanized therapeutic antibodies, intrabodies, peptide inhibitors, peptidomimetics, or small-molecule inhibitors have been employed in cancer therapies and are undergoing clinical trials (Buchwald 2010; Leader *et al.* 2008; Lo *et al.* 2008).

Although therapeutic antibodies usually show a high specificity, they are in general not cell-permeable, thus excluding them as potential drug for targeting the intracellular Cas proteins. Intrabodies, antibodies designed to be expressed intracellularly, circumvent these obstacles and could possibly be directed to distinct subcellular locations (reviewed in Lo *et al.* 2008). It might be feasible to target a specific intracellular antigen e.g. in the nucleus, the endoplasmic reticulum, mitochondria, or at the plasma membrane. This may represent an interesting approach to limit/focus the action of a drug to interfere with certain Cas protein functions.

Small molecules such as peptide inhibitors, peptidomimetics, or small-molecule inhibitors have recently become a focus for researchers to develop novel therapeutics. Great advances in the development of small molecules that modulate PPIs have been achieved (Arkin 2005; Arkin & Wells 2004; Wells & McClendon 2007). In the context of the Cas proteins that mediate their function as adapters by providing docking sites for multiple PPI, progress particularly in developing small-molecule inhibitors to block PPI is of major importance.

Peptide inhibitors represent potent therapeutic agents and over the past decade more than 50 peptides have been approved for the treatment of various diseases and several hundred are in preclinical development and clinical testing (Buchwald 2010). Advantages of peptide inhibitors are the high specificity, low toxicity, and low accumulation in tissues. However, peptide inhibitors exhibit a limited half-life in circulation, frequently possess restricted cell permeability, and are more expensive to produce than traditional small-molecule drugs. Often peptide inhibitors have become the starting point to subsequently develop PPI inhibitors (PPIIs) such as peptidomimetics (small protein-like chain based on a peptide with altered chemical structure designed to adjust the molecular properties to acheive increased stability or biological activity) or small-molecule inhibitors to circumvent these disadvantages.

Advances have been made in targeting PPI utilizing mimetic β-peptides (Kritzer *et al.* 2005), which consist of β amino acids that generally not appear in nature, thus increasing the resistance to proteolysis. Succesfully employed examples are β-peptides that target hDM2 (human double minutes-2, the human homologue of the murine p53 negative regulator MDM2) to prevent its interaction with the tumor suppressor p53 resulting in an upregulation of p53-dependent genes (Harker & Schepartz 2009; Kritzer *et al.* 2004). Importantly, subsequent structural modifications of these β-peptides enhanced their uptake in human coloncarcinoma cells.

In later stages of drug development, the goal would be to develop organic non-peptidic small-molecule inhibitors that are generally less expensive, cell-permeable and can be orally administered. Especially relevant to the CasSD approach, and proof of principle, is the progress made in the development of a small-inhibitory compound targeting the Grb2-HGFR (hepatocye growth factor receptor) interaction. The Grb2 antagonist C90, designed and validated to bind to the Grb2 SH2 domain thereby preventing specifically the association of Grb2 with phosphorylated tyrosine motifs within the HGFR (Atabey *et al.* 2001; Dharmawardana *et al.* 2006). The blockade of the Grb2 and HGFR interaction by the C90 small molecule resulted in the reduction of tumor metastases in two different mouse models (Giubellino *et al.* 2007) and inhibition of angiogenesis *in vivo* (Soriano *et al.* 2004). These studies elegantly demonstrate that small-molecule inhibitors possess the potential to block SH2 domain-mediated PPI with high specificity. Additional examples of small-inhibitory compounds with *in vivo* activity in cancer models include Nutlins (Vassilev 2007; Dickens *et al.* 2010), an inhibitor of MDM2, and the Bcl-2 blockers ABT-737 and ABT-263 (Vogler *et al.* 2009).

To summarize, progress has been made in developing different novel approaches in drug design for targeting cytoplasmic proteins. The successful application of small inhibitory compounds in preclinical and clinical trials shows their potential. Approaches employing small-molecule inhibitors may represent promising strategies to target specific regions and thus particular functions of Cas proteins.

5. Perspectives/Outlook on novel combinatorial adjuvant therapies for breast cancer

Increasingly, women are receiving adjuvant therapies in the form of chemotherapy, hormone- and/or radiation therapy (Yamashita 2008; Nicolini *et al.* 2006). Evidence is mounting that these therapies improve breast cancer survival. Adriamycin is one of the most frequently used agents for effective chemotherapeutic treatment of breast cancer (Gianni *et al.* 2008). Hormonal adjuvant therapy is a more targeted therapy with tamoxifen being a commonly used anti-estrogen for treatment of ERα positive breast cancers. Unfortunately, the use of these agents is limited by toxicity and the evolving resistance as seen for other chemotherapeutic drugs as well. This strongly indicates the need for the development of novel approaches to fight tumor cells and to prevent or reduce drug-resistance in breast cancer.

$p130^{Cas}$ was shown to be associated with tamoxifen (Dorssers *et al.* 2001) and adriamycin (Ta *et al.* 2008) resistance in human breast carcinomas *in vivo* and *in vitro*, respectively. Expression of Src*/CasSD in TAM-R cells re-sensitized TAM-R cells to tamoxifen (Soni *et al.* 2009) and RNAi-mediated depletion of $p130^{Cas}$ in breast cancer cells increased the efficiency of adriamycin treatment (Ta *et al.* 2008). Interestingly, expression of the Src*/CasSD in TAM-R cells attenuated signaling pathways which are also involved in $p130^{Cas}$-mediated adriamycin resistance, suggesting that the Src*/CasSD approach might increase the susceptibility to adriamycin as well. Implementation of the Src*/CasSD approach may potentially enhance the efficiency of other anti-estrogens, such as fulvestrant, or the dual tyrosine kinase inhibitor lapatinib (Tykerb), targeting EGFR and HER2/neu (Medina & Goodin 2008; Azim & Azim, Jr. 2008), as it results in an upregulation of ER alpha and HER2/neu in TAMR-R cells (Soni *et al.* 2009).

Data from these initial studies suggest that a therapeutic agent based on the Src*/CasSD approach may have the potential to open avenues for novel strategies for combinatorial adjuvant treatment of breast cancer in the future.

6. Conclusions/Summary

Although many studies indicate the critical involvement of the Cas family members in breast cancer progression, no therapeutic agents have been developed that target these proteins. Here we reviewed different approaches addressing this issue and presented in detail our SD decoy approach that represents an important novel tool to block endogenous Cas protein functions in mammary cancer. Ongoing studies with the aim to specify the region that is mediating these inhibitory effects may guide in the design of therapeutic agents in the future. As we discussed different future drug designs, small-molecule inhibitor approaches might be favourably suited for clinical applications to target Cas proteins, that may be extended to other PPI domains such as the SH3 and/or CTD, or SER domain.

7. Acknowledgments

The authors regret that there are many other important studies that they were unable to include owing to space limitations. This work was supported by the Public Health Service grants CA106468 and CA143108 from the National Cancer Institute and the Susan G. Komen for the Cure® Breast Cancer Foundation grant KG101208. We thank Dr. Matthew D. Layne for critical reading of the manuscript and for comments.

8. References

Abassi YA, Rehn M, Ekman N, Alitalo K & Vuori K 2003 p130Cas Couples the tyrosine kinase Bmx/Etk with regulation of the actin cytoskeleton and cell migration. *J Biol.Chem.* 278 35636-35643.

Aleshin A & Finn RS 2010 SRC: a century of science brought to the clinic. *Neoplasia.* 12 599-607.

Alexandropoulos K & Baltimore D 1996 Coordinate activation of c-Src by SH3- and SH2-binding sites on a novel p130Cas-related protein, Sin. *Genes Dev.* 10 1341-1355.

Angers-Loustau A, Cote JF, Charest A, Dowbenko D, Spencer S, Lasky LA & Tremblay ML 1999 Protein tyrosine phosphatase-PEST regulates focal adhesion disassembly, migration, and cytokinesis in fibroblasts. *J Cell Biol.* 144 1019-1031.

Arkin M 2005 Protein-protein interactions and cancer: small molecules going in for the kill. *Curr.Opin.Chem.Biol.* 9 317-324.

Arkin MR & Wells JA 2004 Small-molecule inhibitors of protein-protein interactions: progressing towards the dream. *Nat.Rev.Drug Discov.* 3 301-317.

Astier A, Manie SN, Law SF, Canty T, Haghayghi N, Druker BJ, Salgia R, Golemis EA & Freedman AS 1997 Association of the Cas-like molecule HEF1 with CrkL following integrin and antigen receptor signaling in human B-cells: potential relevance to neoplastic lymphohematopoietic cells. *Leuk.Lymphoma* 28 65-72.

Atabey N, Gao Y, Yao ZJ, Breckenridge D, Soon L, Soriano JV, Burke TR, Jr. & Bottaro DP 2001 Potent blockade of hepatocyte growth factor-stimulated cell motility, matrix invasion and branching morphogenesis by antagonists of Grb2 Src homology 2 domain interactions. *J.Biol.Chem.* 276 14308-14314.

Azim H & Azim HA, Jr. 2008 Targeting Her-2/neu in breast cancer: as easy as this! *Oncology* 74 150-157.

Birge RB, Fajardo JE, Reichman C, Shoelson SE, Songyang Z, Cantley LC & Hanafusa H 1993 Identification and characterization of a high-affinity interaction between v-Crk and tyrosine-phosphorylated paxillin in CT10-transformed fibroblasts. *Mol.Cell Biol.* 13 4648-4656.

Biscardi JS, Belsches AP & Parsons SJ 1998 Characterization of human epidermal growth factor receptor and c-Src interactions in human breast tumor cells. *Mol.Carcinog.* 21 261-272.

Bouton AH, Riggins RB & Bruce-Staskal PJ 2001 Functions of the adapter protein Cas: signal convergence and the determination of cellular responses. *Oncogene* 20 6448-6458.

Bridges D & Moorhead GB 2004 14-3-3 proteins: a number of functions for a numbered protein. *Sci.STKE.* 2004 re10.

Briknarova K, Nasertorabi F, Havert ML, Eggleston E, Hoyt DW, Li C, Olson AJ, Vuori K & Ely KR 2005 The serine-rich domain from Crk-associated substrate (p130cas) is a four-helix bundle. *J Biol.Chem.* 280 21908-21914.

Brinkman A, de Jong D, Tuinman S, Azaouagh N, van Agthoven T & Dorssers LC 2009 The substrate domain of BCAR1 is essential for anti-estrogen-resistant proliferation of human breast cancer cells. *Breast Cancer Res.Treat.*

Brinkman A, van der Flier S, Kok EM & Dorssers LC 2000 BCAR1, a human homologue of the adapter protein p130Cas, and antiestrogen resistance in breast cancer cells. *J.Natl.Cancer Inst.* 92 112-120.

Buchwald P 2010 Small-molecule protein-protein interaction inhibitors: therapeutic potential in light of molecular size, chemical space, and ligand binding efficiency considerations. *IUBMB.Life* 62 724-731.

Buday L, Wunderlich L & Tamas P 2002 The Nck family of adapter proteins: regulators of actin cytoskeleton. *Cell Signal.* 14 723-731.

Burnham MR, Bruce-Staskal PJ, Harte MT, Weidow CL, Ma A, Weed SA & Bouton AH 2000 Regulation of c-SRC activity and function by the adapter protein CAS. *Mol.Cell Biol.* 20 5865-5878.

Burnham MR, Harte MT & Bouton AH 1999 The role of SRC-CAS interactions in cellular transformation: ectopic expression of the carboxy terminus of CAS inhibits SRC-CAS interaction but has no effect on cellular transformation. *Mol.Carcinog.* 26 20-31.

Burnham MR, Harte MT, Richardson A, Parsons JT & Bouton AH 1996 The identification of p130cas-binding proteins and their role in cellular transformation. *Oncogene* 12 2467-2472.

Cabodi S, Moro L, Baj G, Smeriglio M, Di Stefano P, Gippone S, Surico N, Silengo L, Turco E, Tarone G & Defilippi P 2004 p130Cas interacts with estrogen receptor alpha and modulates non-genomic estrogen signaling in breast cancer cells. *J Cell Sci.* 117 1603-1611.

Cabodi S, Pilar Camacho-Leal M, Di Stefano P & Defilippi P 2010a Integrin signalling adaptors: not only figurants in the cancer story. *Nat.Rev.Cancer* 10 858-870.

Cabodi S, Tinnirello A, Bisaro B, Tornillo G, Pilar Camacho-Leal M, Forni G, Cojoca R, Iezzi M, Amici A, Montani M, Eva A, Di Stefano P, Muthuswamy SK, Tarone G, Turco E & Defilippi P 2010b p130Cas is an essential transducer element in ErbB2 transformation. *FASEB J* 24 3796-3808.

Cabodi S, Tinnirello A, Di Stefano P, Bisaro B, Ambrosino E, Castellano I, Sapino A, Arisio R, Cavallo F, Forni G, Glukhova M, Silengo L, Altruda F, Turco E, Tarone G & Defilippi P 2006 p130Cas as a new regulator of mammary epithelial cell proliferation, survival, and HER2-neu oncogene-dependent breast tumorigenesis. *Cancer Res.* 66 4672-4680.

Chan YR & Gallo RL 1998 PR-39, a syndecan-inducing antimicrobial peptide, binds and affects p130(Cas). *J Biol.Chem.* 273 28978-28985.

Cote JF, Charest A, Wagner J & Tremblay ML 1998 Combination of gene targeting and substrate trapping to identify substrates of protein tyrosine phosphatases using PTP-PEST as a model. *Biochemistry* 37 13128-13137.

Cowell LN, Graham JD, Bouton AH, Clarke CL & O'Neill GM 2006 Tamoxifen treatment promotes phosphorylation of the adhesion molecules, p130Cas/BCAR1, FAK and Src, via an adhesion-dependent pathway. *Oncogene* 25 7597-7607.

Czernilofsky AP, Levinson AD, Varmus HE, Bishop JM, Tischer E & Goodman HM 1980 Nucleotide sequence of an avian sarcoma virus oncogene (src) and proposed amino acid sequence for gene product. *Nature* 287 198-203.

Defilippi P, Di Stefano P & Cabodi S 2006 p130Cas: a versatile scaffold in signaling networks. *Trends Cell Biol.* 16 257-263.

Dharmawardana PG, Peruzzi B, Giubellino A, Burke TR, Jr. & Bottaro DP 2006 Molecular targeting of growth factor receptor-bound 2 (Grb2) as an anti-cancer strategy. *Anticancer Drugs* 17 13-20.

Di Stefano P, Cabodi S, Boeri EE, Margaria V, Bergatto E, Giuffrida MG, Silengo L, Tarone G, Turco E & Defilippi P 2004 P130Cas-associated protein (p140Cap) as a new tyrosine-phosphorylated protein involved in cell spreading. *Mol.Biol.Cell* 15 787-800.

Dickens MP, Fitzgerald R & Fischer PM 2010 Small-molecule inhibitors of MDM2 as new anticancer therapeutics. *Semin.Cancer Biol.* 20 10-18.

Dolfi F, Garcia-Guzman M, Ojaniemi M, Nakamura H, Matsuda M & Vuori K 1998 The adaptor protein Crk connects multiple cellular stimuli to the JNK signaling pathway. *Proc.Natl.Acad.Sci.U.S.A* 95 15394-15399.

Donaldson JC, Dempsey PJ, Reddy S, Bouton AH, Coffey RJ & Hanks SK 2000 Crk-associated substrate p130(Cas) interacts with nephrocystin and both proteins localize to cell-cell contacts of polarized epithelial cells. *Exp.Cell Res.* 256 168-178.

Donato DM, Ryzhova LM, Meenderink LM, Kaverina I & Hanks SK 2010 Dynamics and mechanism of p130Cas localization to focal adhesions. *J Biol.Chem.* 285 20769-20779.

Dorssers LC, van Agthoven T, Dekker A, van Agthoven TL & Kok EM 1993 Induction of antiestrogen resistance in human breast cancer cells by random insertional mutagenesis using defective retroviruses: identification of bcar-1, a common integration site. *Mol.Endocrinol.* 7 870-878.

Dorssers LC, van der FS, Brinkman A, van Agthoven T, Veldscholte J, Berns EM, Klijn JG, Beex LV & Foekens JA 2001 Tamoxifen resistance in breast cancer: elucidating mechanisms. *Drugs* 61 1721-1733.

Fashena SJ, Einarson MB, O'Neill GM, Patriotis C & Golemis EA 2002 Dissection of HEF1-dependent functions in motility and transcriptional regulation. *J Cell Sci.* 115 99-111.

Fathers KE, Rodrigues S, Zuo D, Murthy IV, Hallett M, Cardiff R & Park M 2010 CrkII transgene induces atypical mammary gland development and tumorigenesis. *Am.J Pathol.* 176 446-460.

Feller SM, Knudsen B & Hanafusa H 1995 Cellular proteins binding to the first Src homology 3 (SH3) domain of the proto-oncogene product c-Crk indicate Crk-specific signaling pathways. *Oncogene* 10 1465-1473.

Feller SM & Lewitzky M 2006 Potential disease targets for drugs that disrupt protein--protein interactions of Grb2 and Crk family adaptors. *Curr.Pharm.Des* 12 529-548.

Feng L, Guedes S & Wang T 2004 Atrophin-1-interacting protein 4/human Itch is a ubiquitin E3 ligase for human enhancer of filamentation 1 in transforming growth factor-beta signaling pathways. *J Biol.Chem.* 279 29681-29690.

Frogne T, Benjaminsen RV, Sonne-Hansen K, Sorensen BS, Nexo E, Laenkholm AV, Rasmussen LM, Riese DJ, de Cremoux P, Stenvang J & Lykkesfeldt AE 2009 Activation of ErbB3, EGFR and Erk is essential for growth of human breast cancer cell lines with acquired resistance to fulvestrant. *Breast Cancer Res.Treat.* 114 263-275.

Garton AJ, Burnham MR, Bouton AH & Tonks NK 1997 Association of PTP-PEST with the SH3 domain of p130cas; a novel mechanism of protein tyrosine phosphatase substrate recognition. *Oncogene* 15 877-885.

Giampieri S, Manning C, Hooper S, Jones L, Hill CS & Sahai E 2009 Localized and reversible TGFbeta signalling switches breast cancer cells from cohesive to single cell motility. *Nat.Cell Biol.* 11 1287-1296.

Gianni L, Herman EH, Lipshultz SE, Minotti G, Sarvazyan N & Sawyer DB 2008 Anthracycline cardiotoxicity: from bench to bedside. *J.Clin.Oncol.* 26 3777-3784.

Giubellino A, Gao Y, Lee S, Lee MJ, Vasselli JR, Medepalli S, Trepel JB, Burke TR, Jr. & Bottaro DP 2007 Inhibition of tumor metastasis by a growth factor receptor bound protein 2 Src homology 2 domain-binding antagonist. *Cancer Res.* 67 6012-6016.

Gotoh T, Cai D, Tian X, Feig LA & Lerner A 2000 p130Cas regulates the activity of AND-34, a novel Ral, Rap1, and R-Ras guanine nucleotide exchange factor. *J Biol.Chem.* 275 30118-30123.

Gotoh T, Hattori S, Nakamura S, Kitayama H, Noda M, Takai Y, Kaibuchi K, Matsui H, Hatase O, Takahashi H &. 1995 Identification of Rap1 as a target for the Crk SH3 domain-binding guanine nucleotide-releasing factor C3G. *Mol.Cell Biol.* 15 6746-6753.

Guy CT, Muthuswamy SK, Cardiff RD, Soriano P & Muller WJ 1994 Activation of the c-Src tyrosine kinase is required for the induction of mammary tumors in transgenic mice. *Genes Dev.* 8 23-32.

Hanahan D & Weinberg RA 2011 Hallmarks of cancer: the next generation. *Cell* 144 646-674.

Harker EA & Schepartz A 2009 Cell-permeable beta-peptide inhibitors of p53/hDM2 complexation. *Chembiochem.* 10 990-993.

Harte MT, Hildebrand JD, Burnham MR, Bouton AH & Parsons JT 1996 p130Cas, a substrate associated with v-Src and v-Crk, localizes to focal adhesions and binds to focal adhesion kinase. *J Biol.Chem.* 271 13649-13655.

Harte MT, Macklem M, Weidow CL, Parsons JT & Bouton AH 2000 Identification of two focal adhesion targeting sequences in the adapter molecule p130(Cas). *Biochim.Biophys.Acta* 1499 34-48.

Hasegawa H, Kiyokawa E, Tanaka S, Nagashima K, Gotoh N, Shibuya M, Kurata T & Matsuda M 1996 DOCK180, a major CRK-binding protein, alters cell morphology upon translocation to the cell membrane. *Mol.Cell Biol.* 16 1770-1776.

Henderson BE & Feigelson HS 2000 Hormonal carcinogenesis. *Carcinogenesis* 21 427-433.

Hiscox S, Morgan L, Barrow D, Dutkowskil C, Wakeling A & Nicholson RI 2004 Tamoxifen resistance in breast cancer cells is accompanied by an enhanced motile and invasive phenotype: inhibition by gefitinib ('Iressa', ZD1839). *Clin.Exp.Metastasis* 21 201-212.

Hoon KD, Jeon CS, Kook S, Kim W & Keun SW 2003 Phosphorylation-dependent cleavage of p130cas in apoptotic rat-1 cells. *Biochem Biophys.Res.Commun.* 300 141-148.

Hornbeck PV, Chabra I, Kornhauser JM, Skrzypek E & Zhang B 2004 PhosphoSite: A bioinformatics resource dedicated to physiological protein phosphorylation. *Proteomics.* 4 1551-1561.

Huang J, Hamasaki H, Nakamoto T, Honda H, Hirai H, Saito M, Takato T & Sakai R 2002 Differential regulation of cell migration, actin stress fiber organization, and cell transformation by functional domains of Crk-associated substrate. *J.Biol.Chem.* 277 27265-27272.

Ikushima H & Miyazono K 2010 TGFbeta signalling: a complex web in cancer progression. *Nat.Rev.Cancer* 10 415-424.

Ishino M, Ohba T, Sasaki H & Sasaki T 1995 Molecular cloning of a cDNA encoding a phosphoprotein, Efs, which contains a Src homology 3 domain and associates with Fyn. *Oncogene* 11 2331-2338.

Izumchenko E, Singh MK, Plotnikova OV, Tikhmyanova N, Little JL, Serebriiskii IG, Seo S, Kurokawa M, Egleston BL, Klein-Szanto A, Pugacheva EN, Hardy RR, Wolfson M, Connolly DC & Golemis EA 2009 NEDD9 promotes oncogenic signaling in mammary tumor development. *Cancer Res.* 69 7198-7206.

Jacobs C & Rubsamen H 1983 Expression of pp60c-src protein kinase in adult and fetal human tissue: high activities in some sarcomas and mammary carcinomas. *Cancer Res.* 43 1696-1702.

Jove R, Kornbluth S & Hanafusa H 1987 Enzymatically inactive p60c-src mutant with altered ATP-binding site is fully phosphorylated in its carboxy-terminal regulatory region. *Cell* 50 937-943.

Kanda H, Mimura T, Hamasaki K, Yamamoto K, Yazaki Y, Hirai H & Nojima Y 1999 Fyn and Lck tyrosine kinases regulate tyrosine phosphorylation of p105CasL, a member of the p130Cas docking protein family, in T-cell receptor-mediated signalling. *Immunology* 97 56-61.

Kim W, Kook S, Kim DJ, Teodorof C & Song WK 2004 The 31-kDa caspase-generated cleavage product of p130cas functions as a transcriptional repressor of E2A in apoptotic cells. *J Biol.Chem.* 279 8333-8342.

Kirsch KH, Kensinger M, Hanafusa H & August A 2002 A p130Cas tyrosine phosphorylated substrate domain decoy disrupts v-crk signaling. *BMC.Cell Biol.* 3 18.

Kirsch KH, Georgescu MM & Hanafusa H 1998 Direct binding of p130(Cas) to the guanine nucleotide exchange factor C3G. *J Biol.Chem.* 273 25673-25679.

Kirsch KH, Georgescu MM, Ishimaru S & Hanafusa H 1999 CMS: an adapter molecule involved in cytoskeletal rearrangements. *Proc.Natl.Acad.Sci.U.S.A* 96 6211-6216.

Klemke RL, Leng J, Molander R, Brooks PC, Vuori K & Cheresh DA 1998 CAS/Crk coupling serves as a "molecular switch" for induction of cell migration. *J.Cell Biol.* 140 961-972.

Kmiecik TE & Shalloway D 1987 Activation and suppression of pp60c-src transforming ability by mutation of its primary sites of tyrosine phosphorylation. *Cell* 49 65-73.

Knowlden JM, Hutcheson IR, Jones HE, Madden T, Gee JM, Harper ME, Barrow D, Wakeling AE & Nicholson RI 2003 Elevated levels of epidermal growth factor receptor/c-erbB2 heterodimers mediate an autocrine growth regulatory pathway in tamoxifen-resistant MCF-7 cells. *Endocrinology* 144 1032-1044.

Konstantinovsky S, Smith Y, Zilber S, Tuft SH, Becker AM, Nesland JM, Reich R & Davidson B 2010 Breast carcinoma cells in primary tumors and effusions have different gene array profiles. *J Oncol.* 2010 969084.

Kritzer JA, Lear JD, Hodsdon ME & Schepartz A 2004 Helical beta-peptide inhibitors of the p53-hDM2 interaction. *J Am.Chem.Soc.* 126 9468-9469.

Kritzer JA, Stephens OM, Guarracino DA, Reznik SK & Schepartz A 2005 beta-Peptides as inhibitors of protein-protein interactions. *Bioorg.Med.Chem.* 13 11-16.

Lakkakorpi PT, Nakamura I, Nagy RM, Parsons JT, Rodan GA & Duong LT 1999 Stable association of PYK2 and p130(Cas) in osteoclasts and their co-localization in the sealing zone. *J Biol.Chem.* 274 4900-4907.

Law SF, Estojak J, Wang B, Mysliwiec T, Kruh G & Golemis EA 1996 Human enhancer of filamentation 1, a novel p130cas-like docking protein, associates with focal adhesion kinase and induces pseudohyphal growth in Saccharomyces cerevisiae. *Mol.Cell Biol.* 16 3327-3337.

Law SF, Zhang YZ, Fashena SJ, Toby G, Estojak J & Golemis EA 1999 Dimerization of the docking/adaptor protein HEF1 via a carboxy-terminal helix-loop-helix domain. *Exp.Cell Res.* 252 224-235.

Law SF, Zhang YZ, Klein-Szanto AJ & Golemis EA 1998 Cell cycle-regulated processing of HEF1 to multiple protein forms differentially targeted to multiple subcellular compartments. *Mol.Cell Biol.* 18 3540-3551.

Leader B, Baca QJ & Golan DE 2008 Protein therapeutics: a summary and pharmacological classification. *Nat.Rev.Drug Discov.* 7 21-39.

Lehmann JM, Riethmuller G & Johnson JP 1990 Nck, a melanoma cDNA encoding a cytoplasmic protein consisting of the src homology units SH2 and SH3. *Nucleic Acids Res.* 18 1048.

Li E, Stupack DG, Brown SL, Klemke R, Schlaepfer DD & Nemerow GR 2000 Association of p130CAS with phosphatidylinositol-3-OH kinase mediates adenovirus cell entry. *J Biol.Chem.* 275 14729-14735.

Liu F, Hill DE & Chernoff J 1996 Direct binding of the proline-rich region of protein tyrosine phosphatase 1B to the Src homology 3 domain of p130(Cas). *J Biol.Chem.* 271 31290-31295.

Liu JF, Chevet E, Kebache S, Lemaitre G, Barritault D, Larose L & Crepin M 1999 Functional Rac-1 and Nck signaling networks are required for FGF-2-induced DNA synthesis in MCF-7 cells. *Oncogene* 18 6425-6433.

Liu X, Elia AE, Law SF, Golemis EA, Farley J & Wang T 2000 A novel ability of Smad3 to regulate proteasomal degradation of a Cas family member HEF1. *EMBO J* 19 6759-6769.

Lo AS, Zhu Q & Marasco WA 2008 Intracellular antibodies (intrabodies) and their therapeutic potential. *Handb.Exp.Pharmacol.* 343-373.

Lu Y, Brush J & Stewart TA 1999 NSP1 defines a novel family of adaptor proteins linking integrin and tyrosine kinase receptors to the c-Jun N-terminal kinase/stress-activated protein kinase signaling pathway. *J Biol.Chem.* 274 10047-10052.

Ma L, Teruya-Feldstein J & Weinberg RA 2007 Tumour invasion and metastasis initiated by microRNA-10b in breast cancer. *Nature* 449 682-688.

Makkinje A, Near RI, Infusini G, Vanden Borre P, Bloom A, Cai D, Costello CE & Lerner A 2009 AND-34/BCAR3 regulates adhesion-dependent p130Cas serine phosphorylation and breast cancer cell growth pattern. *Cell Signal.* 21 1423-1435.

Marcotte R & Muller WJ 2008 Signal transduction in transgenic mouse models of human breast cancer--implications for human breast cancer. *J.Mammary.Gland.Biol.Neoplasia.* 13 323-335.

Matozaki T, Murata Y, Saito Y, Okazawa H & Ohnishi H 2009 Protein tyrosine phosphatase SHP-2: a proto-oncogene product that promotes Ras activation. *Cancer Sci.* 100 1786-1793.

Matsuda M, Tanaka S, Nagata S, Kojima A, Kurata T & Shibuya M 1992 Two species of human CRK cDNA encode proteins with distinct biological activities. *Mol.Cell Biol.* 12 3482-3489.

Mayer EL & Krop IE 2010 Advances in targeting SRC in the treatment of breast cancer and other solid malignancies. *Clin.Cancer Res.* 16 3526-3532.

Medina PJ & Goodin S 2008 Lapatinib: a dual inhibitor of human epidermal growth factor receptor tyrosine kinases. *Clin.Ther.* 30 1426-1447.

Meenderink LM, Ryzhova LM, Donato DM, Gochberg DF, Kaverina I & Hanks SK 2010 P130Cas Src-binding and substrate domains have distinct roles in sustaining focal adhesion disassembly and promoting cell migration. *PLoS.One.* 5 e13412.

Meulmeester E & Ten Dijke P 2011 The dynamic roles of TGF-beta in cancer. *J Pathol.* 223 205-218.

Minegishi M, Tachibana K, Sato T, Iwata S, Nojima Y & Morimoto C 1996 Structure and function of Cas-L, a 105-kD Crk-associated substrate-related protein that is involved in beta 1 integrin-mediated signaling in lymphocytes. *J Exp.Med.* 184 1365-1375.

Minn AJ, Gupta GP, Siegel PM, Bos PD, Shu W, Giri DD, Viale A, Olshen AB, Gerald WL & Massague J 2005 Genes that mediate breast cancer metastasis to lung. *Nature* 436 518-524.

Muthuswamy SK & Muller WJ 1995 Activation of Src family kinases in Neu-induced mammary tumors correlates with their association with distinct sets of tyrosine phosphorylated proteins in vivo. *Oncogene* 11 1801-1810.

Nakamoto T, Sakai R, Honda H, Ogawa S, Ueno H, Suzuki T, Aizawa S, Yazaki Y & Hirai H 1997 Requirements for localization of p130cas to focal adhesions. *Mol.Cell Biol.* 17 3884-3897.

Nakamoto T, Sakai R, Ozawa K, Yazaki Y & Hirai H 1996 Direct binding of C-terminal region of p130Cas to SH2 and SH3 domains of Src kinase. *J Biol.Chem.* 271 8959-8965.

Nakamoto T, Yamagata T, Sakai R, Ogawa S, Honda H, Ueno H, Hirano N, Yazaki Y & Hirai H 2000 CIZ, a zinc finger protein that interacts with p130(cas) and activates the expression of matrix metalloproteinases. *Mol.Cell Biol.* 20 1649-1658.

Nasertorabi F, Tars K, Becherer K, Kodandapani R, Liljas L, Vuori K & Ely KR 2006 Molecular basis for regulation of Src by the docking protein p130Cas. *J Mol.Recognit.* 19 30-38.

Nicolini A, Giardino R, Carpi A, Ferrari P, Anselmi L, Colosimo S, Conte M, Fini M, Giavaresi G, Berti P & Miccoli P 2006 Metastatic breast cancer: an updating. *Biomed.Pharmacother.* 60 548-556.

Nishio H & Suzuki K 2002 Ethanol-induced Cas tyrosine phosphorylation and Fyn kinase activation in rat brain. *Alcohol Clin.Exp.Res.* 26 38S-43S.

Nourry C, Maksumova L, Pang M, Liu X & Wang T 2004 Direct interaction between Smad3, APC10, CDH1 and HEF1 in proteasomal degradation of HEF1. *BMC.Cell Biol.* 5 20.

Okada S & Pessin JE 1996 Interactions between Src homology (SH) 2/SH3 adapter proteins and the guanylnucleotide exchange factor SOS are differentially regulated by insulin and epidermal growth factor. *J Biol.Chem.* 271 25533-25538.

Ottenhoff-Kalff AE, Rijksen G, van Beurden EA, Hennipman A, Michels AA & Staal GE 1992 Characterization of protein tyrosine kinases from human breast cancer: involvement of the c-src oncogene product. *Cancer Res.* 52 4773-4778.

Parsons JT, Martin KH, Slack JK, Taylor JM & Weed SA 2000 Focal adhesion kinase: a regulator of focal adhesion dynamics and cell movement. *Oncogene* 19 5606-5613.

Pellicena P & Miller WT 2001 Processive phosphorylation of p130Cas by Src depends on SH3-polyproline interactions. *J Biol.Chem.* 276 28190-28196.

Petruzzelli L, Takami M & Herrera R 1996 Adhesion through the interaction of lymphocyte function-associated antigen-1 with intracellular adhesion molecule-1 induces tyrosine phosphorylation of p130cas and its association with c-CrkII. *J Biol.Chem.* 271 7796-7801.

Piwnica-Worms H, Saunders KB, Roberts TM, Smith AE & Cheng SH 1987 Tyrosine phosphorylation regulates the biochemical and biological properties of pp60c-src. *Cell* 49 75-82.

Polte TR & Hanks SK 1995 Interaction between focal adhesion kinase and Crk-associated tyrosine kinase substrate p130Cas. *Proc.Natl.Acad.Sci.U.S.A* 92 10678-10682.

Prasad N, Topping RS & Decker SJ 2001 SH2-containing inositol 5'-phosphatase SHIP2 associates with the p130(Cas) adapter protein and regulates cellular adhesion and spreading. *Mol.Cell Biol.* 21 1416-1428.

Provenzano PP, Inman DR, Eliceiri KW, Beggs HE & Keely PJ 2008 Mammary epithelial-specific disruption of focal adhesion kinase retards tumor formation and metastasis in a transgenic mouse model of human breast cancer. *Am.J Pathol.* 173 1551-1565.

Provenzano PP & Keely PJ 2009 The role of focal adhesion kinase in tumor initiation and progression. *Cell Adh.Migr.* 3 347-350.

Ren R, Mayer BJ, Cicchetti P & Baltimore D 1993 Identification of a ten-amino acid proline-rich SH3 binding site. *Science* 259 1157-1161.

Rodrigues SP, Fathers KE, Chan G, Zuo D, Halwani F, Meterissian S & Park M 2005 CrkI and CrkII function as key signaling integrators for migration and invasion of cancer cells. *Mol.Cancer Res.* 3 183-194.

Rucci N, Recchia I, Angelucci A, Alamanou M, Del Fattore A, Fortunati D, Susa M, Fabbro D, Bologna M & Teti A 2006 Inhibition of protein kinase c-Src reduces the incidence of breast cancer metastases and increases survival in mice: implications for therapy. *J Pharmacol.Exp.Ther.* 318 161-172.

Ruest PJ, Shin NY, Polte TR, Zhang X & Hanks SK 2001 Mechanisms of CAS substrate domain tyrosine phosphorylation by FAK and Src. *Mol.Cell Biol.* 21 7641-7652.

Sakai R, Iwamatsu A, Hirano N, Ogawa S, Tanaka T, Mano H, Yazaki Y & Hirai H 1994a A novel signaling molecule, p130, forms stable complexes in vivo with v-Crk and v-Src in a tyrosine phosphorylation-dependent manner. *EMBO J* 13 3748-3756.

Sakai R, Iwamatsu A, Hirano N, Ogawa S, Tanaka T, Nishida J, Yazaki Y & Hirai H 1994b Characterization, partial purification, and peptide sequencing of p130,the main phosphoprotein associated with v-Crk oncoprotein. *J Biol.Chem.* 269 32740-32746.

Sakai R, Nakamoto T, Ozawa K, Aizawa S & Hirai H 1997 Characterization of the kinase activity essential for tyrosine phosphorylation of p130Cas in fibroblasts. *Oncogene* 14 1419-1426.

Sakakibara A & Hattori S 2000 Chat, a Cas/HEF1-associated adaptor protein that integrates multiple signaling pathways. *J Biol.Chem.* 275 6404-6410.

Salgia R, Pisick E, Sattler M, Li JL, Uemura N, Wong WK, Burky SA, Hirai H, Chen LB & Griffin JD 1996 p130CAS forms a signaling complex with the adapter protein CRKL in hematopoietic cells transformed by the BCR/ABL oncogene. *J Biol.Chem.* 271 25198-25203.

Schlaepfer DD, Broome MA & Hunter T 1997 Fibronectin-stimulated signaling from a focal adhesion kinase-c-Src complex: involvement of the Grb2, p130cas, and Nck adaptor proteins. *Mol.Cell Biol.* 17 1702-1713.

Schwartz DE, Tizard R & Gilbert W 1983 Nucleotide sequence of Rous sarcoma virus. *Cell* 32 853-869.

Scibelli A, d'Angelo D, Pelagalli A, Tafuri S, Avallone L, Della MR & Staiano N 2003 Expression levels of the focal adhesion-associated proteins paxillin and p130CAS in canine and feline mammary tumors. *Vet.Res.* 34 193-202.

Shin NY, Dise RS, Schneider-Mergener J, Ritchie MD, Kilkenny DM & Hanks SK 2004 Subsets of the major tyrosine phosphorylation sites in Crk-associated substrate (CAS) are sufficient to promote cell migration. *J.Biol.Chem.* 279 38331-38337.

Shintani Y, Fukumoto Y, Chaika N, Svoboda R, Wheelock MJ & Johnson KR 2008 Collagen I-mediated up-regulation of N-cadherin requires cooperative signals from integrins and discoidin domain receptor 1. *J Cell Biol.* 180 1277-1289.

Simpson KJ, Selfors LM, Bui J, Reynolds A, Leake D, Khvorova A & Brugge JS 2008 Identification of genes that regulate epithelial cell migration using an siRNA screening approach. *Nat.Cell Biol.* 10 1027-1038.

Singh MK, Dadke D, Nicolas E, Serebriiskii IG, Apostolou S, Canutescu A, Egleston BL & Golemis EA 2008 A novel Cas family member, HEPL, regulates FAK and cell spreading. *Mol.Biol.Cell* 19 1627-1636.

Songyang Z, Shoelson SE, Chaudhuri M, Gish G, Pawson T, Haser WG, King F, Roberts T, Ratnofsky S, Lechleider RJ &. 1993 SH2 domains recognize specific phosphopeptide sequences. *Cell* 72 767-778.

Soni S, Lin BT, August A, Nicholson RI & Kirsch KH 2009 Expression of a phosphorylated p130(Cas) substrate domain attenuates the phosphatidylinositol 3-kinase/Akt survival pathway in tamoxifen resistant breast cancer cells. *J Cell Biochem* 107 364-375.

Soriano JV, Liu N, Gao Y, Yao ZJ, Ishibashi T, Underhill C, Burke TR, Jr. & Bottaro DP 2004 Inhibition of angiogenesis by growth factor receptor bound protein 2-Src homology 2 domain bound antagonists. *Mol.Cancer Ther.* 3 1289-1299.

Spencer KS, Graus-Porta D, Leng J, Hynes NE & Klemke RL 2000 ErbB2 is necessary for induction of carcinoma cell invasion by ErbB family receptor tyrosine kinases. *J Cell Biol.* 148 385-397.

Stylli SS, Stacey TT, Verhagen AM, Xu SS, Pass I, Courtneidge SA & Lock P 2009 Nck adaptor proteins link Tks5 to invadopodia actin regulation and ECM degradation. *J Cell Sci.* 122 2727-2740.

Superti-Furga G, Fumagalli S, Koegl M, Courtneidge SA & Draetta G 1993 Csk inhibition of c-Src activity requires both the SH2 and SH3 domains of Src. *EMBO J* 12 2625-2634.

Ta HQ, Thomas KS, Schrecengost RS & Bouton AH 2008 A novel association between p130Cas and resistance to the chemotherapeutic drug adriamycin in human breast cancer cells. *Cancer Res.* 68 8796-8804.

Takeya T & Hanafusa H 1982 DNA sequence of the viral and cellular src gene of chickens. II. Comparison of the src genes of two strains of avian sarcoma virus and of the cellular homolog. *J Virol.* 44 12-18.

ten Hoeve J, Morris C, Heisterkamp N & Groffen J 1993 Isolation and chromosomal localization of CRKL, a human crk-like gene. *Oncogene* 8 2469-2474.

Tikhmyanova N, Little JL & Golemis EA 2010 CAS proteins in normal and pathological cell growth control. *Cell Mol.Life Sci.* 67 1025-1048.

van der Flier S, Brinkman A, Look MP, Kok EM, Meijer-van Gelder ME, Klijn JG, Dorssers LC & Foekens JA 2000 Bcar1/p130Cas protein and primary breast cancer: prognosis and response to tamoxifen treatment. *J.Natl.Cancer Inst.* 92 120-127.

Vassilev LT 2007 MDM2 inhibitors for cancer therapy. *Trends Mol.Med.* 13 23-31.

Verbeek BS, Vroom TM, Adriaansen-Slot SS, Ottenhoff-Kalff AE, Geertzema JG, Hennipman A & Rijksen G 1996 c-Src protein expression is increased in human breast cancer. An immunohistochemical and biochemical analysis. *J Pathol.* 180 383-388.

Vogler M, Dinsdale D, Dyer MJ & Cohen GM 2009 Bcl-2 inhibitors: small molecules with a big impact on cancer therapy. *Cell Death.Differ.* 16 360-367.

Vultur A, Buettner R, Kowolik C, Liang W, Smith D, Boschelli F & Jove R 2008 SKI-606 (bosutinib), a novel Src kinase inhibitor, suppresses migration and invasion of human breast cancer cells. *Mol.Cancer Ther.* 7 1185-1194.

Wang FM, Liu HQ, Liu SR, Tang SP, Yang L & Feng GS 2005 SHP-2 promoting migration and metastasis of MCF-7 with loss of E-cadherin, dephosphorylation of FAK and secretion of MMP-9 induced by IL-1beta in vivo and in vitro. *Breast Cancer Res.Treat.* 89 5-14.

Wang X, Weng LP & Yu Q 2000 Specific inhibition of FGF-induced MAPK activation by the receptor-like protein tyrosine phosphatase LAR. *Oncogene* 19 2346-2353.

Webster MA, Cardiff RD & Muller WJ 1995 Induction of mammary epithelial hyperplasias and mammary tumors in transgenic mice expressing a murine mammary tumor virus/activated c-src fusion gene. *Proc.Natl.Acad.Sci.U.S.A* 92 7849-7853.

Wells JA & McClendon CL 2007 Reaching for high-hanging fruit in drug discovery at protein-protein interfaces. *Nature* 450 1001-1009.

Wendt MK, Smith JA & Schiemann WP 2009 p130Cas is required for mammary tumor growth and transforming growth factor-beta-mediated metastasis through regulation of Smad2/3 activity. *J Biol.Chem.* 284 34145-34156.

Weng LP, Wang X & Yu Q 1999 Transmembrane tyrosine phosphatase LAR induces apoptosis by dephosphorylating and destabilizing p130Cas. *Genes Cells* 4 185-196.

Wheeler DL, Iida M & Dunn EF 2009 The role of Src in solid tumors. *Oncologist.* 14 667-678.

Yamakita Y, Totsukawa G, Yamashiro S, Fry D, Zhang X, Hanks SK & Matsumura F 1999 Dissociation of FAK/p130(CAS)/c-Src complex during mitosis: role of mitosis-specific serine phosphorylation of FAK. *J Cell Biol.* 144 315-324.

Yamashita H 2008 Current research topics in endocrine therapy for breast cancer. *Int.J.Clin.Oncol.* 13 380-383.

Yo K, Iwata S, Hashizume Y, Kondo S, Nomura S, Hosono O, Kawasaki H, Tanaka H, Dang NH & Morimoto C 2009 SHP-2 inhibits tyrosine phosphorylation of Cas-L and regulates cell migration. *Biochem Biophys.Res.Commun.* 382 210-214.

Yu H, Chen JK, Feng S, Dalgarno DC, Brauer AW & Schreiber SL 1994 Structural basis for the binding of proline-rich peptides to SH3 domains. *Cell* 76 933-945.

Zhang Y, Su H, Rahimi M, Tochihara R & Tang C 2009 EGFRvIII-induced estrogen-independence, tamoxifen-resistance phenotype correlates with PgR expression and modulation of apoptotic molecules in breast cancer. *Int.J Cancer* 125 2021-2028.

Zheng M & McKeown-Longo PJ 2002 Regulation of HEF1 expression and phosphorylation by TGF-beta 1 and cell adhesion. *J Biol.Chem.* 277 39599-39608.

5

Red American Ginseng and Breast Cancer

Chong-Zhi Wang, Guang-Jian Du and Chun-Su Yuan
Tang Center for Herbal Medicine Research and Department of Anesthesia & Critical Care, The Pritzker School of Medicine, University of Chicago, Chicago, U.S.A.

1. Introduction

Breast cancer is the most frequently diagnosed form of cancer among women. Breast cancer is the leading cause of cancer death in nearly all developed countries, showing an increased incidence over the last decades, and the expected number of new U.S. patients in 2010 would be 209,060, and the death number will be 40,230 [1]. The clinical management of breast cancer invariably involves diverse conventional modalities, including surgery, chemotherapy, and radiation [2]. The complex characteristics of breast cancer may also require some alternative management to improve the therapeutic efficacy of conventional treatment and the quality of life for cancer patients [3].

American ginseng (*Panax quinquefolius* L.) is a commonly used herb in the United States which belongs to the genus *Panax* L. in family Araliaceae [4]. *Panax* is a small genus, and nearly all species in this genus are important herbal medicines, especially Asian ginseng (*Panax ginseng* C. A. Meyer) [5]. Since Asian ginseng has been used as herbal medicine for a long history in oriental countries, many studies have been conducted on its constituents and its pharmacological effects [6]. Asian ginseng has many reported health benefits including anticancer activities [7-9]. In the 1990s, a case-control study on over a thousand Korean subjects showed that long-term ginseng consumption was associated with a decreased risk for many different cancers compared with those who did not consume ginseng [10,11]. In contrast to many studies on Asian ginseng's anticancer effects, investigation of American ginseng is limited [7], and its mechanisms of action are largely unknown.

American ginseng extracts were found to inhibit the growth of breast cancer cells[12]. We previously investigated the effects of several herbal extracts on reducing chemotherapeutic side effects and found that American ginseng can attenuate cisplatin-induced nausea and vomiting in a rat model, while not affecting its anticancer properties in human cancer cells[13]. In addition, the extract from American ginseng enhanced the antiproliferation effect of cisplatin on human breast cancer cells, suggesting that it possesses its own anticancer activity[13].

In Asia, ginseng root is air-dried into white ginseng or steamed at 100 °C to give red ginseng. It is believed that red ginseng is more pharmacologically effective than white ginseng [14]. The differences in the biological effects of white and red Asian ginseng are attributed to the significant changes in ginsenosides from the steaming treatment [15]. In this study, we treated American ginseng root at various temperatures and heating times. After heat-processing, the root of American ginseng, like Asian ginseng, changes from white to red; steamed *P. quinquefolius* root is therefore referred to as red American ginseng.

Currently, the most popular herbal products are in extract forms. New regulations released by FDA on alternative complementary supplements require the botanical extracts to be standardized [16]. The contents of ginsenosides in the extracts were not assayed before. We treated American ginseng root at various temperatures and heating times. The contents of representative ginsenosides in unsteamed and steamed American ginseng root extracts were determined using HPLC. In addition to the cell line MCF-7, we also used the MDA-MB-230 human breast cancer cells to evaluate the chemopreventive activities of unsteamed and steamed American ginseng root extracts and four ginsenosides. To observe the anticancer mechanisms, the effects of American ginseng extracts and single compounds on apoptosis and cell cycle were evaluated.

2. Materials and methods

2.1 Chemicals

All solvents were of high-performance liquid chromatography (HPLC) grade from Fisher Scientific (Norcross, GA). Milli Q water was supplied by a water purification system (US Filter, Palm Desert, CA). Standards for ginsenosides Rb_1, Rb_2, Rc, Rd, Re, and Rg_1 were obtained from Indofine Chemical Company (Somerville, NJ); ginsenosides Rb3, Rg2, Rg3, Rh1, Rh2 and 20*(R)*-ginsenoside Rg2 (20*R*-Rg2) were obtained from the Delta Information Center for Natural Organic Compounds (Xuancheng, Anhui, China). All standards were of biochemical-reagent grade and at least 95% pure as confirmed by HPLC. All the plastic materials were purchased from Falcon Labware (Franklin Lakes, NJ). Trypsin, RPMI 1640 medium, fetal bovine serum (FBS), and penicillin/streptomycin solution (200×) were obtained from Mediatech, Inc. (Herndon, VA). A CellTiter 96 Aqueous One Solution Cell Proliferation Assay kit was obtained from Promega (Madison, WI). Annexin V-FITC, cyclin A-FITC and cyclin D1-FITC were obtained from BD Biosciences (San Diego, CA).

2.2 Plant materials, processing and extraction

American ginseng roots (*Panax quinquefolius* L.) were obtained from Roland Ginseng, LLC (Wausau, WI). The voucher samples were deposited at the Tang Center for Herbal Medicine Research at University of Chicago (Chicago, IL). For the heat-processing of American ginseng, the roots were steamed at 100 °C and 120 °C for 1 h or at 120 °C for 0.5, 1, 2, 3, and 4 h.

For the HPLC analysis, dried American ginseng sample (0.5 g) was extracted with methanol in a Soxhlet extractor for 8 h. The extract was concentrated, transferred into a 25-ml volumetric flask and diluted to the desired volume with methanol. One millimeter of the solution was purified by solid-phase extraction [17]. Purified solutions were stored at 4 °C until HPLC analysis.

For the *in vitro* anti-cancer studies, the process for the extraction of American ginseng samples was as follows: A root sample, unsteamed or steamed at various temperatures and times, was ground to powder and passed through a 40 mesh screen. Then 25 g of powder was extracted with 500 ml of 70% ethanol for 4 h; the water bath was maintained at 90 °C. When cooled, the solution was filtered with P8 filter paper (Fisher Scientific, Pittsburgh, PA) and the filtrate was collected. The residue was extracted with 500 ml of 70% ethanol once more and then filtered while the solution was cooled. The filtrates were combined and the solvent was evaporated under vacuum. The dried extract was dissolved in 100 ml water and then extracted with water-saturated *n*-butanol. The *n*-butanol phase was evaporated under vacuum and then lyophilized.

The root of *P. quinquefolius* L. was collected from Roland Ginseng, LLC (Wausau, WI, USA).

2.3 HPLC analysis

The HPLC system was a Waters 2960 instrument (Milford, MA) with a quaternary pump, an automatic injector, a photodiode array detector (Model 996), and Waters Millennium 32 software for peak identification and integration. The separation was carried out on a 250×3.2 mm i.d., 5μ, Ultrasphere C18 column (Alltech, Deerfield, IL) with a 7.5×3.2 mm i.d. guard column. For HPLC analysis, a 20-μL sample was injected into the column and eluted at room temperature with a constant flow rate of 1.0 ml/min. For the mobile phase, acetonitrile (solvent A) and water (solvent B) were used. Gradient elution started with 18% solvent A and 82% solvent B. Elution was changed to 21% A for 20 min, then to 26% A for 3 min and held for 19 min. It was then changed to 36% A for 13 min, to 50% A for 9 min, to 95% A for 2 min, and held for 3 min. Lastly elution was changed to 18% A for 3 min and held for 8 min. The detection wavelength was set to 202 nm. All tested solutions were filtered through Millex 0.2-μm nylon membrane syringe filters (Millipore Co., Bedford, MA) before use. The linearity of this method was assayed by analyzing standard solutions in the range of 2-400 μg/ml for the 12 ginsenosides. Calibration curves were constructed from the measured peak areas and the related amount of ginsenosides. Ginsenosides Rb1, Rb2, Rb3, Rc, Rd, Re, Rg1, Rg2, 20*R*-Rg2, Rg3, Rh1 and Rh2 (Figure **1**) in extract samples were identified by comparison of their retention times with those obtained from the chromatograms of mixed ginsenoside standards. The contents of saponins in each sample were calculated using standard curves of ginsenosides.

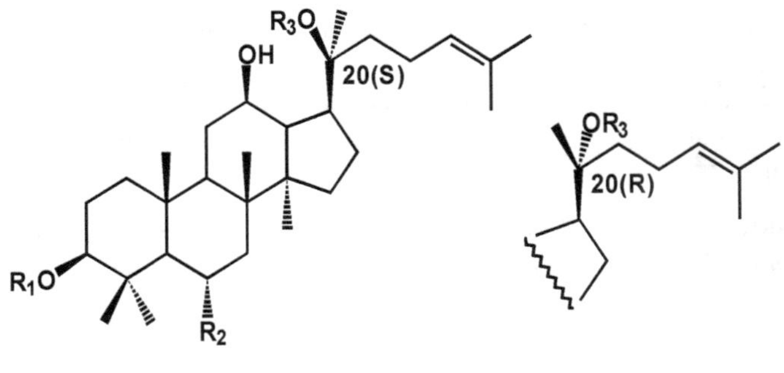

Name	R1	R2	R3
Ginsenoside Rb1	-glc^{2}- ^{1}glc	-H	20(S), -glc^{6}- ^{1}glc
Ginsenoside Rb2	-glc^{2}- ^{1}glc	-H	20(S), -glc^{6}- ^{1}ara(pyr)
Ginsenoside Rb3	-glc^{2}- ^{1}glc	-H	20(S), -glc^{6}- ^{1}xyl
Ginsenoside Rc	-glc^{2}- ^{1}glc	-H	20(S), -glc^{6}- ^{1}ara(fur)
Ginsenoside Rd	-glc^{2}- ^{1}glc	-H	20(S), -glc
Ginsenoside Re	-H	-O-glc^{2}- ^{1}rha	20(S), -glc
Ginsenoside Rg1	-H	-O-glc	20(S), -glc
Ginsenoside Rg2	-H	-O-glc^{2}- ^{1}rha	20(S), -H
20R-ginsenoside Rg2	-H	-O-glc^{2}- ^{1}rha	20(R), -H
Ginsenoside Rg3	-glc^{2}- ^{1}glc	-H	20(S), -H
Ginsenoside Rh1	-H	-O-glc	20(S), -H
Ginsenoside Rh2	-glc	-H	20(S), -H

Fig. 1. Chemical structures of assayed ginsenosides in American ginseng.

Ginsenoside Rg3 increased significantly from 0.5 to 3 h of steaming. Ginsenoside Rh2 is also an active anticancer saponin, however, after steaming treatment, the content of Rh2 was very low (Table **1**).

Ginsenoside	Asian Ginseng	Red Asian Ginseng	American Ginseng	Steaming Time (Red American Ginseng)				
				0.5 h	1 h	2 h	3 h	4 h
Rg1	0.279	0.276	0.133	0.098	0.075	0.017	ND	ND
Re	0.234	0.188	1.750	1.347	0.968	0.221	0.032	ND
Rh1	ND	0.015	ND	0.008	0.017	0.040	0.042	0.049
Rg2	0.031	0.034	0.015	0.154	0.266	0.405	0.444	0.363
20*R*-Rg2	ND	0.022	ND	0.086	0.155	0.388	0.425	0.422
Rb1	0.545	0.462	4.940	3.918	3.252	1.743	0.735	0.177
Rc	0.523	0.294	0.387	0.325	0.278	0.141	0.087	0.018
Rb2	0.443	0.200	0.043	0.042	0.036	0.026	0.018	ND
Rb3	0.067	0.032	0.063	0.064	0.050	0.035	0.017	ND
Rd	0.257	0.073	0.604	0.510	0.460	0.335	0.206	0.097
Rg3	0.004	0.033	0.003	0.143	0.271	0.664	1.053	1.225
Rh2	ND	0.009	0.007	0.007	0.018	0.047	0.057	0.066
Total	**2.38**	**1.64**	**7.95**	**6.70**	**5.85**	**4.05**	**3.11**	**2.42**

n = 3; ND, not detected; values are expressed as percentage of dry weight; RSD (relative standard derivation) are less than 15%.

Table 1. Ginsenoside contents in Asian ginseng, red Asian ginseng and American ginseng which were unsteamed or steamed at 120°C for 0.5-4 h.

2.4 Cell culture

The human breast cancer cell lines MCF-7 and MDA-MB-231 were purchased from American Type Culture Collection, ATCC (Manassas, VA, USA) and grown in RPMI 1640 medium supplemented with 10% FBS and 50 IU penicillin/streptomycin in a humidified atmosphere of 5% CO_2 at 37°C.

2.5 Cell proliferation analysis

Cells were seeded in 96-well plates. After 1 d, various concentrations of extracts/ginsenosides were added to the wells. The final concentration of ethanol was 0.5%. Controls were exposed to culture medium containing 0.5% ethanol without drugs. All experiments were performed in triplicate and repeated 3 times. Cell proliferation was evaluated using an MTS assay according to the manufacturer's instructions. Briefly, at the end of the drug exposure period, the medium was replaced with 100 µl of fresh medium, 20 µl of MTS reagent (CellTiter 96 Aqueous Solution) in each well, and the plate was returned to the incubator for 1-2 h. A 60-µl aliquot of medium from each well was transferred to an ELISA 96-well plate and its absorbance at 490 nm was recorded [4,18]. Results were expressed as percentage of control (ethanol vehicles set at 100%).

2.6 Apoptosis assay

Cells were seeded in 24-well tissue culture plates. After culturing for 1 day, the medium was changed and extracts/ginsenosides were added. After treated for 48 h, cells floating in the medium were collected. The adherent cells were detached with 0.05% trypsin. Then culture medium containing 10% FBS (and floating cells) was added to inactivate trypsin. After being pipetted gently, the cells were centrifuged for 5 min at 1500 g. The supernatant was removed and cells were stained with annexin V-FITC and propidium iodide according to the manufacturer's instructions. Untreated cells were used as control for double staining. Cells were analyzed immediately after staining using a FACScan flow cytometer (Becton Dickinson, Mountain View, CA) and FlowJo 7.1.0 software (Tree Star, Ashland, OR). For each measurement, at least 20,000 cells were counted.

2.7 Cyclin A and cyclin D1 assay

Cells were seeded in 24-well tissue culture plates. On the second day, the medium was changed and cells were treated with extracts. Cells were incubated for 48 h before the cells were harvested. The cells were fixed gently by putting 80% ethanol in freezer for 2 h and were then treated with 0.25% Triton X-100 for 5 min on ice bath. Cells were resuspended in 300 ul of PBS containing 40 µg/ml propidium iodide and 0.1 mg/ml RNase. Then, 20 µl of cyclin A-FITC or cyclin D1-FITC was added to the cell suspension. Then the cells were incubated in a dark room for 20 min at room temperature, and analyzed with a FACScan flow cytometer. For each measurement, at least 20,000 cells were counted.

2.8 Cell cycle assay

After cells were treated with extracts/ginsenosides, the cells were harvested in similar manner to the method used in the cyclins assay. Then, the cells were stained with propidium iodide, and analyzed with a FACScan flow cytometer. For each measurement, at least 20,000 cells were counted.

2.9 Statistical analysis

Data are presented as mean ± standard deviation (SD) with n = 3. A one-way ANOVA determined whether the results had statistical significance. In some cases, Student's t-test was used for comparing two groups. The level of statistical significance was set at $P<0.05$.

3. Results

3.1 Saponin composition changes in extracts during heat-processing

Twelve ginsenosides (Figure 1) were determined in American ginseng using high performance liquid chromatography (HPLC). All the assayed ginsenosides were dammarane glycosides [17,19]. The influence of steaming at 100°C and 120°C on the ginsenoside content of American ginseng was tested. Compared with unsteamed American ginseng, the roots treated at 100°C for 1 h decreased total ginsenoside content slightly, from 7.95% to 7.32%. For the main saponin contents, ginsenoside Rb1 was changed from 4.940% to 4.463%, and Re was from 1.756% to 1.630%; ginsenoside Rg3 increased from 0.003% to 0.048%. Steaming at 120°C for 1 h decreased the total ginsenoside content to 5.85%, as follows: Rb1, 3.252%; Re, 0.968%; and Rg3, 0.271%. Ginsenoside Rg3 increased significantly at 120°C.

Chromatograms of unsteamed and steamed American ginseng roots for 2 and 4 h at 120°C are shown in Figure **2**. The peak areas of Rb1, Rd and Re decreased during the steaming process. On the other hand, ginsenoside Rg3, which is a trace saponin in unsteamed root [17], was augmented during the steaming process (Figure **3**). The content of the 12 ginsenosides in steamed American ginseng roots is shown in Table **1**. During the steaming process, Rg1, Re, Rb1, Rc, Rb2, Rb3, and Rd decreased; Rh1, Rg2, 20R-Rg2, Rg3 and Rh2 increased.

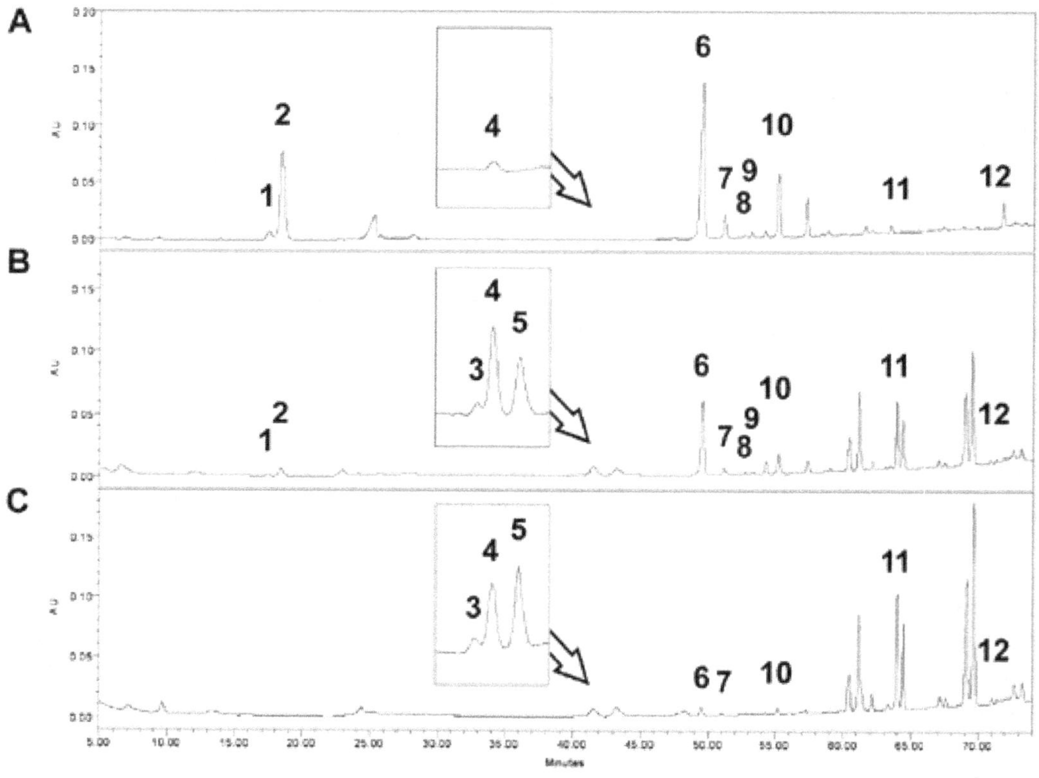

Fig. 2. HPLC analysis of ginsenosides in unsteamed and steamed American ginseng roots. Chromatograms of unsteamed (**A**), or steamed at 120°C for 2 h (**B**) and 4 h (**C**) are shown. Ginsenoside peaks: (**1**) Rg1, (**2**) Re, (**3**) Rh1, (**4**) Rg2, (**5**) 20R-Rg2, (**6**) Rb1, (**7**) Rc, (**8**) Rb2, (**9**) Rb3, (**10**) Rd, (**11**) Rg3, (**12**) Rh2. Peak numbers are not shown if saponins were not detected.

The chemical constituents of white ginseng and red ginseng (*P. ginseng* C. A. Meyer) were also determined. Data shown in Table **1** indicated that for the Asian ginseng, after steaming at 100°C, the contents of the main ginsenosides (Rg1, Re, Rb1, Rb2, Rc and Rd) were decreased. Ginsenoside Rg3 increased from 0.004% to 0.033%. The changes of ginsenoside contents are similar to that of American ginseng steamed at 100°C.

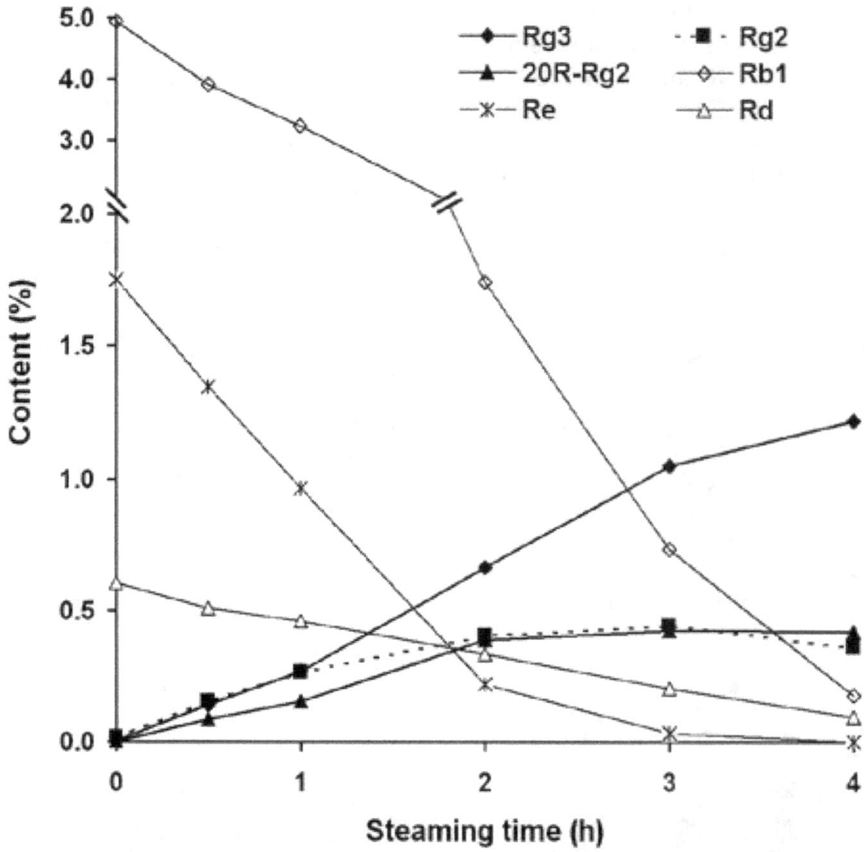

Fig. 3. Saponin content in American ginseng roots steamed at 120 °C for 0-4 h. The content of six major ginsenosides was changed during the steaming process.

3.2 Antiproliferative effects of extracts and ginsenosides on human breast cancer cells

Using two human breast cancer cell lines MCF-7 and MDA-MB-231, the antiproliferative effect of unsteamed and steamed American ginseng root extracts were evaluated. For the MCF-7 cells, at 0.25 mg/ml, unsteamed extract inhibited cell growth by 17.0%. After steaming for 1 h, the extract inhibited cell growth by 60.0% ($P<0.01$ vs. unsteamed extract). Moreover, after cells treated with 2 h steamed extract, cell growth was inhibited absolutely. At 0.5 mg/ml, extracts from 1 h and 2 h steamed roots inhibited cell growth over 99.6% (Figure **4A**). For the MDA-MB-231 cells, at 0.25 mg/ml, extracts from unsteamed and 1 h steamed roots did not show a antiproliferative effect, while extract from 2 h steamed roots showed a very strong effect, as cell growth was inhibited by 99.2% (Figure **4B**). These results suggested that steaming on American ginseng roots increased antiproliferative effects on human breast cancer cells, and the effects of extract from root steamed for 2 h were more potent than that of root steamed for 1 h.

Four representative ginsenosides were used to test for antiproliferative effects on breast cancer cells. Among them, two ginsenosides (Rb1 and Re) were major constituents in unsteamed American ginseng roots, while two other ginsenosides (Rg2 and Rg3) were main constituents in steamed roots. At 30-300 µM, after 72 h treatment, ginsenosides Rb1, Re and Rg2 did not show antiproliferative effects on MCF-7 and MDA-MB-231 cells. Ginsenoside Rg3 showed positive antiproliferative effect on both the cancer cell lines. At 100 µM, ginsenoside Rg3 inhibited cell growth by 49.8% on MCF-7 cells, and by 27.3% on MDA-MB-231 cells (both $P<0.01$ vs. untreated control). At 300 µM, ginsenoside Rg3 almost inhibited cell growth on both the cell lines absolutely (Figure **4C** and **4D**).

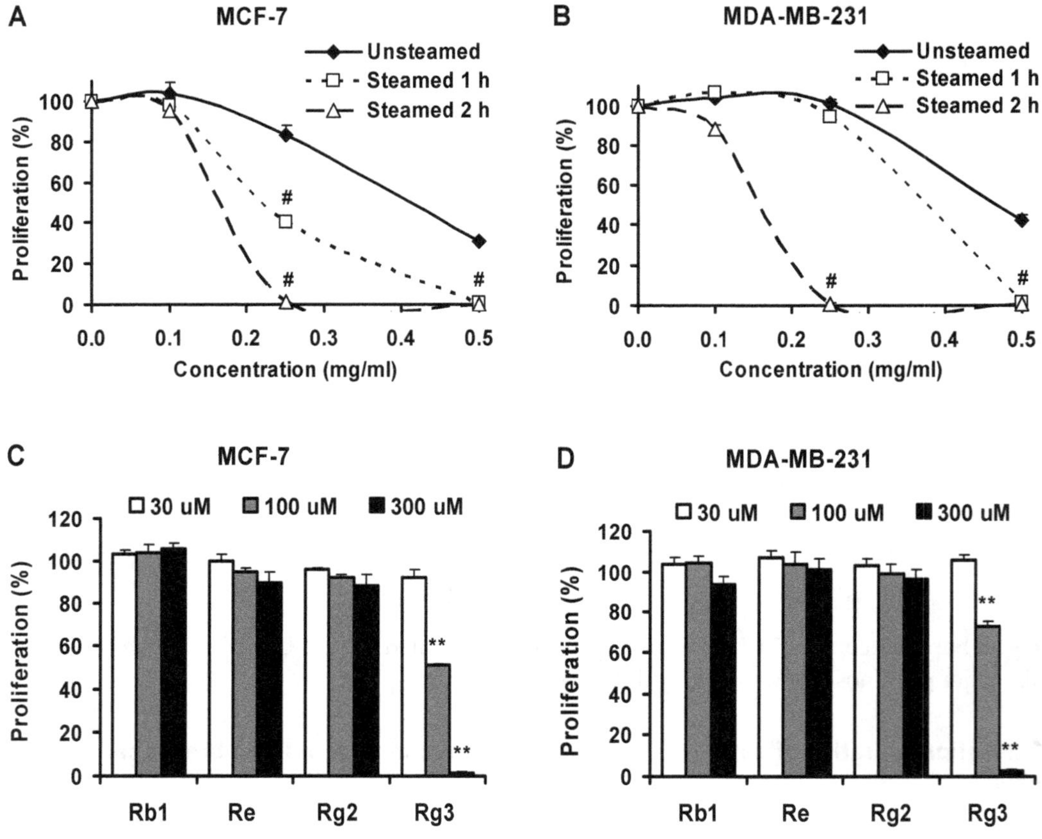

Fig. 4. Effects of American ginseng extracts and ginsenosides on proliferation of MCF-7 (A, C) and MDA-MB-231 (B, D) human breast cancer cells. Cells were treated with extracts (A, B) or ginsenosides (C, D) for 72 h, and then assayed by MTS method. #, $P<0.01$ vs. unsteamed extract; **, $P<0.01$ vs. control.

3.3 Apoptotic effect of extracts and ginsenosides on MCF-7 cells

Apoptosis and necrosis were evaluated in MCF-7 cells using annexin V-FITC, which detects translocation of phosphatidylinositol from the inner to outer cell membrane during early apoptosis, and propidium iodide, which can enter the cell in late apoptosis or necrosis. As shown in Figure **5**, compared to untreated control (early apoptosis 5.7%, late apoptosis/necrosis 6.1%), after treatment with 0.25 mg/ml for 48 h, unsteamed extract increased early apoptosis to 10.3%, but did not influence late apoptosis/necrosis (5.2%). After treatment with extract from 2 h steamed roots, early apoptosis increased slightly

(7.6%), and late apoptosis/necrosis increased significantly to 37.2%. Since early apoptosis is considered real apoptosis, steamed extract did not show obviously activity on early apoptosis. For the viable cells, the control was 88.1%, unsteamed extract was 83.8%, while 2 h steamed extract was 41.5%. Steamed extract significantly decrease the viable cells.

The effects of induction of apoptosis of representative ginsenosides on MCF-7 cells were also determined. Compared to control (5.5%), after treatment with 100-300 μM of ginsenosides Rb1 and Rg3 for 48 h, the percentage of early apoptotic cells were not increased (less than 6.2% and 5.8%, respectively). At the concentration of 300 μM, ginsenoside Re and Rg2 increased the cell percentage of early apoptosis to 13.0% and 9.1%, respectively. Consider both the apoptosis effects of steamed extract and its major ginsenosides Rb1 and Rg3, the MCF-7 cell growth inhibition activity of steamed extract may not be caused by the induction of apoptosis.

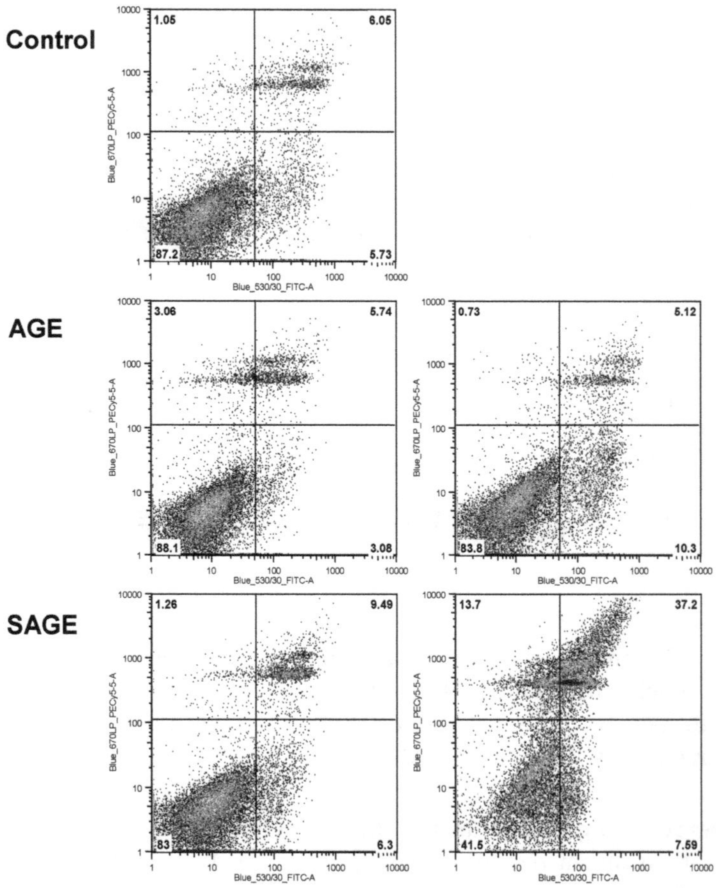

Fig. 5. Apoptosis assay using flow cytometry after annexin V-FITC/propidium iodide (PI) staining. MCF-7 cells were treated with 0.1 and 0.25 mg/ml of unsteamed and 2 h steamed extract for 48 h. Viable cells are in lower left quadrant, early apoptotic cells are in lower right quadrant, late apoptotic or necrotic cells are in upper right quadrant, and non-viable cells which underwent necrosis are in upper left quadrant.

3.4 Effect of extracts on the expression of cyclins on MCF-7 cells

The protein expression of cyclin A and cyclin D1 were evaluated by flow cytometry after staining with cyclin A-FITC and cyclin D1-FITC. For the percentage of cyclin A positive cells, the untreated control was 56.0%. After treatment with 0.1 and 0.25 mg/ml unsteamed extract for 48 h, the cyclin A positive cells were increased to 62.5% and 65.8%, while treated with 0.1 and 0.2 mg/ml 2 h steamed extract, cyclin A positive cells were decreased to 48.4% and 14.5%, respectively (Figure **6A**). For cyclin D1, unsteamed extract did not influence the expression of cyclin D1, while 2 h steamed extract decreased the expression of cyclin D1 significantly (Figure **6B**). Cyclin A and cyclin D1 are important cell cycle regulation proteins. Steamed extract decreased the expression of both cyclins, suggesting that the inhibition of cell growth of steamed extract may caused by the influences of cell cycle.

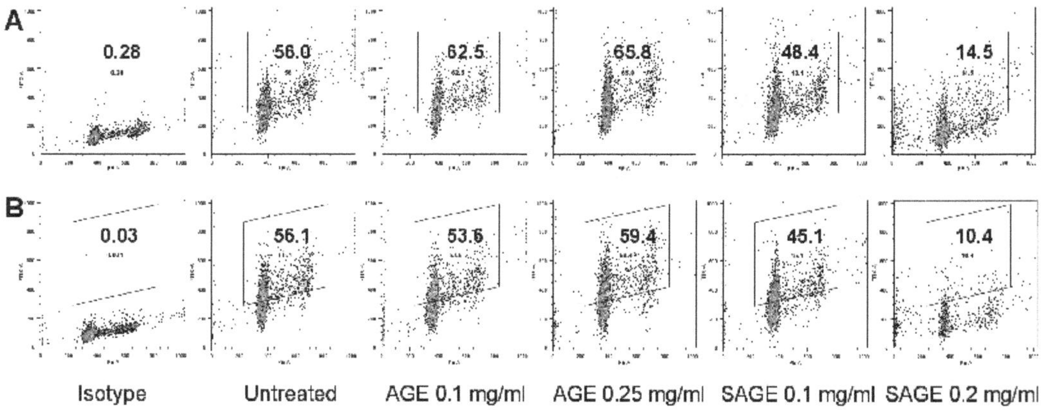

Fig. 6. Cyclins A and D1 analysis of MCF-7 cells using flow cytometry. After treated for 48 h, MCF-7 cells were stained with cyclin A-FITC/PI (A) and cyclin D1/PI (B). Isotype: untreated cells were stained with isotype antibody/PI. The percentage of cyclin A (A) and cyclin D1 (B) positive cells is shown in the gate.

3.5 Effects of extracts and ginsenosides on MCF-7 cell cycle

After treatment with unsteamed and steamed extract for 48 h, cells were stained with propidium iodide (PI) and then assayed by flow cytometry. Unsteamed extract did not influence the cell cycle profile (Figure 7). Compared to untreated control (G1, 68.2%), 0.2 mg/ml 2 h steamed extract increased the percentage of cells in G1 phase to 83.6%. For the single compounds, ginsenosides Rb1, Re and Rg2 almost did not influence the cell cycle. Ginsenoside Rg3, a previously recognized anticancer compound, increased the G1 fraction to 87.4% (Figure 7). Data from this study suggests that both the 2 h steamed extract and ginsenoside Rg3 arrested MCF-7 cells in G1 phase.

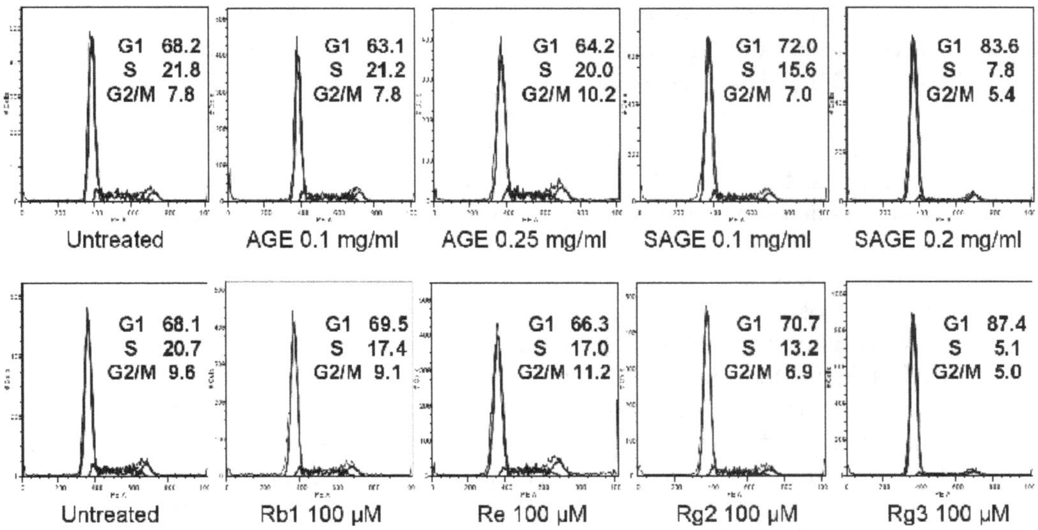

Fig. 7. Effects of extracts and ginsenosides on cell cycle. After MCF-7 cells were treated with extracts or ginsenosides for 48 h, the cells were stained with PI and assayed using flow cytometry. The percentage of cells in G1, S and G2/M phases are indicated.

4. Discussion

Herbal medicines are comprised of a complicated mixture of biologically active compounds. The concentrations of these compounds may vary significantly depending on many intrinsic and extrinsic factors such as genetics, season, geographical distribution, plant growth, and production and extract processes [20]. Thus, herbal medicine identification and analysis are very important issues in the quality assurance of herbal products. Since American ginseng from Wisconsin is a reliable ginseng source [21], in this study, the American ginseng used was from Roland Ginseng, LLC (Wausau, WI). The plant material was identified according to the United States Pharmacopoeia NF 21, monograph: American ginseng (*Panax quinquefolius* L.). The contents of major ginsenosides in different American ginseng extracts were determined using HPLC, which means that our American ginseng extracts were standardized and the quantitative assay data are critical references for future studies.

Heat-processing on American ginseng changes the constituent profiles. We have reported the steaming temperatures and times on the changes of ginsenosides in the crude herb [22]. In this study, the contents of main ginsenosides in the extracts were evaluated. In unsteamed extract, the content of ginsenoside Rb1 was 34.2%, and the summary of six ginsenosides were 63.9%. The content of total ginsenoside in extract was very high, suggesting that the extraction and purification method used in this study are reasonable.

Ginsenoside Rg3, a previously recognized anticancer compound [7], was detected in the unsteamed and steamed extracts. In unsteamed extract, Rg3 was only a trace saponin (0.06%). After 2 h steaming, the content of Rg3 was increased to 5.9%, becoming a main constituent in the extract. Therefore, steaming on American ginseng increased Rg3 content significantly.

Pharmacological studies showed that heat-processing on American ginseng increases the antiproliferative effect significantly. The biological effects of extracts were based on their chemical constituents. We consequently evaluated the antiproliferative activities of representative ginsenosides on human breast cancer cells. Using both cancer cell lines (MCF-7 and MDA-MB-231), ginsenosides Rb1 and Re, taken from unsteamed extract almost had no effect at the concentration range of 30-300 uM. Ginsenoside Rg3, which was taken from steamed extract, showed strong antiproliferative activity. The increase of antiproliferative effect of steam-processing is based on the increase of anticancer constituents.

Apoptosis is considered an important pathway in the inhibition of cancer cells of many anticancer agents [23,24]. In this study, we assayed the induction of apoptosis by American ginseng extracts and single compounds. However, the apoptotic induction activities on MCF-7 cells were not confirmed by current data. The antiproliferative effect of red American ginseng extract on human breast cancer cells may be caused by other mechanisms.

Recent studies found that overexpression of cyclin D1 promotes tumor cell growth, and confers resistance of chemotherapy [23,24]. Cyclins assay found that American ginseng extracts regulated the expression of cyclin A and cyclin D1 on MCF-7 cells. Red American ginseng extract decreased the expression of cyclin A and cyclin D1 significantly. Since cyclins are important regulation proteins in cell cycle, we assayed the influence of extract on cell cycle. Data showed that red American ginseng extract arrested cells in G1 phase, and decrease the percentage of cells in S and G2/M phases. We subsequently studied the influence of representative saponins on the cell cycle. Treatment with 100 μM of ginsenosides Rb1, Re and Rg2 for 48 h, did not influence the cell cycle profile. Ginsenoside Rg3, a main constituent in red American ginseng, arrested cells in G1 phase. This result is similar to that of red American ginseng extract.

At the concentration of 0.25 mg/ml, 2 h steamed extract inhibited cell growth absolutely. The 0.25 mg/ml 2 h steamed extract contains 18.6 μM of ginsenoside Rg3. However, even 30 μM of ginsenoside Rg3 did not show significant antiproliferative activity. From the HPLC chromatogram of 2 h steamed extract, several peaks of unidentified compounds can be found. We expected that other more potent compounds existed in red American ginseng extract, and these compounds have similar effects to Rg3 on cell cycle. This should be focus of future studies.

In summary, analytical and pharmacological data obtained from our observations suggest that steamed American ginseng root significantly augments the content of ginsenoside Rg3 and other unidentified active compounds, which is responsible for the increase in anticancer activity. Red American ginseng, which is the heat-processed root of *P. quinquefolius*, may be a potent anti-breast cancer herbal medicine.

5. Acknowledgements

This work was supported in part by the NIH/NCCAM grants P01 AT004418 and K01 AT005362.

6. References

Jemal A, Siegel R, Xu J, Ward E. Cancer statistics, 2010. *CA Cancer J Clin.* Sep-Oct 2010;60(5):277-300.

Lee MC, Newman LA. Management of patients with locally advanced breast cancer. *Surg Clin North Am.* 2007;87:379-398.

Gerber B, Scholz C, Reimer T, Briese V, Janni W. Complementary and alternative therapeutic approaches in patients with early breast cancer: a systematic review. *Breast Cancer Res Treat.* Feb 2006;95(3):199-209.

Wang CZ, Luo X, Zhang B, et al. Notoginseng enhances anti-cancer effect of 5-fluorouracil on human colorectal cancer cells. *Cancer Chemother Pharmacol.* Jun 2007;60(1):69-79.

Ang-Lee MK, Moss J, Yuan CS. Herbal medicines and perioperative care. *Jama.* Jul 11 2001;286(2):208-216.

Attele AS, Wu JA, Yuan CS. Ginseng pharmacology: multiple constituents and multiple actions. *Biochem Pharmacol.* Dec 1 1999;58(11):1685-1693.

Helms S. Cancer prevention and therapeutics: Panax ginseng. *Altern Med Rev.* Sep 2004;9(3):259-274.

Yoo HH, Yokozawa T, Satoh A, Kang KS, Kim HY. Effects of ginseng on the proliferation of human lung fibroblasts. *Am J Chin Med.* 2006;34(1):137-146.

Koo HN, Jeong HJ, Choi IY, et al. Mountain grown ginseng induces apoptosis in HL-60 cells and its mechanism have little relation with TNF-alpha production. *Am J Chin Med.* 2007;35(1):169-182.

Yun TK, Choi SY. Preventive effect of ginseng intake against various human cancers: a case-control study on 1987 pairs. *Cancer Epidemiol Biomarkers Prev.* Jun 1995;4(4):401-408.

Yun TK, Choi SY. Non-organ specific cancer prevention of ginseng: a prospective study in Korea. *Int J Epidemiol.* Jun 1998;27(3):359-364.

Corbit R, Ebbs S, King ML, Murphy LL. The influence of lead and arsenite on the inhibition of human breast cancer MCF-7 cell proliferation by American ginseng root (Panax quinquefolius L.). *Life Sci.* Feb 16 2006;78(12):1336-1340.

Aung HH, Mehendale SR, Wang CZ, Xie JT, McEntee E, Yuan CS. Cisplatin's tumoricidal effect on human breast carcinoma MCF-7 cells was not attenuated by American ginseng. *Cancer Chemother Pharmacol.* Feb 2007;59(3):369-374.

Takaku T, Kameda K, Matsuura Y, Sekiya K, Okuda H. Studies on insulin-like substances in Korean red ginseng. *Planta Med.* Feb 1990;56(1):27-30.

Kim WY, Kim JM, Han SB, et al. Steaming of ginseng at high temperature enhances biological activity. *J Nat Prod.* Dec 2000;63(12):1702-1704.

Rapaka RS, Coates PM. Dietary supplements and related products: a brief summary. *Life Sci.* Mar 27 2006;78(18):2026-2032.

Wang CZ, Wu JA, McEntee E, Yuan CS. Saponins composition in American ginseng leaf and berry assayed by high-performance liquid chromatography. *J Agr Food Chem.* Mar 22 2006;54(6):2261-2266.

DiPaola RS, Kuczynski WI, Onodera K, et al. Evidence for a functional kit receptor in melanoma, breast, and lung carcinoma cells. *Cancer Gene Ther.* May-Jun 1997;4(3):176-182.

Qi LW, Wang CZ, Yuan CS. American ginseng: potential structure-function relationship in cancer chemoprevention. *Biochem Pharmacol.* Oct 1 2010;80(7):947- 954.

Fong HH, Pauli GF, Bolton JL, et al. Evidence-based herbal medicine: Challenges in efficacy and safety assessments. In: Leung P-C, Fong, H., Xue, C.C., ed. *Current Review of Chinese Medicine, Annals of Traditional Chinese Medicine, Vol. 2.* Singapore: World Scientific; 2006.

Assinewe VA, Baum BR, Gagnon D, Arnason JT. Phytochemistry of wild populations of Panax quinquefolius L. (North American ginseng). *J Agric Food Chem.* Jul 30 2003;51(16):4549-4553.

Wang CZ, Aung HH, Ni M, et al. Red American ginseng: ginsenoside constituents and antiproliferative activities of heat-processed Panax quinquefolius roots. *Planta Med.* Jun 2007;73(7):669-674.

Reed JC, Pellecchia M. Apoptosis-based therapies for hematologic malignancies. *Blood.* Jul 15 2005;106(2):408-418.

Wu WY, Guo HZ, Qu GQ, Han J, Guo DA. Mechanisms of pseudolaric Acid B-induced apoptosis in bel-7402 cell lines. *Am J Chin Med.* 2006;34(5):887-899.

6

Tamoxifen Resistant Breast Cancer and Autophagy

Grey A. Wilkinson, Adam N. Elwi and Sung-Woo Kim
University of Calgary,
Canada

1. Introduction

1.1 Tamoxifen for the treatment of breast cancer

Tamoxifen was originally developed with the hope of becoming a "morning after" contraceptive. During the 1960s, studies showed that tamoxifen and other anti-estrogens have a profound impact on the fertility of laboratory rats and it was believed that tamoxifen could elicit the same effects in humans. Coincidently, in humans, anti-estrogens were found to improve fertility by inducing ovulation (Jordan, 2006).

The use of tamoxifen for the treatment of breast cancer became apparent when early *in vitro* and *in vivo* studies found that tamoxifen inhibited estradiol (E2) binding to estrogen receptors (ERs) in breast tissue (Jordan, 1976; Jordan & Dowse, 1976; Jordan & Koerner, 1975; Nicholson & Golder, 1975). The inhibition of ERs proved to be a significant finding as the estrogen-stimulated growth and the ovarian dependence of some breast cancers had been known since the later part of the eighteenth century (Beatson, 1896). Prior to the 1970s, and the successful development of drug-based endocrine therapies, attempts to reduce estrogen-stimulated growth of breast cancer include the surgical removal of the ovaries and/or pituitary and adrenal glands (Kennedy, 1965). Unfortunately, for years it was not known which breast tumors would respond favorably to ablative surgery, where only 30% of patients would receive a benefit (Jensen *et al.*, 1971; Kennedy, 1965). By examining proteins from breast tumor biopsies, Jensen *et al.* (1971) showed that if the estrogen receptor is present, tumors will respond to ablative surgical treatment, but if absent, the tumors fail to respond.

Fortunately today, endocrine-based surgical procedures for breast cancer are not necessary for most women as drug-based endocrine therapies have advanced with the use of estrogen antagonists and aromatase inhibitors. Estrogen antagonists, such as tamoxifen or fulvestrant competitively inhibit estrogen binding to ERs. Aromatase inhibitors prevent estrogen production, by inhibiting the aromatase class of enzymes, impeding the conversion of androgens to estrogens and thus reducing the bioavailability of estrogen hormones (Jordan, 1994; Mokbel, 2002).

Currently tamoxifen is typically used as an adjuvant treatment option for early and advanced ER-positive (ER^+) breast cancer in pre- and post-menopausal women (Jordan, 1994). Adjuvant treatment with tamoxifen, has significantly improved disease-free survival and reduced the number of deaths from breast cancer (Early Breast Cancer Trialists' Collaborative, 2005). Tamoxifen may also be used in the neoadjuvant setting and as a preventative agent for women at high risk of developing the disease, although some patients may feel that when used as a preventative agent the risks may outweigh the benefits (Cuzick *et al.*, 2003; Waters *et al.*, 2010). The most adverse effect of tamoxifen is the increased propensity to develop endometrial cancer that occurs predominantly in post-menopausal women. To subside this effect, tamoxifen, in the adjuvant setting, is administered for at most 5 years. If longer therapy is required, patients are typically switched to aromatase inhibitors or a different anti-estrogen, such as fulvestrant (Perez, 2007).

In breast tissue, tamoxifen acts as an antagonist, binding to ERα, competitively inhibiting E2, and preventing the expression of mitogen, angiogenic, and apoptotic factors. In other tissues such as the endometrium, tamoxifen acts as an agonist and elicits a response similar to estrogen when bound to ERs, potentially leading to the development of endometrial cancer. 'Pure' anti-estrogens, like fulvestrant bind the ER competitively inhibiting estrogen but have no estrogen like effects. In some women, tamoxifen's agonistic actions have been found to have favorable effects on serum cholesterol and protection against bone loss and cardiovascular disease (Hoskins *et al.*, 2009; Osborne, 1998). The tissue dependent agonist and antagonist actions of tamoxifen classify the drug as a selective estrogen receptor modulator (SERM). SERMs modulate the ER signal transduction pathway in ER target tissues through complex and not completely understood mechanisms (Jordan, 2006), although the agonist and antagonist functions of tamoxifen are thought to be mediated through two distinct transactivation domains of ERα, Activating Function-1 (AF-1) close to the N-terminus, and AF-2, in the ligand binding site. In breast tissue, tamoxifen inhibits AF-2 activation and functions as an antagonist of genes that rely on AF-2 transactivation. In genes where AF-2 function is redundant, tamoxifen may function as an agonist and transcription may be driven solely by the AF-1 domain (McDonnell *et al.*, 1995; Ring & Dowsett, 2004; Tzukerman *et al.*, 1994).

1.2 Estrogen receptors

The primary target of tamoxifen is the ER. The ER is a ligand-activated transcription factor that is a critical regulator of breast epithelial cell proliferation, differentiation, and apoptosis. There are two ER isoforms, ERα and ERβ (Dahlman-Wright *et al.*, 2006). The receptors differ in their cellular function, tissue distribution, as well as ligand binding properties. Both ERα and ERβ are expressed in normal and neoplastic tissues. ERα is expressed in 15-30% of the luminal epithelial cells while ERβ is more ubiquitously expressed throughout the mammary tissue. Estrogen dependent proliferation in non-neoplastic breast epithelial cells is thought to occur through paracrine mechanisms where ERα cells promote the proliferation of adjacent ER negative cells (Riggins *et al.*, 2007). In neoplastic breast tissue, ERα is expressed in a greater proportion of cells and growth is thought to occur through both autocrine and paracrine mechanisms (Riggins *et al.*, 2007). The roll of ERβ in breast cancer development is not well understood. ERβ is often down regulated in malignant cells and its presence is often correlated with a better prognosis (Saji *et al.*, 2005; Sugiura *et al.*, 2007). *In vivo* studies in mice have revealed that ERβ expression prevents tumor formation and angiogenesis (Behrens *et al.*, 2007; Paruthiyil *et al.*, 2004). Indeed ERβ may contribute to the pregnancy/lactation-associated protection from breast cancer by disrupting the formation of tight junctions and altering the expression of β-cantenin, traits that have been associated with malignant phenotypes (Riggins *et al.*, 2007). Moreover, ERβ is a marker of improved response to tamoxifen (Hopp *et al.*, 2004). Thus most endocrine therapies target the actions of ERα.

ERα-positive (ERα+) breast cancers account for at least 75% of the breast cancer patient population. The presence of ERα, assessed immunohistologically, serves as a biomarker for a patient's response to endocrine therapy (Harvey *et al.*, 1999). The majority, 65%, of ERα+ breast cancers also express the progesterone receptor (PR) (Hoskins *et al.*, 2009). The PR, like the ER, is a ligand activated transcription factor that is involved in a wide range of physiological functions, contributing to cell homeostasis and differentiation. A small number of ER-negative but PR-positive tumors also respond favorably to tamoxifen treatment, but this is likely due to a small presence of ERα below the limit of detection (Clarke *et al.*, 2001).

ERα has three distinct pathways of regulating gene expression. The classic model of ERα signaling involves the ligand bound ERα that activates gene expression by direct dimeric binding to DNA response elements in complexes involving co-activators (CoAs) and histone acetyl transferases (HATs). The ER can also influence transcription through protein-protein interactions with other transcription factors, such as activation protein 1 (Ap1) and specific protein 1 (Sp1), which facilitate binding to serum response elements. Lastly, ERs can be activated by downstream signaling events or crosstalk with receptor tyrosine kinases including: epidermal growth factor receptor (EGFR), human epidermal growth factor receptor 2 (HER2, also known as ERBB2), and insulin-like growth factor-1 receptor (IGF-1R) (Kushner *et al.*, 2000; Musgrove & Sutherland, 2009; Ring & Dowsett, 2004; Schiff *et al.*, 2003). Indeed deregulation of estrogen signaling through the estrogen receptors with proliferation through alternative pathways are common mechanisms for tamoxifen resistance (Ali & Coombes, 2002; Musgrove & Sutherland, 2009; Riggins *et al.*, 2007).

1.3 Resistance to tamoxifen

A challenge to nearly all cancer therapies is the development of resistance. Resistance to cancer therapy can be categorized into two major forms, *de novo* and acquired. *De novo* or intrinsic resistance is present in patients that are initially unresponsive to treatment, despite having a phenotypic classification similar to patients that do respond; while acquired resistance is present in patients that respond to treatment initially, but eventually relapse.

Despite tamoxifen's successes, where 70% of ERα+ and/or progesterone receptor positive breast cancer patients respond favorably to treatment, 30-50% of patients will have recurrent disease within 15 years (Clarke *et al.*, 2001; Early Breast Cancer Trialists' Collaborative, 2005). Few strategies besides resorting to invasive chemotherapy, radiation therapy, and surgery have found success in circumventing anti-estrogen resistance. The challenge then, is to identify specific biomarkers that can predict therapeutic response to endrocrine therapies and identify new targets to combat endocrine resistant disease (Musgrove & Sutherland, 2009).

1.4 *De novo* resistance

One of the most prevalent factors contributing to *de novo* tamoxifen resistances is lack of ERα expression (Giacinti *et al.*, 2006). The decreased expression of ERα can be the result of hypermethylation in the CpG islands of the ERα promoter. Studies using MDA-MB-231 ERα-negative breast cancer cells have shown that by re-expressing endogenous ERα with a histone deacelylase (HDAC) inhibitor cells can be re-sensitized to tamoxifen (Sharma *et al.*,

2006). Similar studies have shown that by ectopically expressing ERα in the same cell line, cells do not become sensitive to tamoxifen treatment but have a decreased proliferative and metastatic phenotype when exposed to estrogen (Garcia *et al.*, 1992). Thus, the restoration of ERα appears to be a potential therapy for *de novo* resistance or ERα-negative breast cancers. Candidate therapies include the use of demethylating agents or HDAC inhibitors, which could potentially decrease the hypermethylation of CpG island-s within the ERα promoter (Giacinti *et al.*, 2006).

In addition, Hoskins and collogues identified a pharmacokinetic mechanism behind *de novo* tamoxifen resistance (Hoskins *et al.*, 2009). Patients carrying inactive alleles of cytochrome P450 2D6 (CYP2D6), or are co-administered drugs that inhibit CYP2D6, fail to convert tamoxifen into its active metabolites endoxifen and 4-hydroxytamoxifen, as a result, patients seem to derive little therapeutic benefit. Interestingly, the inactive alleles of CYP2D6 vary among different ethnic groups, suggesting an ethnic based difference in response to tamoxifen treatment. Approximately 20% of East Asian women, 16% of women with African ancestry, and 6-10% of Caucasian women have decreased CYP2D6 metabolism. The ethnic differences emphasize the importance of patient based therapies and the potential employment of CYP2D6 genotyping prior to tamoxifen treatment (Hoskins *et al.*, 2009). Other mechanisms of *de novo* resistance and the mechanisms that lead to lack of ERα expression are not as well understood, although they may be similar to some of the mechanisms that lead to acquired tamoxifen resistance.

1.5 Acquired resistance

Tamoxifen is typically prescribed in the adjuvant setting and administered for a 5 year period. Prolonged exposure may drive the development of acquired resistance that can arise from multiple factors including host-specific differences in immunity, endocrinology, and drug pharmacokinetics. Tumor-specific factors such as alterations in ER isoform ratios or ER transactivation and downstream signaling as well as changes in tyrosine kinases or mitogen growth factor signaling may also contribute to acquired tamoxifen resistance.

In cases where patients acquire resistance to tamoxifen, loss of ERα expression occurs in only 15-20% of breast cancers (Gutierrez *et al.*, 2005). Mutations in ERα are also quite rare occurring in <1% of $ER\alpha^{+}$ tumors (Clarke *et al.*, 2003; Herynk & Fuqua, 2004; Riggins *et al.*, 2007). Indeed, following the development of tamoxifen resistance, many tumors still respond to treatment with aromatase inhibitors or 'pure' anti-estrogens such as fulvestrant, which also block the effects of estrogen but have no estrogen-like effects, unlike tamoxifen. These observations suggest that estrogen still plays a critical role in tamoxifen-resistant tumors and support the idea that endocrine therapies can lead to the activation of novel signaling pathways that circumvent the effects of anti-estrogens (Lewis & Jordan, 2005; Musgrove & Sutherland, 2009; Riggins *et al.*, 2007). In addition, the activation of these pathways may also contribute to *de novo* and acquired resistance to aromatase inhibitors and other anti-estrogens.

In large part, the development of acquired resistance can be attributed to a deregulation of estrogen receptor signaling as well as altered expression and/or modification of several tyrosine kinase growth factor receptors and their downstream signaling targets (Musgrove & Sutherland, 2009; Riggins *et al.*, 2007). Signaling from tyrosine kinase receptors such as EGFR, HER2, as well as the IGF-1 receptor (IGF1R) have been associated with the expression of anti-apoptotic, autophagic, and other pro-survival signaling factors that allow for the

development of endocrine resistance. Others have previously discussed the role of the HER2 and EGFR signaling pathways in relation to tamoxifen resistance (reviewed in: Clarke *et al.*, 2003; Musgrove & Sutherland, 2009; Riggins *et al.*, 2007).
In this chapter, we discuss the significance of IGF signaling and present additional results of a previously published RNA interference (RNAi) tamoxifen resistance screen (Ahn *et al.*, 2010). The screen was used to identify new targets to combat tamoxifen-resistant disease or to identify specific biomarkers that predict response to tamoxifen therapy. One of the identified targets, IGF binding protein 5 (IGFBP5) will be discussed in detail, while the other targets have a role in autophagy which has been shown to be essential for cell survival, differentiation, development, and homeostasis in response to stress and nutrient deprivation (Levine & Kroemer, 2008).

2. Methods

RNAi is a powerful tool to inhibit gene expression at the post-transcriptional level and allows the identification of novel cellular mechanisms that regulate gene expression. As well, its manipulation makes high-throughput genetic screens possible. The silencing of genes within mammalian cells is possible by designing small interfering RNA (siRNA) sequences. The siRNAs can be synthesized chemically, then taken up by the cell. Alternatively siRNAs can be produced within the cell, in the form of short hairpin RNAs (shRNAs) from exogenously introduced vectors.

2.1 siRNAs and shRNAs

Since RNA interference (RNAi) was first discovered in the nematode *Caenorhabditis elegans* it has been used to exploit the function of genes in higher organisms (Fire *et al.*, 1998). In particular, large-scale RNAi based techniques have innovated the existing loss-of-function genetic screens in mammalian cells (Elbashir *et al.*, 2001). The use of chemically-synthesized siRNAs has a couple of key advantages including: the constant quality control of reagents that is important for high-throughput settings; and the diverse modification of siRNA molecules that improves stability and delivery to cells. Vice versa, synthetic siRNAs has disadvantages, including its short-life that results in the transient inhibition of gene expression only, along with difficulty in efficiently delivering siRNAs to non-dividing primary cells and their cost in genome-wide high-throughput screens. To circumvent these limitations, several groups have developed vectors that produce short hairpin RNAs (shRNAs) that are processed within the cell into short duplex RNAs having siRNA-like properties (Brummelkamp *et al.*, 2002). Such vectors provide a renewable source of a gene-silencing reagent that can mediate persistent gene silencing after stable integration of the vector into the host-cell genome. Furthermore, the core silencing 'hairpin' cassette can be readily inserted into retroviral, lentiviral, or adenoviral vectors, facilitating delivery of shRNAs into a broad range of cell types (Brummelkamp *et al.*, 2002; Michiels *et al.*, 2002). Additionally, inducible versions of shRNA vectors have been generated and used successfully in genetic screens (Ngo *et al.*, 2006).

2.2 RNAi-screening in breast cancer

The large collections of RNAi libraries have been used in many different ways to identify genes associated with drugs resistance or specific cellular phenotypes such as migration or invasion that act in a cancer-specific genetic context. A list of published screens performed in breast cancer is presented in Table 1. Using an shRNA library genetic screen, Berns *et al.* (2007) made a significant contribution to breast cancer research when they discovered that PI3K is a determinant in Trastuzumab (Herceptin) resistance for HER2-positive breast cancers. In a siRNA screen with ovarian and breast cancer cells, Swanton *et al.* (2007) revealed that CERT and its client ceramide were integral to paclitaxel-mediated cell death. Furthermore, Swanton and collogues showed that the paclitaxel response metagene is promising as a paclitaxel-specific predictor of pathological complete response in triple-negative breast cancer. Through the genetic screen of tamoxifen resistant breast cancer, Kim and his group identified IGFBP5 as a determinant of its sensitivity (Ahn *et al.*, 2010).

Screening for	**Cell line used**	**shRNA set used**	**Genes identified**	**Reference**
Herceptin resistance	BT-474	Retroviral shRNAs	PI3K pathway	(Berns *et al.*, 2007)
Paclitaxel resistance	MDA-MB-231, MDA-MB-468	siRNAs	PPM1D, CENP, IGF1..	(Bauer *et al.*, 2010)
Paclitaxel resistance	MDA-MB-231, SKOV-3	siRNAs	Ceramide metabolism regulators	(Juul *et al.*, 2010; Swanton *et al.*, 2007)
Tamoxifen resistance	MCF-7	Retroviral shRNAs	IGFBP5	(Ahn *et al.*, 2010)

Table 1. Application of RNAi library screens in breast cancer.

Overall, genetic RNAi screening holds promise in accelerating the development of drug-specific therapeutics or predictive biomarkers, since they target cancer-specific genetic alterations.

2.3 Screening strategies

The screening strategy is shown in schematic form in Fig. 1. Several breast cancer cells, including MCF-7, BT-474 and MDA-MB-231 cells were cultured in DMEM supplemented with 10% fetal bovine serum and treated with tamoxifen (5 μM) to find out which cell line is most sensitive. MCF-7 cells were selected for the RNAi screening as they were shown to be the most sensitive to the drug (Fig. 2). Tamoxifen-resistant MCF-7 cells were established by culturing for 4 wks in 10 μM 4-hydroxytamoxifen. Three shRNA oligonucleotides against each of 8,000 genes were designed and cloned into retroviral vector (pRS) containing a shRNA cassette.

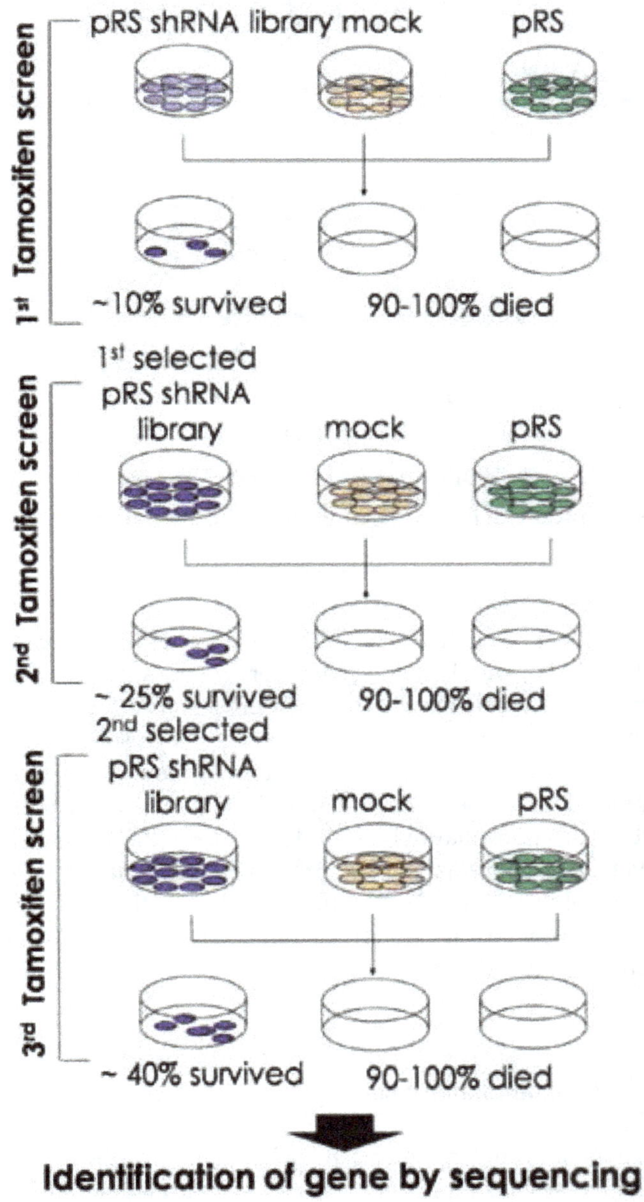

Fig. 1. The screening strategy employed for the identification of tamoxifen resistant genes.

MCF-7 cells were infected with pRS-shRNA library or pRS or mock-infected, selected with puromycin (1 µg/mL) for 2 weeks, and cultured in the presence or absence of tamoxifen (5 µM). After 6 days, genomic DNA was isolated and shRNA inserts were sub-cloned into a pRS vector. Screening was done for two additional rounds to enrich for targets. Targeted genes were identified by sequencing shRNA inserts.

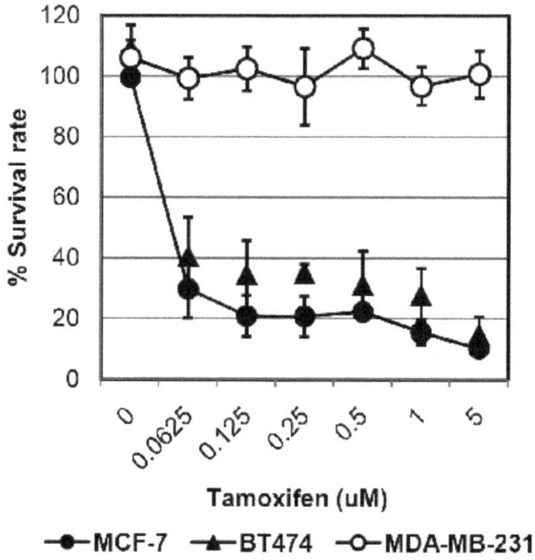

Fig. 2. Various breast cancer cell lines treated with 4-hydroxytamoxifen.

3. Results

Our screen revealed that loss of IGFBP5 contributed to tamoxifen resistance (Ahn *et al.*, 2010). In addition to IGFBP5, we identified several other genes that have a role in regulating autophagy or have a function in the downstream effects of autophagy. Autophagy is the regulated turnover of large components of the cell (e.g., cytosol and organelles) through engulfment in double-membrane sacs, termed autophagosomes, followed by fusion with lysosomes for degradation. These genes include: Vacuolar protein sorting 15 (Vps15), a regulatory subunit of the phosphatidyl inositide 3-kinase (PI3K) complex subunit Vps34 (Lindmo *et al.*, 2008); regulatory-associated protein of mammalian target of rapamycin (mTOR) (Raptor), an inhibitor of mTOR complex kinase activity (Kim *et al.*, 2002); and, interleukin 6 (IL-6), a pro-senescent cytokine (Kuilman *et al.*, 2008). The significance of each of the identified genes will be discussed below.

4. Discussion

4.1 The role of IGFBP5 in tamoxifen resistance

The IGF signaling pathway has important roles in regulating energy metabolism, cellular proliferation, differentiation, and apoptosis (Gluckman *et al.*, 1992; Valentinis & Baserga, 2001). The IGF axis involves a complex regulatory network that operates at a physiological, cellular and sub-cellular level (Pollak *et al.*, 2004). The relationship between IFG signaling and neoplasia has been well documented but the correlation between IGF signaling and endrocrine resistance is not as well understood (Pollak, 2008; Pollak *et al.*, 2004). In general, deregulation of IGF signaling may also correlate with the higher incidences of cancer, in particular breast cancer, among affluent nations due to higher incidences of obesity and a preference for a sedentary lifestyle. Both estrogen and IGFs have a synergistic effect on cell proliferation in MCF-7 breast cancer cell lines. Crosstalk between these two pathways has been implicated in the development of resistance to endocrine therapy and cancer recurrence.

The IGF signaling pathway consists of two peptide growth factors, IGF-1 and IGF-2, which can have characteristics of both circulating hormones and tissue growth factors. IGF-1 and IGF-2 can bind their cell surface receptors, IGF-1R and IGF-2R, as well as six different IGF-binding proteins, IGFBP1 to 6 that influence the binding of IGFs to their receptors. The IGF axis is further regulated by IGFBP proteases, and the proteins involved in intracellular signaling distal to IGF-1R which include members of the insulin receptor substrate family, AKT, the target of rapamycin (TOR), and S6 kinase (Pollak *et al.*, 2004).

Compared to HER2 and EGFR, the role of IGF signaling in anti-estrogen resistance is not as well understood and unlike HER2 and EGFR, data is mixed as to whether IGF-1R levels are elevated or decreased in resistant tumors and cell lines (Brockdorff *et al.*, 2003; Gee *et al.*, 2005; Knowlden *et al.*, 2005). Expression of the ER is controlled by IGF-1 in breast cancer cells (Lee *et al.*, 1997). Conversely, genomic and non-genomic interactions of ER can activate the mitogen-inducing signals of the IGF pathway (Fagan & Yee, 2008). Estrogen signaling also causes the expression of insulin receptor substrate 1 (IRS-1), a scaffolding molecule, which activates downstream signaling of IGF-1 and potentiates its proliferative abilities. Salerno *et al.* (1999) suggest that anti-estrogens, like tamoxifen, down regulated IRS-1 and that this down regulation may be one of the possible mechanisms involved in anti-estrogen response. The importance of IGF-1R is further illustrated with studies that show IGF-1R, in ER-negative MDA-MB-231 breast cancer cells, regulates the migration and adhesion abilities of these cells whereas in ER positive MCF-7 breast cancer cells, IGF-1R can modulate mitogenic stimulation (Bartucci *et al.*, 2001). Crosstalk between the IGF signaling pathway and the ER pathway is not only important in breast cancer development but may allow for the development of therapeutics that targets the interactions and communications between the two signaling pathways.

In our own studies, when screening for genes that confer resistance to tamoxifen, we identified IGFBP5 (Ahn *et al.*, 2010). IGFBP5 is a secreted protein and known to inhibit growth factor binding and signaling through IGF-1R (Beattie *et al.*, 2006). In addition, IGFBP5 has recently been shown to play a critical role in breast cancer progression and metastasis, although the exact mechanism remains obscure (Akkiprik *et al.*, 2008). We showed that knock-down of IGFBP5 resulted in resistance to tamoxifen treatment in MCF-7 cells and in mice tumor xenografts. The IGFBP5 knockdown-induced resistance to tamoxifen occurred potentially via altered IGF signaling and loss of ER expression (Bunone *et al.*, 1996; Kato *et al.*, 1995; Lee *et al.*, 1997). We found that treatment with recombinant IGFBP5 reversed *in vitro* and *in vivo* tamoxifen resistance. We also demonstrated, with a cohort of 153 breast cancer patients, that low IGFBP5 expression is associated with shorter overall survival after tamoxifen therapy. *In vitro,* others have shown that with tamoxifen or fulvestrant treated MCF-7 cells, growth inhibition is associated with increased expression of IGFBP5 and increased IGFBP5 secretion into the cell culture media (Huynh *et al.*, 1996; Parisot *et al.*, 1999; Pratt & Pollak, 1993). Preliminary evidence, in addition to some microarray data, supports the idea that IGFBP5 expression level determines tamoxifen responsiveness (Becker *et al.*, 2005).

4.2 Interleukin-6

Results from our screen indicate that reduced expression of IL-6 can confer tamoxifen resistance *in vitro*. IL-6 is a pleiotropic cytokine that has been found to have both tumor-promoting and tumor-inhibiting functions in breast cancer development (Knupfer & Preiss, 2007). Cytokines can be defined as small protein signaling molecules that tend to be glycosylated and exert their biological function at low concentrations (pg to ng/mL). Cytokines are secreted predominantly by lymphocytes and macrophages and exert their effect by binding to receptors on the target cell surface, altering the function of the target cell by either paracrine or autocrine signaling. The effects of different cytokines can be additive, synergistic, or antagonistic, and the integration of these effects determines the overall outcome and function of a particular cytokine.

Recently, Gilbert *et al.* (Gilbert & Hemann, 2010) have identified IL-6 as a mediator in the development of chemotherapeutic-resistant niches, a novel physiological mechanism behind drug-resistant lymphoma and a likely contributor to the development of cancer recurrence. Specifically, IL-6 along with metallopeptidase inhibitor 1 (Timp-1) were released from the thymus in response to chemotherapy-induced DNA damage, creating a "chemo-resistant niche". The niche helps promote the survival of undetectable residual disease, serving as a reservoir for eventual tumor relapse. Currently it is not known if chemo-resistant niches are present in other cancers or if tamoxifen can elicit the development of such niches.

Notwithstanding, in breast cancer cells, tumor necrosis factor alpha (TNFα) can induce the expression of IL-6 along with IL-11, promoting osteoclast formation and mediating osteolysis at the site of breast cancer bone metastases (Suarez-Cuervo *et al.*, 2003). IL-6 has also been implicated in mediating oncogene-induced cellular senescence (Kuilman *et al.*, 2008). Cellular senescence, where cells continue to be metabolically active but generally lose their ability to divide may act as a safeguard against a variety of cellular insults, including anti-estrogen therapy. Interestingly, Young *et al.* (2009) identified autophagy as a new effector mechanism of senescence by allowing for rapid protein turnover and cellular re-modeling that occurs when a cell transitions form a proliferative to a senescent state. How knockdown of IL-6 confers resistance to tamoxifen therapy is unclear. The pleiotropic actions of IL-6 complicate our understanding of its role in anti-estrogen resistance and highlight a limitation of RNAi based screens, in that one gene may confer multiple phenotypes.

4.3 Raptor, Vps15, and autophagy

Several gene targets identified in our RNA interference screen for tamoxifen resistance were found to be involved directly in macroautophagy, including Raptor and Vps15. Macroautophagy, hereafter referred to as autophagy, involves the delivery of cytoplasmic cargo, such as long-lived proteins and organelles, sequestered inside double-membrane vesicles, termed autophagosomes, to the lysosomes for degradation. Digested components are recycled back to the cell; therefore, autophagy is a cellular process essential for tissue development and homeostasis, and as an adaptive response to stress and nutrient deprivation (Levine & Kroemer, 2008).

The mTOR, a central regulator of cell growth, is activated through signaling by receptor tyrosine kinase-mediated PI3K activation (Efeyan & Sabatini, 2009). Two distinct protein complexes of mTOR mediate its effects on controlling the rate of cell growth and timing of cell cycle progression including, mTORC1 and mTORC2, respectively (Efeyan & Sabatini, 2009). The mTORC1 complex consists of mTOR, Raptor, and mLST8 and activation leads to increased protein translation, ribosome biogenesis and inhibition of autophagy, the combined effects resulting in increased cell growth (Efeyan & Sabatini, 2009). Raptor participates in mTORC1 complex as a key scaffolding protein to bind mTOR substrates such as eukaryotic initiation factor 4E binding protein 1 (4EBP1) and p70 S6 kinease α (p70α), facilitating phosphorylation and activation by mTOR (Hara *et al.*, 2002; Kim *et al.*, 2002).

Under nutrient-replete conditions mTOR-Raptor association is weak but is stabilized by nutrient deprivation resulting in inhibition of mTOR kinase activity (Hara *et al.*, 2002; Kim *et al.*, 2002). Raptor-mediated inhibition of mTORC1 is particularly relevant for its role in autophagy as Raptor inhibition of mTOR phosphorylation of ULK1/2 kinase complex leads to ULK1/2 dephosphorylation and activation to initiate autophagosome formation by Atg family of proteins (Kroemer *et al.*, 2010).

Recent attention to development and application of mTOR inhibitors in cancer therapy, including breast cancer, highlights the significance of our finding that loss of Raptor contributes to tamoxifen resistance (Dancey, 2010). In the context of autophagy, loss of Raptor may lead to mTOR phosphorylation of ULK1/2 and autophagy inactivation. In breast cancer, inhibition of mTOR activity has been found to restore tamoxifen sensitivity in breast cancer (deGraffenried *et al.*, 2004).

Vps15 is a putative serine/threonine protein kinase (Stack & Emr, 1994), required for Vps34 activity, a Class III PI3K that produces phosphatidylinositol-3-phophate (Backer, 2008; Schu *et al.*, 1993; Volinia *et al.*, 1995). Vps34 lipid kinase activity has recognized critical functions in early endosome fusion (Christoforidis *et al.*, 1999), maturation (Futter *et al.*, 2001), vesicular trafficking (Stack & Emr, 1994) and starvation-induced autophagy (Takahashi *et al.*, 2007). *In vitro*, Vps15 enhances Vps34 lipid kinase activity (Panaretou *et al.*, 1997); however, Vps34 does not appear to be a substrate of Vps15. Further, Vps15 deletion leads to loss of phosphatidylinositol-3-phosphate production and vesicular trafficking (Stack & Emr, 1994). Lastly, regulation of Vps34 activity by autophagy-related proteins or nutrients requires Vps15 (Yan *et al.*, 2009). The Beclin-1 complex containing Beclin 1, Vps34, Vps15, UVRAG, Atg14L and Rubicon orchestrates demarcation of sites for formation of double membrane organelles associated with Atg5 and Atg12, termed autophagosomes (Zhong *et al.*, 2009). Vps15 regulation of Vp34 activity is necessary for marking sites of autophagosome formation and eventual autophagic removal of protein aggregates (Lindmo *et al.*, 2008).

While little is known about Vps15 in breast cancer, Vps34 function appears to have a pro-survival function mediated through promotion of autophagy. First, increased Vps34 expression levels and tyrosine phosphorylation by pp60c-Scr contributes to enhanced tumorigenic activity in breast cancer cells (Hirsch *et al.*, 2010). Second, in MCF-7 cells, knockdown of Vps34 by RNA interference reduced cytoprotective autophagy mediated by Bcl-2 homology domain 3 (BH3) mimetic gossypol and potentiated apoptosis induction (Gao *et al.*, 2010). Lastly, Vps34 has tumor suppressor function in MCF-7 mouse xenograft tumors mediated through distinct Beclin-1 binding and enhancement of starvation-induced autophagy (Furuya *et al.*, 2005). These studies corroborate lines of evidence demonstrating that PI3K/AKT/mTOR pathway, implicated in cell survival, contributes to anti-estrogen resistance (Musgrove & Sutherland, 2009).

In contrast, our studies have identified loss of Vps15 and Raptor as candidate gene target for mediating breast cancer tamoxifen resistance *in vitro*, suggesting that Vps15- or Raptor-mediated autophagy promotes cell death mediated by tamoxifen. In support of this, inhibitors of each of PI3K, Akt, and mTOR are in clinical trials (Dancey, 2010) and inhibition of mTOR activity is thought to restore tamoxifen sensitivity in breast cancer (deGraffenried *et al.*, 2004). Also, others have also demonstrated that tamoxifen and anti-estrogen-binding site ligands induce autophagic cell death in human breast cancer cells (de Medina *et al.*, 2009; Payre *et al.*, 2008). Tamoxifen-induced cell death through autophagy was associated with cholesterol accumulation. Interestingly, our laboratory's RNA interference screen also identified several genes involved in cholesterol metabolism including Niemann-Pick C 2

(NPC2) protein, reportedly involved NPC disease, in which cells accumulate sterols in multilamellar bodies resulting in onset of autophagy (Pacheco *et al.*, 2007). Furthermore, an ectopic over-expression screen identified a small heat-shock protein family member, which limited autophagic cell death mediated by tamoxifen (Gonzalez-Malerva *et al.*, 2011).

Controversy remains as to whether autophagy limits or promotes tumor malignancy, including drug resistance. Genetic inactivation of autophagy is known to promote tumorigenesis and constitutes a new category of tumor suppressors including Beclin 1. And while oncogenes including PI3K/AKT/mTOR and Bcl-2 inhibit autophagy and hence the ability of tumor cells to proliferate, other oncogenes including Ras and myc stimulate autophagy (Kondo *et al.*, 2005). These variegated effects could represent the significance of autophagy at different stages of tumor progression. Further investigation into the impact of autophagy inactivation on clinical tamoxifen resistance is warranted, specifically on the candidate targets Vps15 and Raptor.

5. Final remarks

Over the last several decades the therapeutic use of tamoxifen has undoubtedly saved countless lives. However, predicting responsiveness and understanding resistance is critical to advances in treatment. Although this chapter has focused on tamoxifen, future studies investigating the mechanisms of resistance to aromatase inhibitors and other anti-estrogens will likely reveal similar mechanisms as the clinical data and experience with these drugs matures. Progress towards better treatment and understanding resistance may be made by further examining the role of IGF signaling and crosstalk with the ER and the role of autophagy.

6. References

Ahn, B. Y., Elwi, A. N., Lee, B., Trinh, D. L., Klimowicz, A. C., Yau, A., et al. (2010). Genetic screen identifies insulin-like growth factor binding protein 5 as a modulator of tamoxifen resistance in breast cancer. *Cancer Res*, 70, 3013-3019.

Akkiprik, M., Feng, Y., Wang, H., Chen, K., Hu, L., Sahin, A., et al. (2008). Multifunctional roles of insulin-like growth factor binding protein 5 in breast cancer. *Breast Cancer Res*, 10, 212.

Ali, S., & Coombes, R. C. (2002). Endocrine-responsive breast cancer and strategies for combating resistance. *Nat Rev Cancer*, 2, 101-112.

Backer, J. M. (2008). The regulation and function of class iii pi3ks: Novel roles for vps34. *Biochem J*, 410, 1-17.

Bartucci, M., Morelli, C., Mauro, L., Ando, S., & Surmacz, E. (2001). Differential insulin-like growth factor i receptor signaling and function in estrogen receptor (er)-positive mcf-7 and er-negative mda-mb-231 breast cancer cells. *Cancer Res*, 61, 6747-6754.

Bauer, J. A., Ye, F., Marshall, C. B., Lehmann, B. D., Pendleton, C. S., Shyr, Y., et al. (2010). Rna interference (rnai) screening approach identifies agents that enhance paclitaxel activity in breast cancer cells. *Breast Cancer Res*, 12, R41.

Beatson, G. (1896). On the treatment of inoperable cases of carcinoma of the mamma: Suggestions for a new method of treatment, with illustrative cases. *The Lancet*, 148, 162-165.

Beattie, J., Allan, G. J., Lochrie, J. D., & Flint, D. J. (2006). Insulin-like growth factor-binding protein-5 (igfbp-5): A critical member of the igf axis. *Biochem J*, 395, 1-19.

Becker, M., Sommer, A., Kratzschmar, J. R., Seidel, H., Pohlenz, H. D., & Fichtner, I. (2005). Distinct gene expression patterns in a tamoxifen-sensitive human mammary carcinoma xenograft and its tamoxifen-resistant subline maca 3366/tam. *Mol Cancer Ther*, 4, 151-168.

Behrens, D., Gill, J. H., & Fichtner, I. (2007). Loss of tumourigenicity of stably erbeta-transfected mcf-7 breast cancer cells. *Mol Cell Endocrinol*, 274, 19-29.

Berns, K., Horlings, H. M., Hennessy, B. T., Madiredjo, M., Hijmans, E. M., Beelen, K., et al. (2007). A functional genetic approach identifies the pi3k pathway as a major determinant of trastuzumab resistance in breast cancer. *Cancer Cell*, 12, 395-402.

Brockdorff, B. L., Heiberg, I., & Lykkesfeldt, A. E. (2003). Resistance to different antiestrogens is caused by different multi-factorial changes and is associated with reduced expression of igf receptor ialpha. *Endocr Relat Cancer*, 10, 579-590.

Brummelkamp, T. R., Bernards, R., & Agami, R. (2002). A system for stable expression of short interfering rnas in mammalian cells. *Science*, 296, 550-553.

Bunone, G., Briand, P. A., Miksicek, R. J., & Picard, D. (1996). Activation of the unliganded estrogen receptor by egf involves the map kinase pathway and direct phosphorylation. *EMBO J*, 15, 2174-2183.

Christoforidis, S., Miaczynska, M., Ashman, K., Wilm, M., Zhao, L., Yip, S. C., et al. (1999). Phosphatidylinositol-3-oh kinases are rab5 effectors. *Nat Cell Biol*, 1, 249-252.

Clarke, R., Leonessa, F., Welch, J. N., & Skaar, T. C. (2001). Cellular and molecular pharmacology of antiestrogen action and resistance. *Pharmacol Rev*, 53, 25-71.

Clarke, R., Liu, M. C., Bouker, K. B., Gu, Z., Lee, R. Y., Zhu, Y., et al. (2003). Antiestrogen resistance in breast cancer and the role of estrogen receptor signaling. *Oncogene*, 22, 7316-7339.

Cuzick, J., Powles, T., Veronesi, U., Forbes, J., Edwards, R., Ashley, S., et al. (2003). Overview of the main outcomes in breast-cancer prevention trials. *Lancet*, 361, 296-300.

Dahlman-Wright, K., Cavailles, V., Fuqua, S. A., Jordan, V. C., Katzenellenbogen, J. A., Korach, K. S., et al. (2006). International union of pharmacology. Lxiv. Estrogen receptors. *Pharmacol Rev*, 58, 773-781.

Dancey, J. (2010). Mtor signaling and drug development in cancer. *Nat Rev Clin Oncol*, 7, 209-219.

de Medina, P., Payre, B., Boubekeur, N., Bertrand-Michel, J., Terce, F., Silvente-Poirot, S., et al. (2009). Ligands of the antiestrogen-binding site induce active cell death and autophagy in human breast cancer cells through the modulation of cholesterol metabolism. *Cell Death Differ*, 16, 1372-1384.

deGraffenried, L. A., Friedrichs, W. E., Russell, D. H., Donzis, E. J., Middleton, A. K., Silva, J. M., et al. (2004). Inhibition of mtor activity restores tamoxifen response in breast cancer cells with aberrant akt activity. *Clin Cancer Res*, 10, 8059-8067.

Early Breast Cancer Trialists' Collaborative, G. (2005). Effects of chemotherapy and hormonal therapy for early breast cancer on recurrence and 15-year survival: An overview of the randomised trials. *Lancet*, 365, 1687-1717.

Efeyan, A., & Sabatini, D. M. (2009). Mtor and cancer: Many loops in one pathway. *Curr Opin Cell Biol*, 22, 169-176.

Elbashir, S. M., Harborth, J., Lendeckel, W., Yalcin, A., Weber, K., & Tuschl, T. (2001). Duplexes of 21-nucleotide rnas mediate rna interference in cultured mammalian cells. *Nature*, 411, 494-498.

Fagan, D. H., & Yee, D. (2008). Crosstalk between igf1r and estrogen receptor signaling in breast cancer. *J Mammary Gland Biol Neoplasia*, 13, 423-429.

Fire, A., Xu, S., Montgomery, M. K., Kostas, S. A., Driver, S. E., & Mello, C. C. (1998). Potent and specific genetic interference by double-stranded rna in caenorhabditis elegans. *Nature*, 391, 806-811.

Furuya, N., Yu, J., Byfield, M., Pattingre, S., & Levine, B. (2005). The evolutionarily conserved domain of beclin 1 is required for vps34 binding, autophagy and tumor suppressor function. *Autophagy*, 1, 46-52.

Futter, C. E., Collinson, L. M., Backer, J. M., & Hopkins, C. R. (2001). Human vps34 is required for internal vesicle formation within multivesicular endosomes. *J Cell Biol*, 155, 1251-1264.

Gao, P., Bauvy, C., Souquere, S., Tonelli, G., Liu, L., Zhu, Y., et al. (2010). The bcl-2 homology domain 3 mimetic gossypol induces both beclin 1-dependent and beclin 1-independent cytoprotective autophagy in cancer cells. *J Biol Chem*, 285, 25570-25581.

Garcia, M., Derocq, D., Freiss, G., & Rochefort, H. (1992). Activation of estrogen receptor transfected into a receptor-negative breast cancer cell line decreases the metastatic and invasive potential of the cells. *Proc Natl Acad Sci U S A*, 89, 11538-11542.

Gee, J. M., Robertson, J. F., Gutteridge, E., Ellis, I. O., Pinder, S. E., Rubini, M., et al. (2005). Epidermal growth factor receptor/her2/insulin-like growth factor receptor signalling and oestrogen receptor activity in clinical breast cancer. *Endocr Relat Cancer*, 12 Suppl 1, S99-S111.

Giacinti, L., Claudio, P. P., Lopez, M., & Giordano, A. (2006). Epigenetic information and estrogen receptor alpha expression in breast cancer. *Oncologist*, 11, 1-8.

Gilbert, L. A., & Hemann, M. T. (2010). DNA damage-mediated induction of a chemoresistant niche. *Cell*, 143, 355-366.

Gluckman, P., Klempt, N., Guan, J., Mallard, C., Sirimanne, E., Dragunow, M., et al. (1992). A role for igf-1 in the rescue of cns neurons following hypoxic-ischemic injury. *Biochem Biophys Res Commun*, 182, 593-599.

Gonzalez-Malerva, L., Park, J., Zou, L., Hu, Y., Moradpour, Z., Pearlberg, J., et al. (2011). High-throughput ectopic expression screen for tamoxifen resistance identifies an atypical kinase that blocks autophagy. *Proc Natl Acad Sci U S A*, 108, 2058-2063.

Gutierrez, M. C., Detre, S., Johnston, S., Mohsin, S. K., Shou, J., Allred, D. C., et al. (2005). Molecular changes in tamoxifen-resistant breast cancer: Relationship between estrogen receptor, her-2, and p38 mitogen-activated protein kinase. *J Clin Oncol*, 23, 2469-2476.

Hara, K., Maruki, Y., Long, X., Yoshino, K., Oshiro, N., Hidayat, S., et al. (2002). Raptor, a binding partner of target of rapamycin (tor), mediates tor action. *Cell*, 110, 177-189.

Harvey, J. M., Clark, G. M., Osborne, C. K., & Allred, D. C. (1999). Estrogen receptor status by immunohistochemistry is superior to the ligand-binding assay for predicting response to adjuvant endocrine therapy in breast cancer. *J Clin Oncol*, 17, 1474-1481.

Herynk, M. H., & Fuqua, S. A. (2004). Estrogen receptor mutations in human disease. *Endocr Rev*, 25, 869-898.

Hirsch, D. S., Shen, Y., Dokmanovic, M., & Wu, W. J. (2010). Pp60c-src phosphorylates and activates vacuolar protein sorting 34 to mediate cellular transformation. *Cancer Res*, 70, 5974-5983.

Hopp, T. A., Weiss, H. L., Parra, I. S., Cui, Y., Osborne, C. K., & Fuqua, S. A. (2004). Low levels of estrogen receptor beta protein predict resistance to tamoxifen therapy in breast cancer. *Clin Cancer Res*, 10, 7490-7499.

Hoskins, J. M., Carey, L. A., & McLeod, H. L. (2009). Cyp2d6 and tamoxifen: DNA matters in breast cancer. *Nat Rev Cancer*, 9, 576-586.

Huynh, H., Yang, X. F., & Pollak, M. (1996). A role for insulin-like growth factor binding protein 5 in the antiproliferative action of the antiestrogen ici 182780. *Cell Growth Differ*, 7, 1501-1506.

Jensen, E. V., Block, G. E., Smith, S., Kyser, K., & DeSombre, E. R. (1971). Estrogen receptors and breast cancer response to adrenalectomy. *Natl Cancer Inst Monogr*, 34, 55-70.

Jordan, V. C. (1976). Effect of tamoxifen (ici 46,474) on initiation and growth of dmba-induced rat mammary carcinomata. *Eur J Cancer*, 12, 419-424.

Jordan, V. C. (1994). The development of tamoxfen for breast cancer therapy. In V. C. Jordan (Ed) *Long-term tamoxifen treatment for breast cancer* pp. 3-26). Madison: University of Wisconsin Press.

Jordan, V. C. (2006). Tamoxifen (ici46,474) as a targeted therapy to treat and prevent breast cancer. *Br J Pharmacol*, 147 Suppl 1, S269-276.

Jordan, V. C., & Dowse, L. J. (1976). Tamoxifen as an anti-tumour agent: Effect on oestrogen binding. *J Endocrinol*, 68, 297-303.

Jordan, V. C., & Koerner, S. (1975). Tamoxifen (ici 46,474) and the human carcinoma 8s oestrogen receptor. *Eur J Cancer*, 11, 205-206.

Juul, N., Szallasi, Z., Eklund, A. C., Li, Q., Burrell, R. A., Gerlinger, M., et al. (2010). Assessment of an rna interference screen-derived mitotic and ceramide pathway metagene as a predictor of response to neoadjuvant paclitaxel for primary triple-negative breast cancer: A retrospective analysis of five clinical trials. *Lancet Oncol*, 11, 358-365.

Kato, S., Endoh, H., Masuhiro, Y., Kitamoto, T., Uchiyama, S., Sasaki, H., et al. (1995). Activation of the estrogen receptor through phosphorylation by mitogen-activated protein kinase. *Science*, 270, 1491-1494.

Kennedy, B. J. (1965). Hormone therapy for advanced breast cancer. *Cancer*, 18, 1551-1557.

Kim, D. H., Sarbassov, D. D., Ali, S. M., King, J. E., Latek, R. R., Erdjument-Bromage, H., et al. (2002). Mtor interacts with raptor to form a nutrient-sensitive complex that signals to the cell growth machinery. *Cell*, 110, 163-175.

Knowlden, J. M., Hutcheson, I. R., Barrow, D., Gee, J. M., & Nicholson, R. I. (2005). Insulin-like growth factor-i receptor signaling in tamoxifen-resistant breast cancer: A supporting role to the epidermal growth factor receptor. *Endocrinology*, 146, 4609-4618.

Knupfer, H., & Preiss, R. (2007). Significance of interleukin-6 (il-6) in breast cancer (review). *Breast Cancer Res Treat*, 102, 129-135.

Kondo, Y., Kanzawa, T., Sawaya, R., & Kondo, S. (2005). The role of autophagy in cancer development and response to therapy. *Nat Rev Cancer*, 5, 726-734.

Kroemer, G., Marino, G., & Levine, B. (2010). Autophagy and the integrated stress response. *Mol Cell*, 40, 280-293.

Kuilman, T., Michaloglou, C., Vredeveld, L. C., Douma, S., van Doorn, R., Desmet, C. J., et al. (2008). Oncogene-induced senescence relayed by an interleukin-dependent inflammatory network. *Cell*, 133, 1019-1031.

Kushner, P. J., Agard, D. A., Greene, G. L., Scanlan, T. S., Shiau, A. K., Uht, R. M., et al. (2000). Estrogen receptor pathways to ap-1. *J Steroid Biochem Mol Biol*, 74, 311-317.

Lee, A. V., Weng, C. N., Jackson, J. G., & Yee, D. (1997). Activation of estrogen receptor-mediated gene transcription by igf-i in human breast cancer cells. *J Endocrinol*, 152, 39-47.

Levine, B., & Kroemer, G. (2008). Autophagy in the pathogenesis of disease. *Cell*, 132, 27-42.

Lewis, J. S., & Jordan, V. C. (2005). Selective estrogen receptor modulators (serms): Mechanisms of anticarcinogenesis and drug resistance. *Mutat Res*, 591, 247-263.

Lindmo, K., Brech, A., Finley, K. D., Gaumer, S., Contamine, D., Rusten, T. E., et al. (2008). The pi 3-kinase regulator vps15 is required for autophagic clearance of protein aggregates. *Autophagy*, 4, 500-506.

McDonnell, D. P., Clemm, D. L., Hermann, T., Goldman, M. E., & Pike, J. W. (1995). Analysis of estrogen receptor function in vitro reveals three distinct classes of antiestrogens. *Mol Endocrinol*, 9, 659-669.

Michiels, F., van Es, H., van Rompaey, L., Merchiers, P., Francken, B., Pittois, K., et al. (2002). Arrayed adenoviral expression libraries for functional screening. *Nat Biotechnol*, 20, 1154-1157.

Mokbel, K. (2002). The evolving role of aromatase inhibitors in breast cancer. *Int J Clin Oncol*, 7, 279-283.

Musgrove, E. A., & Sutherland, R. L. (2009). Biological determinants of endocrine resistance in breast cancer. *Nat Rev Cancer*, 9, 631-643.

Ngo, V. N., Davis, R. E., Lamy, L., Yu, X., Zhao, H., Lenz, G., et al. (2006). A loss-of-function rna interference screen for molecular targets in cancer. *Nature*, 441, 106-110.

Nicholson, R. I., & Golder, M. P. (1975). The effect of synthetic anti-oestrogens on the growth and biochemistry of rat mammary tumours. *Eur J Cancer*, 11, 571-579.

Osborne, C. K. (1998). Tamoxifen in the treatment of breast cancer. *N Engl J Med*, 339, 1609-1618.

Pacheco, C. D., Kunkel, R., & Lieberman, A. P. (2007). Autophagy in niemann-pick c disease is dependent upon beclin-1 and responsive to lipid trafficking defects. *Hum Mol Genet*, 16, 1495-1503.

Panaretou, C., Domin, J., Cockcroft, S., & Waterfield, M. D. (1997). Characterization of p150, an adaptor protein for the human phosphatidylinositol (ptdins) 3-kinase. Substrate presentation by phosphatidylinositol transfer protein to the p150.Ptdins 3-kinase complex. *J Biol Chem*, 272, 2477-2485.

Parisot, J. P., Leeding, K. S., Hu, X. F., DeLuise, M., Zalcberg, J. R., & Bach, L. A. (1999). Induction of insulin-like growth factor binding protein expression by ici 182,780 in a tamoxifen-resistant human breast cancer cell line. *Breast Cancer Res Treat*, 55, 231-242.

Paruthiyil, S., Parmar, H., Kerekatte, V., Cunha, G. R., Firestone, G. L., & Leitman, D. C. (2004). Estrogen receptor beta inhibits human breast cancer cell proliferation and tumor formation by causing a g2 cell cycle arrest. *Cancer Res*, 64, 423-428.

Payre, B., de Medina, P., Boubekeur, N., Mhamdi, L., Bertrand-Michel, J., Terce, F., et al. (2008). Microsomal antiestrogen-binding site ligands induce growth control and differentiation of human breast cancer cells through the modulation of cholesterol metabolism. *Mol Cancer Ther*, 7, 3707-3718.

Perez, E. A. (2007). Safety profiles of tamoxifen and the aromatase inhibitors in adjuvant therapy of hormone-responsive early breast cancer. *Ann Oncol*, 18 Suppl 8, viii26-35.

Pollak, M. (2008). Insulin and insulin-like growth factor signalling in neoplasia. *Nat Rev Cancer*, 8, 915-928.

Pollak, M., Schernhammer, E. S., & Hankinson, S. E. (2004). Insulin-like growth factors and neoplasia. *Nat Rev Cancer*, 4, 505-518.

Pratt, S. E., & Pollak, M. N. (1993). Estrogen and antiestrogen modulation of mcf7 human breast cancer cell proliferation is associated with specific alterations in accumulation of insulin-like growth factor-binding proteins in conditioned media. *Cancer Res*, 53, 5193-5198.

Riggins, R. B., Schrecengost, R. S., Guerrero, M. S., & Bouton, A. H. (2007). Pathways to tamoxifen resistance. *Cancer Lett*, 256, 1-24.

Ring, A., & Dowsett, M. (2004). Mechanisms of tamoxifen resistance. *Endocr Relat Cancer*, 11, 643-658.

Saji, S., Hirose, M., & Toi, M. (2005). Clinical significance of estrogen receptor beta in breast cancer. *Cancer Chemother Pharmacol*, 56 Suppl 1, 21-26.

Salerno, M., Sisci, D., Mauro, L., Guvakova, M. A., Ando, S., & Surmacz, E. (1999). Insulin receptor substrate 1 is a target for the pure antiestrogen ici 182,780 in breast cancer cells. *Int J Cancer*, 81, 299-304.

Schiff, R., Massarweh, S., Shou, J., & Osborne, C. K. (2003). Breast cancer endocrine resistance: How growth factor signaling and estrogen receptor coregulators modulate response. *Clin Cancer Res*, 9, 447S-454S.

Schu, P. V., Takegawa, K., Fry, M. J., Stack, J. H., Waterfield, M. D., & Emr, S. D. (1993). Phosphatidylinositol 3-kinase encoded by yeast vps34 gene essential for protein sorting. *Science*, 260, 88-91.

Sharma, D., Saxena, N. K., Davidson, N. E., & Vertino, P. M. (2006). Restoration of tamoxifen sensitivity in estrogen receptor-negative breast cancer cells: Tamoxifen-bound reactivated er recruits distinctive corepressor complexes. *Cancer Res*, 66, 6370-6378.

Stack, J. H., & Emr, S. D. (1994). Vps34p required for yeast vacuolar protein sorting is a multiple specificity kinase that exhibits both protein kinase and phosphatidylinositol-specific pi 3-kinase activities. *J Biol Chem*, 269, 31552-31562.

Suarez-Cuervo, C., Harris, K. W., Kallman, L., Vaananen, H. K., & Selander, K. S. (2003). Tumor necrosis factor-alpha induces interleukin-6 production via extracellular-regulated kinase 1 activation in breast cancer cells. *Breast Cancer Res Treat*, 80, 71-78.

Sugiura, H., Toyama, T., Hara, Y., Zhang, Z., Kobayashi, S., Fujii, Y., et al. (2007). Expression of estrogen receptor beta wild-type and its variant erbetacx/beta2 is correlated with better prognosis in breast cancer. *Jpn J Clin Oncol*, 37, 820-828.

Swanton, C., Marani, M., Pardo, O., Warne, P. H., Kelly, G., Sahai, E., et al. (2007). Regulators of mitotic arrest and ceramide metabolism are determinants of sensitivity to paclitaxel and other chemotherapeutic drugs. *Cancer Cell*, 11, 498-512.

Takahashi, Y., Coppola, D., Matsushita, N., Cualing, H. D., Sun, M., Sato, Y., et al. (2007). Bif-1 interacts with beclin 1 through uvrag and regulates autophagy and tumorigenesis. *Nat Cell Biol*, 9, 1142-1151.

Tzukerman, M. T., Esty, A., Santiso-Mere, D., Danielian, P., Parker, M. G., Stein, R. B., et al. (1994). Human estrogen receptor transactivational capacity is determined by both cellular and promoter context and mediated by two functionally distinct intramolecular regions. *Mol Endocrinol*, 8, 21-30.

Valentinis, B., & Baserga, R. (2001). Igf-i receptor signalling in transformation and differentiation. *Mol Pathol*, 54, 133-137.

Volinia, S., Dhand, R., Vanhaesebroeck, B., MacDougall, L. K., Stein, R., Zvelebil, M. J., et al. (1995). A human phosphatidylinositol 3-kinase complex related to the yeast vps34p-vps15p protein sorting system. *EMBO J*, 14, 3339-3348.

Waters, E. A., Cronin, K. A., Graubard, B. I., Han, P. K., & Freedman, A. N. (2010). Prevalence of tamoxifen use for breast cancer chemoprevention among u.S. Women. *Cancer Epidemiol Biomarkers Prev*, 19, 443-446.

Yan, Y., Flinn, R. J., Wu, H., Schnur, R. S., & Backer, J. M. (2009). Hvps15, but not ca2+/cam, is required for the activity and regulation of hvps34 in mammalian cells. *Biochem J*, 417, 747-755.

Young, A. R., Narita, M., Ferreira, M., Kirschner, K., Sadaie, M., Darot, J. F., et al. (2009). Autophagy mediates the mitotic senescence transition. *Genes Dev*, 23, 798-803.

Zhong, Y., Wang, Q. J., Li, X., Yan, Y., Backer, J. M., Chait, B. T., et al. (2009). Distinct regulation of autophagic activity by atg14l and rubicon associated with beclin 1-phosphatidylinositol-3-kinase complex. *Nat Cell Biol*, 11, 468-476.

7

Legume-Derived Bioactive Compounds for the Prevention and Treatment of Breast Cancer

Graziella Joanitti, Sonia Freitas and Ricardo Azevedo
University of Brasilia,
Brazil

1. Introduction

Breast cancer is one of the most prevalent cancer types among women worldwide (Jemal et al., 2011); however, its incidence rates among populations are heterogeneous. Epidemiologic studies have shown that breast cancer incidence in Asian women is 40% lower than in Caucasian women (Goldin et al., 1986). A reasonable explanation for the difference in the cancer incidence rates could be related to intrinsic biological characteristics present in each population. For example, in general, breast cancer growth requires the presence of estrogen and it is known that Asian women have lower estrogen serum levels than Caucasian women (Shimizu et al., 1990). Nevertheless, epidemiologic studies have reported that when Asian women moved to western countries the breast cancer incidence of their subsequent generations were similar to the Caucasian women (Wu et al., 1996). Therefore, it seems that other factors have been influencing breast cancer incidence rates in each population.

In fact, it is known that only 10-15% of all breast cancers cases are caused by genetic predisposition such as BRCA and Li-Fraumeni mutations; whereas the remaining 85-90% of cases are attributed to environmental, reproductive, lifestyle factors including radiation, chemicals, late pregnancy, early menarche, nulliparity, diet and reduced physical activity (Colditz et al., 1995). The diet is an important factor affecting breast cancer incidence rates and is estimated to be correlated with 50% of new diagnosed cases (Willett, 1995). It has been described that diets based on the consumption of garlic, onion, tomato, vegetables, fruits and legumes are associated with reduced breast cancer risk. One of the major differences between western and Asian populations is their diet. The consumption of legumes (soy, beans, peas) in Asian populations is expressively higher than in western populations. These disparities on breast cancer risk and on legume intake have attracted the attention of scientists and since then this topic has been the goal of innumerable researches (Messina et al., 2006).

In addition to their importance as a nutritive food source, legumes and their bioactive compounds have also been described to show protective and therapeutic effects not only in breast cancer, but also in symptoms of menopause, heart disease and osteoporosis. On the other hand, findings suggesting no effects or possible risks in legume intake and breast cancer have also been published (Messina et al., 2008). Therefore, the evaluation of the effects of legume consumption on women at high risk for breast cancer and breast cancer patients is an important public health goal (Messina et al., 2006). In this chapter, we provide a comprehensive review of the biological, nutritional and economic background on legumes and gather the current knowledge regarding the benefits and risks of their bioactive molecules in breast cancer prevention and treatment.

2. Legumes - biological, nutritional and economic aspects

The legumes are classified in the family Fabacea (or Leguminosae) - including around 700 legume genera and 20,000 species - and are the third largest flowering plant family (Doyle et al., 2003; Gepts et al., 2005). They present a large range of variation and are also well adapted to several temperatures and climates (Doyle et al., 2003). Despite the large number of species, only a few legumes are generally known due to their use as feeds and foods. Clovers (*Trifolium* sp.), vetches (*Vicia faba*) and alfafa (*Medicago sativa*) are mainly grown for animal feeding; while beans (*Phaseolus vulgaris*), soybeans (*Glycine max*), lentils (*Lens esculenta*), peas (*Pisum sativum*), and peanuts (*Arachis hypogaea*) are the main species grown for food (Doyle et al., 2003; Gepts et al., 2005).

Legumes nutritional profile includes dietary fibers, low glycemic indexes, no cholesterol, low levels of fat (2- 5%), and high amounts of carbohydrates (55- 60%). In addition, essential minerals and vitamins for human health are also present (Rochfort et al., 2007). High protein content (20-40%) is another notable feature of legumes which is known to be 2-3 times higher than cereals. Along with their high protein content, they also produce a good balance of all essential aminoacids, with the exception of methionine (Rochfort et al., 2007).

Among legumes, soybeans have not only the highest protein content but also the highest protein digestibility, which is typically 90%. Soybeans and peanuts are considered an exception among legumes in terms of nutritional profile. Despite producing high protein contents, they are low in carbohydrates but high in fat (40% total energy) (Messina et al., 2010). In addition, soy is a component widely used to fortify school breakfast and lunch programs and is also present in upwards 60% of processed foods (Patisaul et al., 2010).

Some legumes produce antinutritional factors which have shown to induce allergy and intestinal disturbance when eaten raw. However, the majority of these toxins can be eliminated through heating or other industrially processing (Gepts et al., 2005).

The intake rates of legumes vary dramatically among populations worldwide. In Asian countries, legumes have been consumed for centuries representing ~50% of their diet which achieve and even surpass the minimum intake recommended. On the other hand, the rates of legume consumption by North American and European countries are low (Messina, 2010).

A few decades ago researchers have reported that some compounds produced by legumes could promote protective and therapeutic effects on human health. This new vision of legumes as functional foods has induced a profound impact in sales and consumption of legumes in countries which had low consumption rates as the EUA and European countries (Messina et al., 2001; Messina, 2010; Patisaul et al., 2010).

3. Legume bioactive compounds and breast cancer

Hypothesis regarding protective and therapeutic effects of legumes in breast cancer have been formulated mainly based on epidemiological studies suggesting a negative correlation between legume intake and breast cancer incidence among populations worldwide. Asian women, who traditionally consume high amounts of legumes daily, are 4 to 10 times less likely to be diagnosed with and die from breast cancer than are people in the United States

(Fournier et al., 1998). Interestingly, genetic variations do not seem to be the main factors involved in this disparity since Asian women who immigrate to the United States and adopted a "Western" lifestyle, particularly a diet poor in legumes, develop breast cancer risk comparable to Caucasian women within two generations (Wu et al., 1996).
These evidences have triggered several researches seeking for the identification of potential legume molecules involved in breast cancer prevention and treatment. Isoflavones, protease inhibitors and peptides are the main legume bioactive compounds evaluated in this field. In the next sections, their anticancer properties as well as synergistic effects are discussed.

4. Isoflavones

Legumes produce large amounts and several isoflavones isoforms which are assumed to have antimicrobial activity and to play an important role in plant protection (Rochfort et al., 2007). In particular, soybeans produce 12 isoforms of isoflavones and contain the highest dietary-relevant amounts of these compounds among legumes (Franke et al., 1998). For example, each gram of soy protein in soybeans contains approximately 3.5 mg of isoflavones; while no significant amounts are present in lentils (Murphy et al., 1999). For this reason, the majority of published data regarding their activities in breast cancer involve isoflavones found in soy.

4.1 Structural and bioavailability

The isoflavones are a subclass of flavonoids and belong to the group of naturally occurring heterocyclic phenols. Their basic structure is composed of 2 benzene rings linked through a heterocyclic pyrane ring. Isoflavones are named glycoside (inactive form) when conjugated to glucose or carbohydrate moieties and glycone (active form) when unconjugated (Franke et al., 1998) (Fig.1).

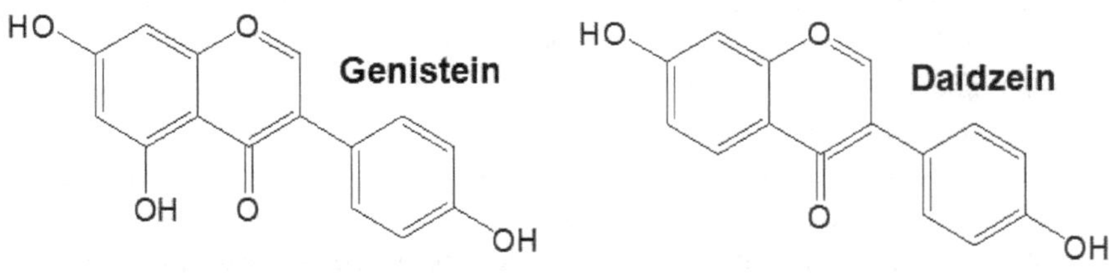

Fig. 1. Chemical structures of the genistein (4', 5, 7-trihydroxyisoflavone) and daidzein (4', 7-dihydroxyisoflavone), the most abundant isoflavones found in soy. The figure was drawn by ChemDraw (Cambridge Soft, version 9.0).

The primary isoflavones found in soybeans are the glycones genistein (4',5,7-trihydroxyisoflavone), daidzein (4',7-dihydroxyisoflavone) and glycitein (7,49- dihydroxy-6-methoxyisoflavone), and their respective glycosides genistin, daidzin and glycitin (Messina et al., 2001). Genistein and daidzein are the most abundant isoflavones in soybeans representing 50% and 40% of the total isoflavone content respectively (Rochfort et al., 2007). The majority of isoflavones found in raw soybeans are almost entirely as glycosides (genistin, daidzin, and glycitin) while only 1 - 3% account for their active form glycone (Murphy et al., 1999). After ingestion, they are rapidly absorbed entering systemic circulation predominantly as conjugated forms (95%) with limited bioavailability (Messina et al., 2006). Isoflavones then are further deconjugated by the action of glucosidases produced in intestinal bacteria. Interestingly, there is considerable inter-individual variation in intestinal bacteria metabolism of genistein and daidzein. The bioconvertion of daidzein to one of its metabolites (equol) is performed by a very specific type of intestinal bacteria which have been found only in 30–50% of individuals (Patisaul et al., 2010).

The resulting isoflavone metabolites are widely biodistributed and their serum levels can reach the low micromolar range according to the amount ingested (Messina et al., 2001). Soy isoflavones have half-lives of approximately 8 hours and are nearly all excreted within 24 hours after consumption (Messina et al., 2006).

4.2 Exploring isoflavones biological effects on breast cancer

4.2.1 Estrogen-receptor dependent properties

Breast cancer development is significantly influenced by the exposure to estrogens. These hormones have been described to induce proliferation of malignant breast cells contributing to breast cancer promotion and progression. Therefore, the control of estrogen exposure is a key factor in breast cancer chemoprevention (Bouker et al., 2000).

The structures of soy isoflavones are similar to mammalian estrogens (Messina et al., 2001). By the early 1960s, isoflavones were characterized as ligands of estrogen receptors and thus labelled as phytoestrogens (Cheng et al., 1953). These findings led to an initial enthusiasm mainly based on the possibility that isoflavones might exert antiestrogenic effects on breast tissue as other known estrogen antagonists such as tamoxifen (Messina et al., 2001).

Folman & Pope were the first to conduct assays establishing the relative binding affinity isoflavones for the estrogen receptor (ER) (Folman et al., 1966). There are two major ER subtypes in mammals, ER-α and ER-β presenting different tissue distributions. Soy isoflavones have singular affinities for each ER and for this reason are classified as selective estrogen receptor modulators (SERMs) (Messina et al., 2006). Genistein is 7- to 48-fold more selective for ER-β than Er-α and is 1,000-fold more potent at triggering transcriptional activity with ER-β than Er-α (Kuiper et al., 1998). However, isoflavones are considered to be weak estrogens, showing binding affinity to ER-α and ER-β of nearly 20- and 5-fold less than estradiol, respectively (Kuiper et al., 1998).

There are some evidences suggesting that activation of ER-β inhibits proliferation in breast cells (Patisaul et al., 2010). Because genistein preferentially binds to ER-β, it may induce antiestrogenic effects through this receptor (Bouker et al., 2000). Moreover, soy isoflavones can act as an antiestrogen through other mechanisms. Genistein has the ability to inhibit the enzyme 17β-hydroxysteroid oxidoreductase type 1 (HSOR-1), which is necessary for estradiol secretion from the ovaries in premenopausal women and is essential for the reduction of estrone to estradiol in the adipose tissues. Isoflavones are also involved in the inhibition of the aromatase enzyme, which is responsible for the conversion of androgens to estrone in peripheral (adipose) tissues (Bouker et al., 2000). Thus, the inhibition of estrogen-metabolizing enzymes can lead to a decreased total estradiol level and intensify isoflavones antiestrogen effects. It is important to highlight that complex feedback mechanisms associated with the hypothalamic/ pituitary/gonadal axis are involved in controlling the levels of estrogen and that the effects of isoflavones in this network are unclear and demand further studies (Bouker et al., 2000).

The main biological effects of soy isoflavones in breast cancer cells involve cell growth arrest and induction of apoptosis (Lamartiniere et al., 1998). Genistein have been shown to inhibit growth factor- and cytokine -stimulated growth of breast cancer cells (Peterson et al., 1996). Indeed, at the molecular level, this isoflavone can influence the regulation of cell cycle molecules by inducing significant up-regulation of p21/WAF1 expression (cell cycle inhibitor) in the treatment of breast cancer cells (Banerjee et al., 2008). In addition, the treatment of breast cancer cells with genistein influences the regulation of apoptotic molecules such as down-regulating anti-apoptotic molecules (Bcl-2, Bcl-xL, and HER-2/neu) and up-regulating pro-apoptotic ones (Bax and caspases). It has been suggested that genistein could also induce the regulation of those genes through the inhibition of proteasome. Overall, these findings suggest that ER stress, cell cycle arrest and apoptosis induction may represent part of the molecular mechanism by which isoflavones exert their anticarcinogenic effects (Banerjee et al., 2008).

4.2.2 Estrogen-receptor independent properties

Interestingly, the effects of soy isoflavones on cell cycle arrest and apoptosis has been detected not only in ER-positive but also in ER-negative breast cancer cells (Theil et al., 2010) suggesting that isoflavones anticancer activity might also occur independently of ER modulation. Indeed, several non-estrogenic targets for isoflavones have been described.

Isoflavones have been described as specific inhibitors of protein-tyrosine kinase (PTK), which is an enzyme frequently overexpressed in cancer cells. PTKs are crucial molecules for tumor development and thus soy isoflavones can potentially slow tumorigenesis by inhibiting their mediated signalling mechanisms (Banerjee et al., 2008; Patisaul et al., 2010).

Isoflavones can modulate and block the activity of several molecules involved in breast cancer cell growth and survival pathways such as topoisomerase I and II, mitogen activated protein kinases (MAPK), urokinase- type plasminogen activator (uPA), and nuclear factor-κB (NF-κB). Isoflavones are also implicated in the growth inhibition of various cancer cells through the regulation of gene activity by modulating epigenetic events that are intimately related to the regulation of cell cycle and apoptosis such as DNA methylation and/or histone acetylation (Messina et al., 2001; Banerjee et al., 2008).

Furthermore, soy isoflavones are able to inhibit invasion, metastasis, and angiogenesis *in vitro* and *in vivo* in a number of cancers including breast cancer. Genistein was described to inhibit the secretion of matrix metalloproteinases (crucial enzymes for invasion and metastasis) in MDA-MB-435 breast cancer cells and blocked invasion of a highly meta-static subline of BALB/c mammary carcinoma cells (Bouker et al., 2000; Messina et al., 2001).

Antioxidant activity is also included among the described effects of soy isoflavones. They are able to protect cells against reactive oxygen species by scavenging free radicals and inhibiting the expression of stress-response related genes which is an interesting approach for cancer prevention (Ruiz-Larrea et al., 1997).

Overall, it is clear that when evaluating biological effects of isoflavones it is necessary to look beyond the estrogen receptor and consider their non-hormone-related activities (Messina et al., 2001).

4.2.3 Dose-dependent effects

Soy isoflavones can induce different effects on breast cancer cells according to the dose used. For example, the effects of soy isoflavones in MCF-7 and BT20 breast cancer cells were only observed in the highest dose tested (50 μg/mL) (Theil et al., 2010). Similar effects were reported showing that isoflavone doses higher than 10 μM could inhibit the growth of breast cancer cells (Wang et al., 1996). In particular, the IC50 values of genistein able to induce growth arrest in both hormone-dependent and hormone-independent breast cancer cells have been described to range from 10 to 50 µM (Messina et al., 2001).

Some researchers question the relevance of these results by claiming that the high isoflavone concentrations used *in vitro* would not be achieved after ingestion in an *in vivo* system. Most Asians or Caucasians that consume a diet rich in soy have serum genistein levels smaller than 1 µM (Bouker et al., 2000). In order to address these claims, several assays evaluated the effects of isoflavones in low concentrations and, surprisingly, showed a different outcome. Low doses (0.01–1 µM) of genistein were shown to stimulate proliferation in human breast cancer cell lines (Bouker et al., 2000; Messina et al., 2001).

In animal studies, soy isoflavones also induce different activities according not only to the dose but to the animal model and the route of administration used (Barnes et al., 1997). Injections of 0.8 mg genistein in rats significantly reduced MNU-induced tumor multiplicity and marginally reduced tumor incidence. Similarly, a high dose of daidzein (0.8 mg) decreased tumor multiplicity without affecting incidence, whereas a low dose (0.4 mg) was ineffective. Other study showed that rats fed with a low dose of biochanin A (10 mg/kg), which is an isoflavone that is converted to genistein *in vivo*, significantly reduced tumor multiplicity and that a higher dose (50 mg/kg) also reduced tumor incidence (Barnes et al., 1997).

Conversely, instead of decreasing tumor growth as previously commented, soy isoflavones have also been described to stimulate breast tumor growth *in vivo* (Helferich et al., 2008; Bouker et al., 2000; Allred et al., 2004). The effects of dietary level of genistein were studied in an athymic BALB/c ovariectomized mice model subcutaneously injected with human estrogen-dependent cells (MCF-7). They found that in mice fed with a standard (control) AIN-93G diet, tumors reduced completely; however, mice fed with diets containing either isoflavone-rich isolated soy protein or isoflavone extracts had tumor growth stimulated (Hsieh et al., 1998). The use of a non-ovariectomized athymic mice model injected with ER-negative breast cancer cells to evaluate the effects of high dietary levels of soy isoflavones intake showed that daidzein increased while genistein decreased mammary tumor growth by 38 and 33% respectively. In addition, daidzein increased lung and heart metastases while genistein decreased bone and liver metastases. Combined soy isoflavones did not affect primary tumor growth but increased metastasis to all organs tested, which include lung, liver, heart, kidney, and bones (Martinez-Montemayor et al., 2010).

In general, the evidences indicate that at lower concentrations isoflavones exert estrogen-like effects while at higher concentrations other non-estrogen receptor-mediated effects are induced (Messina et al., 2001). Data from *in vivo* studies suggest that in a low-estrogen environment (as exists in postmenopausal women), genistein is estrogenic and has a proliferative effect on breast tissue. However, in a high estrogen environment (similar to that in premenopausal women), it has an antiproliferative and possibly antiestrogenic effect (Hsieh et al., 1998; Allred et al., 2004). Therefore, isoflavones can both inhibit or stimulate proliferation of breast cancer cells showing a biphasic effect according to the dose (Bouker et al., 2000).

Several hypothesis and discussion about experimental models limitations/weaknesses have been elaborated to address these conflicting results (Messina et al., 2008). First, considering that both estrogen and soy isoflavones bind to ER, differences in endogenous estrogen levels may interfere in the results. Premenopausal women have high levels of estrogen while basal levels of estrogen are found in postmenopausal women. Thus, *in vitro* estrogen-depleted conditions and ovariectomized animals (with no basal estrogen levels) would not be suitable models because there are no sufficient estrogen levels to promote or even to maintain estrogen-dependent tumors. Even weak estrogenic compounds, such as isoflavones, could stimulate the growth of estrogen-sensitive mammary tumors in such environment (Messina et al., 2006). Thus, these models would not accurately reflect conditions in either premenopausal or postmenopausal women (Messina et al., 2008). Researchers have supported this hypothesis showing that although genistein stimulated proliferation of MCF-7 cells and enhanced expression of the estrogen-responsive pS2 gene in an estrogen-depleted *in vitro* environment, it inhibited estrogen-induced proliferation and reduced pS2 expression of MCF-7 breast cancer cells when in the presence of a maintained level of estrogen (Wang et al., 1996; So et al., 1997). Nevertheless, breast tumor growth stimulation by both dietary and subcutaneously injected genistein has still been noted in animal models in which estrogen levels were more similar to the amounts of pre and postmenopausal women (Messina et al., 2006).

The second critique addresses the use of mice lacking the immune properties (athymic or nude). This animal feature is a necessary element of these models in order to allow the growth of human tumor cells in a murine environment. However, the lack of immune function may eliminate a potential mechanism by which soy isoflavones reduce tumor development (Messina et al., 2008). A recent research in B6C3F1 mice showed that enhanced immune function resulting from pre-treatment with genistein (20 ppm) is correlated with protection against chemically-induced mammary tumors (Guo et al., 2007).

The third critique relates to isoflavone dose. In many studies, breast cancer cells and animals are exposed to high amounts of genistein (750 ppm) which exceeds typical dietary intake. In Japan, adults consume about 15–20 mg genistein daily (total average isoflavone intake is approximately 40 mg), which equates to a dietary concentration of about 30–40 ppm (Messina et al., 2008). However, it is important to highlight that isoflavone biodistribution is not homogeneous. Isoflavone concentrations in breast tissue are two- to threefold higher than paired serum concentrations. It suggests that breast tissue may be exposed to higher levels of biologically active isoflavones than was previously thought (Pasqualini et al., 2005) and supports investigations of high concentrations of isoflavones.

Another aspect of oral doses of isoflavones relies in the amount of free (unconjugated) isoflavones processed by intestinal bacteria. The rodent gut bacteria are able to convert daidzein to the metabolite equol more effectively than humans. Furthermore, even in humans who are classified as equol producers, genistein is the predominant serum isoflavone in response to the ingestion of soy or mixed isoflavones, whereas equol predominates in most other species, including both rodents and monkeys (Gu et al., 2006).

The fourth consideration is based on the fact that it is not clear to what extent the existing MCF-7 xenoplants in nude mice resemble tumors in human breast cancer. These tumors are fully transformed and composed of cells that are extremely sensitive to the growth-stimulating effects of estrogen (Messina et al., 2008). Thus, a better comprehension of the current existing animal models and the development of new ones would contribute to the interpretation and translation of isoflavone effects in humans.

Given the conflicting data and limited *in vitro* and *in vivo* models, the controversy about the effects of isoflavones either from soy foods or supplements would be unlikely solved by additional animal research (Messina et al., 2009). Then, epidemiologic data should be another alternative to study and conclude about isoflavone intake and breast cancer. Current data discussing this topic is provided in the next section.

4.2.4 Aspects of isoflavone intake in humans

Women with high risk of breast cancer, breast cancer patients and survivors are among the group of consumers who have embraced soy products, isoflavone supplements and isoflavone-enriched foods, seeking for their health-promoting properties. Nevertheless, the estrogenic/antiestrogenic effects of these molecules and the disparities of *in vitro* and *in vivo* data have led to considerable controversy and misinterpretation among health professionals and consumers over the use of soy by this group of women. Due to the phytoestrogenic nature of isoflavone, several oncologists often discourage and even prohibit its intake by breast cancer patients, particularly those with ER-positive tumors (Messina et al., 2001).

As previously discussed, early epidemiologic studies have reported that high isoflavone intake was related to low cancer rates regardless of intrinsic genetic and biological differences among populations worldwide (Wu et al., 1996). Since then, more researchers have attempted to refine the knowledge of this matter and further investigate the correlations of isoflavone intake among breast cancer biomarkers, time of exposition, and age.

Soy intake was found to be significantly associated with a decreased risk of death from breast cancer and/or recurrence when evaluated in 5,042 Chinese women aged from 25 to 75 followed for 5 years (Shu et al., 2009). These benefits remained significant even after adjusting the results for 17 factors including tumor, node, metastasis stage, ER, progesterone receptor status and the type of treatment received. It was also observed that women who had the highest level of soyfood intake and did not take tamoxifen had a lower risk of mortality and a lower recurrence rate than women who had the lowest level of soyfood intake and used tamoxifen (Shu et al., 2009; Messina et al., 2010). The association of decreased breast cancer risk and soy isoflavone intake has been observed even in Asian-American women, both pre- and postmenopausal, living in the West (Wu et al., 1996). Overall, evidences show that for Asian women the risk of developing breast cancer reduces as soy intake rises. Even a soy intake of as little as 10 mg per day was sufficient to decrease breast cancer risk by 12% (Patisaul et al., 2010).

Effects of isoflavone intake have also been investigated in non-Asian populations. In a US study, it was observed that breast cancer survivors (n= 1,954; followed for 6.3 years) had reduced risk of cancer recurrence with increasing amounts of isoflavone among postmenopausal women and tamoxifen users. Interestingly, more pronounced effects were observed in women with ER-positive breast cancer (Guha et al., 2009). Beneficial effects of isoflavone intake were also observed in a Dutch study, which compared serum isoflavone concentrations in women with and without breast cancer. It was observed that high plasma concentrations of genistein were associated with a 32% reduction in breast cancer risk (Verheus et al., 2007). Furthermore, it was reported that isoflavone intake was associated with a reduced risk of all-cause mortality during the 5-y follow-up period among postmenopausal U.S. breast cancer patients (Fink et al., 2007).

Conversely, other investigations have failed in detecting benefits in soy isoflavone intake. One of them did not find significant differences in soy daidzein or genistein intake between breast cancer cases and their controls in Shanghai (Zheng et al., 1999). Other investigation showed that soy food intake was unrelated to survival of Chinese breast cancer patients during the 5.2-y follow-up period (Boyapati et al., 2005). Several other researchers have also suggested that soy consumption is not associated with a reduced risk of breast cancer; however, no harmful effects were found in these studies (Bouker et al., 2000).

Breast tissue density has been used as a non-invasive breast cancer biomarker to evaluate isoflavone intake. It was observed that both intervention and epidemiologic studies have not shown evidence of neither harm or benefit of isoflavone on breast cancer density (Messina et al., 2006). Analysis of breast cell proliferation has also been used as a biomarker of potential tumor promotion. Comparison of biopsies taken before and after exposure to soy products did not show increased cell proliferation in any of the four different trials involving breast cancer patients, healthy subjects, and women undergoing breast biopsy or definitive surgery for breast cancer. Daily isoflavone intake in these trials ranged from 36 to more than 100 mg, with study periods ranging from 2 weeks to one year (Messina et al., 2009). Another study examining more than one breast cancer biomarker found no statistically significant differences in cell proliferation (Ki67 index), histology (hyperplasia with or without atypia), or ER expression in 6 and 12 months of soy intake (Messina et al., 2006). Conversely, a study evaluating the effects of soy consumption (38 g soy protein isolate, 80 mg isoflavones) over 5 months showed an association of isoflavone intake and a two- to sixfold increase in breast nipple aspirate fluid (NAF) secretion of premenopausal but not postmenopausal women (Petrakis et al., 1996).

The effects of isoflavone intake in serum estrogen and androgen levels have been widely investigated. The consumption of textured vegetable (i.e., soy) protein for 2 weeks elicited an ER-mediated response detected by increased pS2 levels (protein expressed in response to estrogen) in breast biopsies taken from premenopausal women (Hargreaves et al., 1999). However, high levels of soy products have been described to induce no changes or even decrease plasma estradiol concentrations in premenopausal women. None of these effects were observed in postmenopausal women (Bouker et al., 2000). These contrasting findings could be partially explained by the observation that, despite binding to ERs, isoflavones are also able to inhibit enzymes related to estrogen synthesis and metabolism. Therefore, it has been hypothesized that the presence of other additional simultaneous stimuli may result in either reduced or increased circulating estradiol concentrations (Bouker et al., 2000).

Isoflavone intake has been implicated to interfere in serum levels of other menstrual cycle hormones, such as progesterone. Studies have reported that isoflavone intake was associated with a significant reduction in serum progesterone levels and in luteal phase lengths (Lu et al., 2000). These findings suggest that isoflavones may reduce the probability of neoplastic transformation and breast cancer development since breast cells are more proliferative during the luteal phase of the menstrual cycle, when progesterone concentrations are the highest (Lu et al., 2000).

Overall, inconsistent results about isoflavone intake and breast cancer are also present in epidemiological studies. Indeed, researchers have highlighted the difficulties of comparing clinical studies since several variables are not properly considered. In a meta-analysis by Trock et al., 18 studies (12 case-control and 6 cohort) published between 1978 and 2004 were evaluated. After making several assumptions, the authors showed that there is a small inverse correlation between soy intake and breast cancer for both pre- and postmenopausal women; however data limitations cannot exclude the possibility that this result could be an artifact of the analysis (Trock et al., 2006).

An important variable to be considered when evaluating risks and benefits of soy isoflavone intake comprises the extent and the period of life in which women are exposed to soy food. Studies attempting to address this topic are discussed in the next section.

4.2.5 Lifetime exposition of isoflavones

Throughout the life span, estrogens can induce mammary cell proliferation or cell differentiation depending on the overall hormonal environment. Since isoflavones present estrogenic or antiestrogenic activities, they may have a different impact on the breast if the exposure occurs in utero; during childhood, puberty, or pregnancy; premenopausally; or during postmenopause (Bouker et al., 2000). Studies have been carried out to determine if the putative preventive effects of soy isoflavones are related to the lifetime period of exposition.

Different outcomes have been shown from perinatal/neonatal exposure of isoflavones in animals. The offspring of pregnant rats receiving subcutaneously administration of high doses of genistein exhibited abnormal mammary gland development and higher susceptibility to develop 7,12-dimethylbenz[a]anthracene (DMBA)- induced mammary tumorigenesis (Padilla-Banks et al., 2006; Patisaul et al., 2010). Conversely, it was reported that rat pups born to mothers consuming high levels of genistein during gestation and lactation developed fewer breast tumors (Fritz et al., 1998). Protective effects of isoflavones were also reported when soy exposure occurred perinatally. Rats receiving genistein through diet or subcutaneously during the first days postpartum showed lower tumor incidence after DMBA mammary tumor induction (Lamartiniere, 2000).

The period between puberty and a first full-term pregnancy is when the breast is particularly vulnerable to the effects of carcinogens. During this time, there are a high percentage of indiferentiated breast cells, named terminal end buds (TEBs), actively proliferating. Several investigations in animal models have shown protective effects of prepubertal isoflavone exposure on mammary tumorigenesis induced by DMBA (Murrill et al., 1996; Lamartiniere et al., 1998).

Epidemiological studies support *in vivo* findings showing that isoflavone intake during adolescence and adulthood is correlated with low risk of breast cancer. Shu et al. reported that women consuming tofu (11 g soy protein/day) during their teenage years (13–15 years) were less likely to develop premenopausal and postmenopausal breast cancer as adults (Shu et al., 2001). Other epidemiologic studies have supported these results when protective effects with reductions in risk of breast cancer ranging from 28 to 60% were observed (Messina, 2010).

Investigations on mammary gland morphology and cell differentiation were carried out in animal models to understand how isoflavone exerts the described protective effects. The results indicated that isoflavones might have been exerting its chemoprotective effect by stimulating early cell differentiation leading to a reduction in the number of least differentiated structures in the breast tissue (TEBs) which are susceptible to chemical carcinogens (Bouker et al., 2000; Lamartiniere, 2000).

Therefore, animal and epidemiological studies are consistent with the hypothesis that childhood and/or adolescence is the critical period for isoflavone of exposure (Messina et al., 2006) and also corroborates with speculations that Asian low breast cancer rates is derived from early exposure to soy products, including during pregnancy (Lamartiniere, 2000).

4.2.6 Variables influencing inconsistent outcomes

To better interpret and understand data about isoflavone intake and breast cancer it is important to consider the strengths and weaknesses of a wide variety of experimental models and designs (Messina et al., 2006). As commented previously, the major sources of limitation in those studies are the inappropriate experimental designs and incomplete or unclear information provided about food isoflavone content, patient description, serum isoflavone levels, time of exposition, and isoflavone metabolism. There are studies in which some variables are not even considered. Differences in these factors can considerably difficult comparisons among studies generating misinterpretations of data and are probably related to the majority of inconsistent results in the literature.

Epidemiologic studies should take into consideration that the amounts of isoflavones are not equal in all soy foods. Indeed, there are notably differences in soy food preparations and isoflavone content. Raw soybeans contain nearly 1.0 mg/g (range of 0.4 -2.4 mg/g of total isoflavones while traditional soy foods (i.e., tofu, miso, natto) typically contain 0.2- 0.4 mg/g (Messina et al., 2001). In addition, the content and structure of isoflavones are altered when soy food undergo processing, which was shown to potentially affect the effects on breast cancer (Murphy et al., 1999; Allred et al., 2004).

Moreover, soy isoflavone content can vary according to local, weather, seed maturation, and breeding conditions. It was observed that during the process of seed maturation the contents of isoflavones decrease, whereas sprouting led to a continuing increase of isoflavone content. Interestingly, the protein extracts from the developing seeds showed clearly opposite effects on cell viability and inhibition of foci formation compared with those from sprouting seeds (Park et al., 2005).

Individual differences in the absorption and metabolism of ingested isoflavones are another variable not usually addressed on breast cancer studies. To evaluate the potential risks and benefits of phytochemicals to human health, it is important to know the physiological behavior of these compounds after ingestion (Hsieh et al., 2010). As previously commented, isoflavones are metabolized by intestinal microorganisms, which may be heterogeneous among individuals. This variability may have large contributing effects on the serum levels of free isoflavones and correspondent metabolites and thereby on the resulting physiologic effects. Furthermore, differences in isoflavone metabolism and bioavaiability should also be considered when analyzing data from rodent animal models since a higher percentage of both genistein and daidzein appear in the free or glycone form in rats (Gu et al., 2006).

Individual variabilities should also be considered when analyzing the effects of isoflavone intake in estrogen and progesterone serum levels. Menstrual cycle length varies significantly among women and analysis of reproductive hormone levels in single periods may not provide accurate data on isoflavone effects. In this case, it would be more appropriate to measure the hormone levels during the whole menstrual cycle (Lu et al., 2000). Different times of isoflavone exposition are yet another type of limitation that influences data interpretation. For example, short periods of exposition (such as 2 weeks) may provide data regarding only the acute effects of soy isoflavone intake on breast cancer, thus, limiting comparisons with long-term studies.

Other potential source of variability in clinical studies includes incomplete patient description. Different and more specific correlations would be obtained whether patients were also addressed in subgroups by ER status, serum estrogen levels, and type of treatment being received (e.g. tamoxifen) for example. Those detailed patient information should also be used as valuable adjustment parameters for raw data in order to improve interpretation accurateness (Shu et al., 2009; Messina et al., 2010).

Clearly, there is a need to encourage further detailed studies to reduce the heterogeneity of soy exposure data (Rochfort et al., 2007). Several recommendations have been made to improve study conditions and data interpretation such as: provide clear information about the isoflavone content (including glycone amount) on test products; include detailed description of products, concentrations, and amounts used; relate study conditions to usual soy and isoflavone intakes and/or tissue levels of isoflavones; consider the risks and benefits of research findings for human health; and outline the benefits and limitations of the model system used when conducting cell culture or animal studies (Erdman et al., 2004).

5. Protease Inhibitors

5.1 Structure and bioavalability

Protease inhibitors (PIs) have been isolated from black-eyed peas (*Vigna unguiculata*), soy (*Glycine max*), brazilian pink bean (*Phaseolus vulgaris*), pea (*Pisum sativum*) and lentil (*Lens culinaris*) (Losso, 2008). In seeds, these molecules are involved in the regulation of endogenous proteases and in defense-related strategies against seed-eating insects and microorganisms (Ryan, 1990). The concentration of PIs is affected by the stage of seed development and sprouting. For example, soy-derived BBI content increases during the process of seed maturation while it decreases with soaking time during sprouting (Park et al., 2005).

PIs are classified in more than 20 families according to their inhibitory activity and structural features (Laskowski et al., 2000; Joanitti et al., 2006). The primary families found in legumes are the Kunitz and the Bowman-Birk which are involved in the inhibition of serine proteases (Joanitti et al., 2006; Losso, 2008). Kunitz PIs consist of proteins with molecular mass ranging from 6-20 kDa. These inhibitors are cross-linked by 2-3 disulfide bonds and have one reactive site that generally binds to trypsin. Bowman-Birk PIs are small proteins (6-15 kDa) presenting 5-7 disulfide bonds and 2 different and independent reactive sites located at opposite regions of the molecule (Fig. 2). Due to this double-headed configuration, these inhibitors can interact with 2 enzymes simultaneously (e.g. trypsin and chymotrypsin or trypsin and trypsin (Freitas et al., 1999; Ventura et al., 1966)). The disulfide bonds content of Kunitz and Bowman-Birk PIs are responsible for their remarkable structural stability (Joanitti et al., 2006). It has been reported that the inhibitory activity of these molecules is preserved after being exposed to a wide range of temperatures (up to 100ºC) and pHs (2-13) (Silva et al., 2001; Ho et al., 2008; Ye et al., 2009).

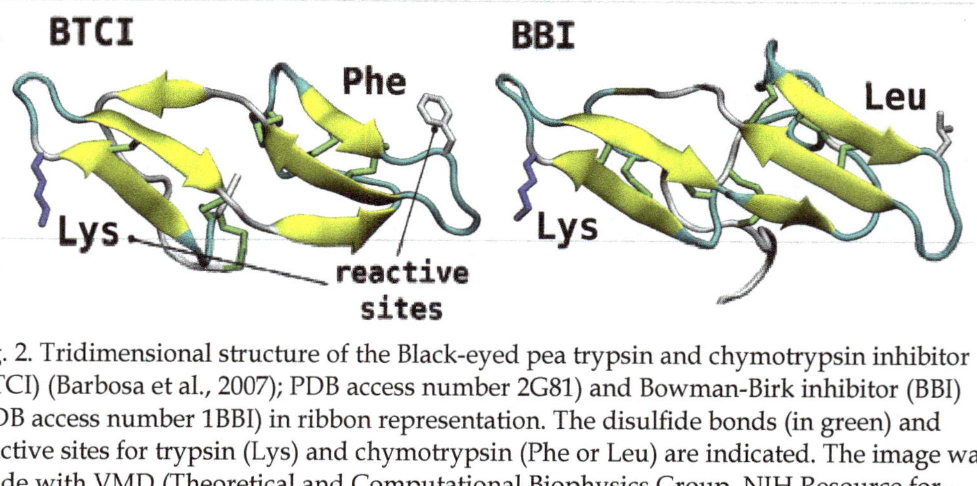

Fig. 2. Tridimensional structure of the Black-eyed pea trypsin and chymotrypsin inhibitor (BTCI) (Barbosa et al., 2007); PDB access number 2G81) and Bowman-Birk inhibitor (BBI) (PDB access number 1BBI) in ribbon representation. The disulfide bonds (in green) and reactive sites for trypsin (Lys) and chymotrypsin (Phe or Leu) are indicated. The image was made with VMD (Theoretical and Computational Biophysics Group, NIH Resource for Macromolecular Modeling and Bioinformatics, Beckman Institute, University of Illinois, Urbana-Champaign).

Because Kunitz and Bowman-Birk PIs are involved in the inhibition of serine proteases, these molecules have been considered as antinutritional factors able to impair digestion. Proper thermal seed processing have been described to eliminate the majority of legume antinutritional factors (Lajolo et al., 2002); nevertheless, some Kunitz and Bowman-Birk PIs are able to resist both acidic conditions and the action of proteolytic enzymes and pass through the stomach and small intestine without major degradation (Clemente et al., 2010). The metabolism and absorption of a soy Bowman-Birk PI (termed BBI) have been well characterized following oral administrations. After ingestion, BBI are rapidly metabolized and absorbed. BBI can resist stomach and small intestine conditions permitting the reach of significant amounts to the large intestine in the active form to exert their reported anticancer and anti-inflammatory properties (Kennedy, 1998). This PI is widely distributed throughout the body including breast tissue (Kennedy, 1998). In mice, BBI metabolites can be found in the liver, serum, and kidneys of mice 1.5 hours after ingestion (Wang et al., 2000). In humans, BBI excretion rates reach the peak within 6 hours and decrease to baseline levels within 12-24 hours (Wan et al., 2000).

PIs have been viewed as toxic agents inhibiting the growth of young animals and, perhaps, contributing to the development of pancreatic cancer. However, the effect on the promotion of atypical growth in rat pancreata, is not expected to occur in humans (Kennedy, 1998). Despite preserving their biological activity after passing through the gastrointestinal tract, it seems that these inhibitors do not act as antinutritional factors since they are not implicated in significant side effects even when ingested in concentrations far higher than the therapeutic dose (Kennedy, 1998).

5.2 Effects on breast cancer

PIs have been considered promising compounds in several economic and clinical areas. These inhibitors are multiple functional molecules with properties varying from insecticide to therapeutical activity in fields as immune systems, microorganism and viral infections, hemostasis, and cancer (Joanitti et al., 2006). PIs have shown promising anticancer effects on the prevention and suppression of cancer in several organ systems and tissue types (e.g. colon, liver, lung, esophagus, oral epithelium, ovarian, prostate, hematopoietic cells, and connective tissue), *in vitro* and *in vivo* (Kennedy, 1998). Particularly, BBI (Bowman-Birk Inhibitor from soy) was recognized as an investigational new drug by the Food and Drug Administration (FDA) and is currently being evaluated in clinical trials against pre-malignant oral cancer lesions, showing successful results on the reduction of cancer lesions with low or no side effects (Armstrong et al., 2000). Despite having their anticancer activity being widely investigated on different tumor types, few studies have addressed the effects of Kunitz and Bowman-Birk PIs specifically on breast cancer.

The effects of soy BBI on DMBA-induced transformation were investigated using an *in vitro* whole organ culture system of mouse mammary glands. It was observed that soy BBI and its palmitic acid conjugate (Pal-BBI) were effective in preventing DMBA-induced transformation, especially when added to the medium during the developing period after the exposure of mammary glands to DMBA, showing 35.9 and 53.4% prevention, respectively. Pal-BBI was also effective in decreasing the transformation incidence (32.2%) while BBI was not (10.3%) when only present in the medium before the promotion period. Possibly, the high lipophilicity of Pal-BBI increased its tissue retention and resulted in higher chemopreventive effects (Du et al., 2001).

An interesting *in vivo* study reported the effects of one year-long feeding of field bean meal (a rich source of PIs with 24% protein content), on mouse mammary tumor virus (MMTV)-induced mammary tumorigenesis in mice. The animals were fed chow with 2%, 4%, and 8% field bean protein (FBP) for 49 weeks and the incidence of mammary tumors was recorded in 58 weeks. A suppressive effect on mammary tumorigenesis was observed with increased FBP intake as mice fed with 2%, 4%, and 8% FBP showed significant tumor incidence reduction of 68%, 75% and 81% respectively. Adverse growth effects were observed only in mice receiving the 8% FBP-fed group (Fernandes et al., 1997).

In addition to chemopreventive properties, PI effects on the viability of breast cancer cells have also been reported. A Bowman-Birk PI isolated from Hokkaido large black soybeans seeds and a Kunitz PI isolated from Chinese black soybean seeds have been described to suppress the proliferation of breast cancer cells (MCF-7) *in vitro* (Ho et al., 2008; Ye et al., 2009). Similar effects were observed in MCF-7 cells treated with Bowman-Birk PIs derived from soy or black-eyed peas (Zhang et al., 1999; Joanitti et al., 2010). Conversely, it was described that soy BBI was not able to induce anticancer effects on ER-negative breast cancer cell MDA-MB 231 (Hsieh et al., 2010). It has been suggested that additional investigations should be made to determine whether tumor cell types and their specific carcinogenesis pathways may be determinants of the cancer chemopreventive properties of BBI (Hsieh et al., 2010).

PIs have been described to act on different cancer stages and activities impairing malignant cell transformation, altered gene expression and proteolytic activity, tumor growth, angiogenesis, and metastasis. These effects have been suggested to be linked to their protease inhibition activity (Kennedy, 1998; Joanitti et al., 2006). Nevertheless, the precise mechanisms by which PIs exerts their preventive and suppressive anticancer effects are not completely elucidated on breast cancer.

One of the main effects observed in tumor cells treated with PIs is a reduction on cell proliferation rates (Wan et al., 1998; Zhang et al., 1999; Chen et al., 2005). In 2005, Chen et al. reported a landmark research study revealing some clues about the mechanisms involved in this growth inhibition. They observed that the soy-derived BBI was able to inhibit proteasome activity, specifically the chymotrypsin-like domain, *in vitro* and *in vivo* in MCF-7 breast cancer cells. Proteasomes are large protein complexes acting in the degradation of misfolded proteins and regulation of particular proteins levels involved in intracellular pathways. Proteasome inhibition by BBI resulted in an accumulation of ubiquitinated proteins and proteasome substrates, such as cell cycle inhibitors p21Cip1/WAF1 and p27Kip1, inducing cell cycle arrest at G1/S phase. Furthermore, an up-regulation of MAP kinase phosphatase-1 (MKP-1) accompanied by a decrease of phosphorylated extracellular signal-related kinases (ERK1/2), which is a pathway involved in cell division, was also observed (Chen et al., 2005).

In addition to tumor growth inhibition, the BBI found in black-eyed peas (termed BTCI) was also shown to induce death on MCF-7 cells (Joanitti et al., 2010). The treatment of cells with BTCI induced significant reduction of the cell proliferation (arrest in S and G2/M phase) accompanied by significative DNA fragmentation, mitochondrial swelling, morphologic alterations, annexin-V+ cell number increase, and mitochondrial membrane potential reduction. These cytotoxic effects at first suggested that BTCI induced apoptosis cell death on MCF-7 cell. However, other features observed such as large lysosomes presenting weak acidification pattern followed by an increase in cytoplasmic acidification indicated another cell death pathway related to lysosomes: the lysosomal membrane permeabilization (LMP).

LMP is characterized by a perturbation of lysosomal membrane function leading to the translocation of lysosomal hydrolases from the lysosomal lumen to the cell cytoplasm. Therefore, the authors suggested that BTCI was able to induce both LMP and apoptosis processes on breast cancer cells (Joanitti et al., 2010).

The ability to induce tumor growth inhibiton and or cell death might be determined by PIs structural features, especially on the reactive sites, leading to different affinities to the targets. Moreover, variations in the dose and time of exposure are also important factors to be considered. For example, low Bowman-Birk PIs concentrations (10-40 μM) and long incubation periods (6-14 days) are frequently associated with proliferation inhibition (Wan et al., 1998; Zhang et al., 1999); while high concentration (200 μM) and short incubation periods (3 days) has been described to induce both tumor growth inhibition and cell death (Joanitti et al., 2010). Overall, these findings indicate that PIs are promising anticancer molecules and encourage more studies of these compounds on breast cancer.

6. Peptides

6.1 Structure and bioavailability

Among bioactive peptides found in legumes, a peptide isolated from soybean cotyledon has stand out as a potential anticancer agent. Lunasin is a 43-amino acid peptide with structurally conserved helix region containing Arg- Gly-Asp (RGD) cell adhesion motif followed by 9 aspartic acid residues at the carboxyl end. This peptide exhibits the primary sequence, SKWQHQQDSCRKQLQGVNLTPCEKHIMEKIQGRGDDDDDDDDD (Hernandez-Ledesma et al., 2009).

Lunasin has been identified in several soybean varieties with concentrations ranging from 4.4 to 70.5 mg lunasin/g protein (Gonzalez de Mejia et al., 2004; Hernandez-Ledesma et al., 2008). These concentrations are affected by the stage of seed development and sprouting. A notable increase of lunasin content is observed during seed maturation while the opposite occurs during sprouting. Breeding conditions (light and dark cycles) do not seem to affect the content of this peptide (Park et al., 2005). Large-scale processing of soy also influences lunasin concentration which was observed to vary from 12 to 44 mg lunasin/g of flour among different U.S. commercially available soy proteins (Gonzalez de Mejia et al., 2004).

Besides presenting heat stability, *in vitro* digestibility studies have shown that lunasin is digested by pancreatin (Galvez et al. 2001). However, animal studies indicate that when lunasin is ingested in combination with soy protein extract, it survives digestion and about 35% of the total oral dose is absorbed within 3 hours (de Lumen, 2005). These findings suggest that other components of soy are protecting lunasin from degradation (see section 7). Lunasin is biodistributed in various tissues including lung, liver, mammary gland, prostate and even the brain within 6 hours after administration. In addition, analysis of the liver and blood showed that this peptide was present in an intact and bioactive form (Jeong et al., 2007; Hsieh et al., 2010).

6.2 Effects on breast cancer

Lunasin was first discovered during studies regarding soy seed development. Early soybean seed development is characterized by orchestrated events of rapid cell division and differentiation. It was observed that the stage of seed cell expansion (massive synthesis of storage molecules) began after cell division had ceased and that a temporal production of lunasin coincided with this mitotic arrest. This data led to the hypothesis that lunasin could also be involved in the disruption of mammalian cell division such as cancer cells. Indeed, lunasin was shown to block mitosis in mammalian cells by binding to chromatin and impairing the formation of the kinetochore complex in the centromere. These effects lead to the failure of microtubules to attach the centromeres and thereby to mitotic arrest and cell death (Galvez et al., 1999).

The mechanism of action for lunasin in the prevention of cell malignant transformation is related to chromatin binding. The dynamics of histone acetylation and deacetylation in non-cancerous cells is involved in chromatin remodelling which is implicated in cell cycle control (Hernandez-Ledesma et al., 2009). These processes are tightly regulated by tumor suppressor molecules which have among other activities the function to keep the histone core in a deacetylated (repressed) state. Nevertheless, during cell malignant transformation, many tumor suppressor molecules are inactivated by chemical and viral carcinogens which lead to the exposure of histones core. At this stage, lunasin is able to inhibit histone acetylation by binding deacetylated histones which prevents transcription and represses cell cycle progression (Galvez et al., 1999; Hernandez-Ledesma et al., 2009). In this context, lunasin can act as a surrogate tumor suppressor. Therefore, it has been suggested that lunasin selectively kills cells that are being transformed by disrupting the dynamics of histone acetylation-deacetylation when a transforming event occurs (Hernandez-Ledesma et al., 2008).

The RGD motif also contributes to the anticancer effects of lunasin. Since RGD motif is implicated in the attachment of tumor cells to the extracellular matrix, peptides containing this motif have been described to prevent metastasis of tumor cells by competitive adhesion to the extracellular matrix. Furthermore, it has been suggested that the internalization of lunasin in MCF-7 cells would be mediated by a functional RGD motif (Galvez et al., 1999).

In *in vitro* studies, lunasin was shown to suppress colony formation induced by the ras-oncogene in MCF-7 cells (Jeong et al., 2003). The *in vivo* effects of lunasin were investigated on an ER-negative MDA-MB-231 breast cancer model in which athymic mice received intraperitoneal injections of lunasin (4 or 20 mg/kg body weight) for 2 months prior to tumor implantation. After 7 weeks, mice treated with lunasin showed a significant reduction in breast tumor incidence and a delay in the appearance of tumors. In addition, histologic analysis revealed low proliferation and high apoptosis indexes in tumors of lunasin-treated mice (Hsieh et al., 2010).

7. Combined effects of bioactive compounds

The combination of therapies has emerged as an interesting approach for cancer prevention and treatment. This alternative strategy is based on synergistic effects of 2 or more anticancer compounds able to act in multiple targets resulting in a more efficacious treatment. Moreover, the combination of agents can result in significant activity at concentrations where the single agent is inactive. Thus, there is possibility to regulate an optimal dose and reduce unwanted side-effects (Lane, 2006).

As extensively commented here, legumes are rich sources of anticancer compounds including not only isoflavones, protease inhibitors and peptides but also saponins, phytic acid, and inositol phosphates. These molecules have different mechanisms of action on cancer cells, which suggests that their combination would result in synergistic effects. For example, a soy extract containing isoflavones and saponins significantly reduced the incidence of mammary tumour induced by DMBA (Gallo et al., 2001; Jin et al., 2002).

Inhibition of both breast tumor growth and metastasis was observed in animals treated with isolated soy proteins and isoflavones (Yan et al., 2002). Supplementation of isoflavone-containing crude soy protein to a transgenic mouse model for mmammary tumor significantly prolonged the latency period of tumour development (Jin et al., 2002).

The effects of combining legume bioactive compounds with other dietary molecules have also been studied. The combination of soy phytochemicals at a low dietary level with tea showed synergistic effects on inhibiting the growth of MCF-7 tumours (Zhou et al., 2004). Velie et al. undertook a large diet-based cohort study (40,559 postmenopausal women) and found that the only diet with significant negative correlation with invasive breast cancer was the traditional southern diet, which comprises high legume intake, low mayonnaise intake, and potentially cabbage intake (Velie et al., 2005).

The potential synergisms among legume bioactive compounds provide a clue to explain the different effects observed between studying the bioactive compound alone and evaluating a specific bioactive compound often associated with other anticancer molecules present in the legume. Therefore, researchers should consider the characterization of each legume extract or food not only in terms of quantity of the studied molecule but also in terms of identifying the presence of other potential bioactive compounds. This approach should improve data quality and allow more reliable comparisons and conclusions regarding the benefits and risks of legume intake.

In addition, the elucidation of these synergistic mechanisms may be useful to clarify the real effect of each bioactive compound and, based on this knowledge, aid in the design of novel preventive/therapeutic approaches and dietary guidelines. Chiesa et al. compared the breast tumor development of mice receiving a diet with different concentrations of isoflavones and soy protein and concluded that only animals receiving an isoflavone-poor soy protein concentrate diet showed reduction in tumor progression rates and metastasis development (Chiesa et al., 2008). Another study aimed to elucidate the synergistic effects between the major bioactive components present in a soy extract termed "Bowman-Birk Inhibitor Concentrate" (BBIC). BBIC was developed for use in large-scale human cancer-prevention trials and has been extensively studied for its bioactivity against several cancer types (Kennedy, 1998). Its anticancer effects have been mainly attributed to the soy-derived BBI, which is present in high concentrations in this extract (Kennedy, 1998). In addition to BBI, lunasin peptide is also present and both represent 44% of total protein in BBIC. BBI and lunasin peptide were administered intraperitoneally and separately in mice for 2 months prior to the implantation of MDA-MB-231 breast cancer cells. Surprisingly, it was observed that only lunasin was effective in inducing significant chemopreventive and therapeutic effects. In this context, BBI and other PIs present in BBIC complement lunasin activity in other manner. Since lunasin is easily degraded by gastrointestinal enzymes when ingested in a pure form, it has been reported that those PIs protect lunasin from digestion and make this peptide bioavailable (Hsieh et al., 2010).

Approaches of combining legumes bioactives compounds with conventional chemotherapeutic drugs have been shown promising results. Ito et al. reported that the combination of 10% miso diet (soy food) with 2.5 mg/kg tamoxifen resulted in a significant reduction in the incidence and multiplicity of MNU-induced mammary carcinomas mice (Ito et al., 1996). The combination of tamoxifen and soy protein isolate provided a better protection than using the components alone. The tumor incidence in DMBA-induced mammary carcinogenesis mice was reduced 29% by tamoxifen, 37% by soy protein isolate and 62% by the combination (Constantinou et al., 2001).

The high intake of soy isoflavones was associated with reduced risk of ER-positive breast cancer recurrence in patients receiving anastrozole treatment (aromatase inhibitor). In addition, it was suggested that the observed effect might be related to a synergistic inhibitory effect of isoflavones and anastrozole on the synthesis of estrogen (Kang et al., 2010). Another interesting combination with centchroman (selective estrogen receptor modulator) and soy intake was investigated on DMBA-induced mammary carcinogenesis. The doses and periods of treatment were optimized and a maximum tumor regression of 98.6% were achieved with centchroman 5 mg/kg per day, alone/in combination with soy 3×10^4 mg/kg per day at 5 weeks treatment period (Mishra et al., 2010).

8. Conclusion

Undoubtedly, plant species are notable sources of compounds essential to human health not only in terms of nutrition but also in a therapeutic aspect. In particular, the variety of legume-derived bioactive compounds has attracted the attention of researchers for their health-promoting properties on breast cancer. Encouraging results have identified the preventive and treatment effects of these compounds on breast cancer in *in vitro, in vivo* and epidemiological studies. However, other data sets indicate harmful or neutral outcomes. Therefore, the discussed data do not allow conclusive statements regarding the effects of legumes and their bioactive compounds on humans, especially on women at high risk for breast cancer and breast cancer patients.

Re-evaluation of current data and further studies are crucial to elucidate such doubts. Nevertheless, in order to provide expressive contributions and to make studies comparable, the design and interpretation of new experiments should be considered. In this context, the influences of variables, such as dose and time of exposition, and potential synergisms or antagonisms among compounds need to be investigated. Indeed, further studies on the effects and mechanisms of action of these molecules on breast cancer will provide a better comprehension regarding the safety of legume intake and the elaboration of suitable dietary guidelines.

The conclusive characterization of legumes as preventive and therapeutic anticancer compounds would lead to interesting future perspectives. Among other options, it would be possible to develop therapies based on legumes compounds; to improve their bioavailability by the use of drug delivery systems; to use them as templates in the process of rational design of new anticancer drugs; and even to control the amounts of specific bioactive compounds produced by genetically engineered legume crops.

9. Acknowledgment

We would like to thank Alexandre Ferreira de Souza Dias for his important comments during the preparation of this chapter. We also would like to thank the financial support provided by the Pós-Graduação em Biologia Molecular/CEL - University of Brasilia, Brazil.

10. References

Allred, C. D.; Allred, K. F.; Ju, Y. H.; Goeppinger, T. S.; Doerge, D. R. & Helferich, W. G. (2004). Soy processing influences growth of estrogen-dependent breast cancer tumors. *Carcinogenesis,* Vol. 25, No. 9, (September 2004), pp. 1649-1657. ISSN 0143-3334.

Armstrong, W. B.; Kennedy, A. R.; Wan, X. S.; Taylor, T. H.; Nguyen, Q. A.; Jensen, J.; Thompson, W.; Lagerberg, W. & Meyskens, F. L., Jr. (2000). Clinical modulation of oral leukoplakia and protease activity by Bowman-Birk inhibitor concentrate in a phase IIa chemoprevention trial. *Clinical Cancer Research,* Vol. 6, No. 12, (December 2000), pp. 4684-4691. ISSN 1078-0432.

Banerjee, S.; Li, Y.; Wang, Z. & Sarkar, F. H. (2008). Multi-targeted therapy of cancer by genistein. *Cancer Letters,* Vol. 269, No. 2, (October 2008), pp. 226-242. ISSN 1872-7980.

Barbosa, J. A.; Silva, L. P.; Teles, R. C.; Esteves, G. F.; Azevedo, R. B.; Ventura, M. M. & de Freitas, S. M. (2007). Crystal structure of the Bowman-Birk Inhibitor from Vigna unguiculata seeds in complex with beta-trypsin at 1.55 A resolution and its structural properties in association with proteinases. *Biophysical Journal,* Vol. 92, No. 5, (March 2007), pp. 1638-1650. ASSN 1542-0086.

Barnes, S. (1997). The chemopreventive properties of soy isoflavonoids in animal models of breast cancer. *Breast cancer research and treatment,* Vol. 46, No. 2-3, (November 1997), pp. 169-179. ASSN 0167-6806.

Bouker, K. B. & Hilakivi-Clarke, L. (2000). Genistein: does it prevent or promote breast cancer? *Environmental health perspectives,* Vol. 108, No. 8, (August 2000), pp. 701-708. ISSN 0091-6765.

Boyapati, S. M.; Shu, X. O.; Ruan, Z. X.; Dai, Q.; Cai, Q.; Gao, Y. T. & Zheng, W. (2005). Soyfood intake and breast cancer survival: a followup of the Shanghai Breast Cancer Study. *Breast cancer research and treatment,* Vol. 92, No. 1, (July 2005), pp. 11-17. ISSN 0167-6806.

Chen, Y. W.; Huang, S. C.; Lin-Shiau, S. Y. & Lin, J. K. (2005). Bowman-Birk inhibitor abates proteasome function and suppresses the proliferation of MCF7 breast cancer cells through accumulation of MAP kinase phosphatase-1. *Carcinogenesis,* Vol. 26, No. 7, (July 2005), pp. 1296-1306. ISSN 0143-3334.

Cheng, E.; Story, C. D.; Yoder, L.; Hale, W. H. & Burroughs, W. (1953). Estrogenic activity of isoflavone derivatives extracted and prepared from soybean oil meal. *Science,* Vol. 118, No. 3058, (August 1953), pp. 164-165. ISSN 0036-8075.

Chiesa, G.; Rigamonti, E.; Lovati, M. R.; Disconzi, E.; Soldati, S.; Sacco, M. G.; Cato, E. M.; Patton, V.; Scanziani, E.; Vezzoni, P.; Arnoldi, A.; Locati, D. & Sirtori, C. R. (2008). Reduced mammary tumor progression in a transgenic mouse model fed an isoflavone-poor soy protein concentrate. *Molecular nutrition & food research,* Vol. 52, No. 10, (October 2008), pp. 1121-1129. ISSN 1613-4133.

Colditz, G. A. & Frazier, A. L. (1995). Models of breast cancer show that risk is set by events of early life: prevention efforts must shift focus. *Cancer Epidemiology, Biomarkers & Prevention,* Vol. 4, No. 5, (July 1995), pp. 567-571. ISSN 1055-9965.

Constantinou, A.; Lantvit, D.; Lim, E.; Xu, H. & Pezzuto, J. M. (2001). Consumption of soy products may enhance tamoxifen's breast cancer preventive effects. *Proceedings of the American Association for Cancer Research,* Vol. 42, No. 2001), pp. 826.

de Lumen, B. O. (2005). Lunasin: a cancer-preventive soy peptide. *Nutrition reviews,* Vol. 63, No. 1, (January 2005), pp. 16-21. ISSN 0029-6643.

Doyle, J. J. & Luckow, M. A. (2003). The rest of the iceberg. Legume diversity and evolution in a phylogenetic context. *Plant Physiology,* Vol. 131, No. 3, (March 2003), pp. 900-910. ISSN 0032-0889.

Du, X.; Beloussow, K. & Shen, W. C. (2001). Bowman-Birk protease inhibitor and its palmitic acid conjugate prevent 7,12-dimethylbenz[a]anthracene-induced transformation in cultured mouse mammary glands. *Cancer Letters,* Vol. 164, No. 2, (March 2001), pp. 135-141. ISSN 0304-3835.

Erdman, J. W.; Badger, T. M.; Lampe, J. W.; Setchell, K. D. R. & Messina, M. (2004). Not All Soy Products Are Created Equal: Caution Needed in Interpretation of Research Results. *Journal of Nutrition,* Vol. 134, No. (May 2004), pp. 1229S-1233S. ISSN

Fernandes, A. O. & Banerji, A. P. (1997). Long-term feeding of field bean protein containing protease inhibitors suppresses virus-induced mammary tumors in mice. *Cancer Letters,* Vol. 116, No. 1, (June 1997), pp. 1-7. ISSN 0304-3835.

Fink, B. N.; Steck, S. E.; Wolff, M. S.; Britton, J. A.; Kabat, G. C.; Gaudet, M. M.; Abrahamson, P. E.; Bell, P.; Schroeder, J. C.; Teitelbaum, S. L.; Neugut, A. I. & Gammon, M. D. (2007). Dietary flavonoid intake and breast cancer survival among women on Long Island. *Cancer Epidemiology, Biomarkers & Prevention,* Vol. 16, No. 11, (November 2007), pp. 2285-2292. ISSN 1055-9965.

Folman, Y. & Pope, G. S. (1966). The interaction in the immature mouse of potent oestrogens with coumestrol, genistein and other utero-vaginotrophic compounds of low potency. *The Journal of endocrinology,* Vol. 34, No. 2, (February 1966), pp. 215-225. ISSN 0022-0795.

Fournier, D. B.; Erdman, J. W., Jr. & Gordon, G. B. (1998). Soy, its components, and cancer prevention: a review of the in vitro, animal, and human data. *Cancer Epidemiology, Biomarkers & Prevention,* Vol. 7, No. 11, (November 1998), pp. 1055-1065. ISSN 1055-9965.

Franke, A. A.; Custer, L. J.; Wang, W. & Shi, C. Y. (1998). HPLC analysis of isoflavonoids and other phenolic agents from foods and from human fluids. *Proceedings of the Society for Experimental Biology and Medicine,* Vol. 217, No. 3, (March 1998), pp. 263-273. ISSN 0037-9727.

Freitas, S.M.; Ikemoto, H. & Ventura, M.M. (1999). Thermodynamics of the binding of chymotrypsin with the black-eyed pea trypsin and chimotrypsin inhibitor (BTCI). *Journal of Protein Chemistry,* Vol. 18, No. 3. (April 1999), pp 307–313. ISSN 0277-8033.

Fritz, W. A.; Coward, L.; Wang, J. & Lamartiniere, C. A. (1998). Dietary genistein: perinatal mammary cancer prevention, bioavailability and toxicity testing in the rat. *Carcinogenesis,* Vol. 19, No. 12, (December 1998), pp. 2151-2158. ISSN 0143-3334.

Gallo, D.; Giacomelli, S.; Cantelmo, F.; Zannoni, G. F.; Ferrandina, G.; Fruscella, E.; Riva, A.; Morazzoni, P.; Bombardelli, E.; Mancuso, S. & Scambia, G. (2001). Chemoprevention of DMBA-induced mammary cancer in rats by dietary soy. *Breast cancer research and treatment,* Vol. 69, No. 2, (September 2001), pp. 153-164. ISSN 0167-6806.

Galvez, A. F. & de Lumen, B. O. (1999). A soybean cDNA encoding a chromatin-binding peptide inhibits mitosis of mammalian cells. *Nature Biotechnology,* Vol. 17, No. 5, (May 1999), pp. 495-500. ISSN 1087-0156.

Gepts, P.; Beavis, W. D.; Brummer, E. C.; Shoemaker, R. C.; Stalker, H. T.; Weeden, N. F. & Young, N. D. (2005). Legumes as a model plant family. Genomics for food and feed report of the Cross-Legume Advances Through Genomics Conference. *Plant Physiology,* Vol. 137, No. 4, (April 2005), pp. 1228-1235. ISSN 0032-0889.

Goldin, B. R.; Adlercreutz, H.; Gorbach, S. L.; Woods, M. N.; Dwyer, J. T.; Conlon, T.; Bohn, E. & Gershoff, S. N. (1986). The relationship between estrogen levels and diets of Caucasian American and Oriental immigrant women. *The American journal of clinical nutrition,* Vol. 44, No. 6, (December 1986), pp. 945-953. ISSN 0002-9165.

Gonzalez de Mejia, E.; Vasconez, M.; de Lumen, B. O. & Nelson, R. (2004). Lunasin concentration in different soybean genotypes, commercial soy protein, and isoflavone products. *Journal of agricultural and food chemistry,* Vol. 52, No. 19, (September 2004), pp. 5882-5887. ISSN 0021-8561.

Gu, L.; House, S. E.; Prior, R. L.; Fang, N.; Ronis, M. J.; Clarkson, T. B.; Wilson, M. E. & Badger, T. M. (2006). Metabolic phenotype of isoflavones differ among female rats, pigs, monkeys, and women. *The Journal of nutrition,* Vol. 136, No. 5, (May 2006), pp. 1215-1221. ISSN 0022-3166.

Guha, N.; Kwan, M. L.; Quesenberry, C. P., Jr.; Weltzien, E. K.; Castillo, A. L. & Caan, B. J. (2009). Soy isoflavones and risk of cancer recurrence in a cohort of breast cancer survivors: the Life After Cancer Epidemiology study. *Breast cancer research and treatment,* Vol. 118, No. 2, (November 2009), pp. 395-405. ISSN 1573-7217.

Guo, T. L.; Chi, R. P.; Hernandez, D. M.; Auttachoat, W. & Zheng, J. F. (2007). Decreased 7,12-dimethylbenz[a]anthracene-induced carcinogenesis coincides with the induction of antitumor immunities in adult female B6C3F1 mice pretreated with genistein. *Carcinogenesis,* Vol. 28, No. 12, (December 2007), pp. 2560-2566. ISSN 1460-2180.

Hargreaves, D. F.; Potten, C. S.; Harding, C.; Shaw, L. E.; Morton, M. S.; Roberts, S. A.; Howell, A. & Bundred, N. J. (1999). Two-week dietary soy supplementation has an estrogenic effect on normal premenopausal breast. *The Journal of clinical endocrinology and metabolism,* Vol. 84, No. 11, (November 1999), pp. 4017-4024. ISSN 0021-972X.

Helferich, W. G.; Andrade, J. E. & Hoagland, M. S. (2008). Phytoestrogens and breast cancer: a complex story. *Inflammopharmacology,* Vol. 16, No. 5, (October 2008), pp. 219-226. ISSN 0925-4692.

Hernandez-Ledesma, B. & de Lumen, B. O. (2008). Lunasin: a novel cancer preventive seed Peptide. *Perspectives in medicinal chemistry,* Vol. 2, pp. 75-80. ISSN 1177-391X.

Hernandez-Ledesma, B.; Hsieh, C. C. & de Lumen, B. O. (2009). Lunasin, a novel seed peptide for cancer prevention. *Peptides,* Vol. 30, No. 2, (February 2009), pp. 426-430. ISSN 0196-9781.

Ho, V. S. & Ng, T. B. (2008). A Bowman-Birk trypsin inhibitor with antiproliferative activity from Hokkaido large black soybeans. *Journal of Peptide Science,* Vol. 14, No. 3, (March 2008), pp. 278-282. ISSN 1075-2617.

Hsieh, C. C.; Hernandez-Ledesma, B.; Jeong, H. J.; Park, J. H. & de Lumen, B. O. (2010). Complementary roles in cancer prevention: protease inhibitor makes the cancer preventive peptide lunasin bioavailable. *PLoS One,* Vol. 5, No. 1, pp. e8890. ISSN 1932-6203.

Hsieh, C. Y.; Santell, R. C.; Haslam, S. Z. & Helferich, W. G. (1998). Estrogenic effects of genistein on the growth of estrogen receptor-positive human breast cancer (MCF-7) cells in vitro and in vivo. *Cancer Research,* Vol. 58, No. 17, (September 1998), pp. 3833-3838. ISSN 0008-5472.

Ito, A.; Goto, T.; Okamoto, T.; Yamada, K. & Roy, G. (1996). A combined effect of tamoxifen (Tam) and miso for the development of mammary tumors induced with MNU in SD rats. *Proceedings of the American Association for Cancer Research,* Vol. 37, pp. 271.

Jemal, A.; Bray, F.; Center, M. M.; Ferlay, J.; Ward, E. & Forman, D. (2011). Global cancer statistics. *CA: a cancer journal for clinicians,* Vol. 61, No. 2, (March 2011), pp. 69-90. ISSN 1542-4863.

Jeong, H. J.; Jeong, J. B.; Kim, D. S. & de Lumen, B. O. (2007). Inhibition of core histone acetylation by the cancer preventive peptide lunasin. *Journal of agricultural and food chemistry,* Vol. 55, No. 3, (February 2007), pp. 632-637. ISSN 0021-8561.

Jeong, H. J.; Park, J. H.; Lam, Y. & de Lumen, B. O. (2003). Characterization of lunasin isolated from soybean. *Journal of agricultural and food chemistry,* Vol. 51, No. 27, (December 2003), pp. 7901-7906. ISSN 0021-8561.

Jin, Z. & MacDonald, R. S. (2002). Soy isoflavones increase latency of spontaneous mammary tumors in mice. *The Journal of nutrition,* Vol. 132, No. 10, (October 2002), pp. 3186-3190. ISSN 0022-3166.

Joanitti, G. A.; Azevedo, R. B. & Freitas, S. M. (2010). Apoptosis and lysosome membrane permeabilization induction on breast cancer cells by an anticarcinogenic Bowman-Birk protease inhibitor from Vigna unguiculata seeds. *Cancer Letters,* Vol. 293, No. 1, (July 2010), pp. 73-81. ISSN 1872-7980.

Joanitti, G. A.; Freitas, S. M. & Silva, L. P. (2006). Proteinaceous Protease Inhibitors: Structural Features and Multiple Functional Faces. *Current Enzyme Inhibition,* Vol. 2, No. 3, (August 2006), pp. 199-217. ISSN

Kang, X.; Zhang, Q.; Wang, S.; Huang, X. & Jin, S. (2010). Effect of soy isoflavones on breast cancer recurrence and death for patients receiving adjuvant endocrine therapy. *Canadian Medical Association Journal,* Vol. 182, No. 17, (November 2010), pp. 1857-1862. ISSN 1488-2329.

Kennedy, A. R. (1998). The Bowman-Birk inhibitor from soybeans as an anticarcinogenic agent. *The American journal of clinical nutrition,* Vol. 68, No. 6 Suppl, (December 1998), pp. 1406S-1412S. ISSN 0002-9165.

Kuiper, G. G.; Lemmen, J. G.; Carlsson, B.; Corton, J. C.; Safe, S. H.; van der Saag, P. T.; van der Burg, B. & Gustafsson, J. A. (1998). Interaction of estrogenic chemicals and phytoestrogens with estrogen receptor beta. *Endocrinology,* Vol. 139, No. 10, (October 1998), pp. 4252-4263. ISSN 0013-7227.

Lajolo, F. M. & Genovese, M. I. (2002). Nutritional significance of lectins and enzyme inhibitors from legumes. *Journal of agricultural and food chemistry,* Vol. 50, No. 22, (October 2002), pp. 6592-6598. ISSN 0021-8561.

Lamartiniere, C. A. (2000). Protection against breast cancer with genistein: a component of soy. *The American journal of clinical nutrition,* Vol. 71, No. 6 Suppl, (June 2000), pp. 1705S-1707S. ISSN 0002-9165.

Lamartiniere, C. A.; Murrill, W. B.; Manzolillo, P. A.; Zhang, J. X.; Barnes, S.; Zhang, X.; Wei, H. & Brown, N. M. (1998). Genistein alters the ontogeny of mammary gland development and protects against chemically-induced mammary cancer in rats. *Proceedings of the Society for Experimental Biology and Medicine,* Vol. 217, No. 3, (March 1998), pp. 358-364. ISSN 0037-9727.

Lane, D. (2006). Designer combination therapy for cancer. *Nature Biotechnology,* Vol. 24, No. 2, (February 2006), pp. 163-164. ISSN 1087-0156.

Laskowski, M., & M. A. Qasim (2000). What can the structures of enzyme-inhibitor complexes tell us about the structures of enzyme substrate complexes? *Biochimica et Biophysica Acta,* Vol. 1477, (March 2000), pp. 324–337. ISSN 0006-3002.

Losso, J. N. (2008). The biochemical and functional food properties of the bowman-birk inhibitor. *Critical reviews in food science and nutrition,* Vol. 48, No. 1, (January 2008), pp. 94-118. ISSN 1040-8398.

Lu, L. J.; Anderson, K. E.; Grady, J. J.; Kohen, F. & Nagamani, M. (2000). Decreased ovarian hormones during a soya diet: implications for breast cancer prevention. *Cancer Research,* Vol. 60, No. 15, (August 2000), pp. 4112-4121. ISSN 0008-5472.

Martinez-Montemayor, M. M.; Otero-Franqui, E.; Martinez, J.; De La Mota-Peynado, A.; Cubano, L. A. & Dharmawardhane, S. (2010). Individual and combined soy isoflavones exert differential effects on metastatic cancer progression. *Clinical & experimental metastasis,* Vol. 27, No. 7, (October 2010), pp. 465-480. ISSN 1573-7276.

Messina, M. (2010). Insights gained from 20 years of soy research. *The Journal of nutrition,* Vol. 140, No. 12, (December 2010), pp. 2289S-2295S. ISSN 1541-6100.

Messina, M.; Abrams, D. I. & Hardy, M. (2010). Can clinicians now assure their breast cancer patients that soyfoods are safe? *Womens Health,* Vol. 6, No. 3, (May 2010), pp. 335-338. ISSN 1745-5065.

Messina, M.; McCaskill-Stevens, W. & Lampe, J. W. (2006). Addressing the soy and breast cancer relationship: review, commentary, and workshop proceedings. *Journal of the National Cancer Institute,* Vol. 98, No. 18, (September 2006), pp. 1275-1284. ISSN 1460-2105.

Messina, M. & Wu, A. H. (2009). Perspectives on the soy-breast cancer relation. *The American journal of clinical nutrition,* Vol. 89, No. 5, (May 2009), pp. 1673S-1679S. ISSN 1938-3207.

Messina, M. J. & Loprinzi, C. L. (2001). Soy for breast cancer survivors: a critical review of the literature. *The Journal of nutrition,* Vol. 131, No. 11, (November 2001), pp. 3095S-3108S. ISSN 0022-3166.

Messina, M. J. & Wood, C. E. (2008). Soy isoflavones, estrogen therapy, and breast cancer risk: analysis and commentary. *Nutrition journal,* Vol. 7, No. 2008), pp. 17. ISSN 1475-2891.

Mishra, R.; Tiwari, A.; Bhadauria, S.; Mishra, J.; Murthy, P. K. & Murthy, P. S. (2010). Therapeutic effect of centchroman alone and in combination with glycine soya on 7,12-dimethylbenz[alpha]anthracene-induced breast tumor in rat. *Food and Chemical Toxicology,* Vol. 48, No. 6, (June 2010), pp. 1587-1591. ISSN 1873-6351.

Murphy, P. A.; Song, T.; Buseman, G.; Barua, K.; Beecher, G. R.; Trainer, D. & Holden, J. (1999). Isoflavones in retail and institutional soy foods. *Journal of agricultural and food chemistry,* Vol. 47, No. 7, (July 1999), pp. 2697-2704. ISSN 0021-8561.

Murrill, W. B.; Brown, N. M.; Zhang, J. X.; Manzolillo, P. A.; Barnes, S. & Lamartiniere, C. A. (1996). Prepubertal genistein exposure suppresses mammary cancer and enhances gland differentiation in rats. *Carcinogenesis,* Vol. 17, No. 7, (July 1996), pp. 1451-1457. ISSN 0143-3334.

Padilla-Banks, E.; Jefferson, W. N. & Newbold, R. R. (2006). Neonatal exposure to the phytoestrogen genistein alters mammary gland growth and developmental programming of hormone receptor levels. *Endocrinology,* Vol. 147, No. 10, (October 2006), pp. 4871-4882. ISSN 0013-7227.

Park, J. H.; Jeong, H. J. & de Lumen, B. O. (2005). Contents and bioactivities of lunasin, bowman-birk inhibitor, and isoflavones in soybean seed. *Journal of agricultural and food chemistry,* Vol. 53, No. 20, (October 2005), pp. 7686-7690. ISSN 0021-8561.

Pasqualini, J. R. & Chetrite, G. S. (2005). Recent insight on the control of enzymes involved in estrogen formation and transformation in human breast cancer. *The Journal of steroid biochemistry and molecular biology,* Vol. 93, No. 2-5, (February 2005), pp. 221-236. ISSN 0960-0760.

Patisaul, H. B. & Jefferson, W. (2010). The pros and cons of phytoestrogens. *Frontiers in neuroendocrinology,* Vol. 31, No. 4, (October 2010), pp. 400-419. ISSN 1095-6808.

Peterson, G. & Barnes, S. (1996). Genistein inhibits both estrogen and growth factor-stimulated proliferation of human breast cancer cells. *Cell Growth & Differentiation,* Vol. 7, No. 10, (October 1996), pp. 1345-1351. ISSN 1044-9523.

Petrakis, N. L.; Barnes, S.; King, E. B.; Lowenstein, J.; Wiencke, J.; Lee, M. M.; Miike, R.; Kirk, M. & Coward, L. (1996). Stimulatory influence of soy protein isolate on breast secretion in pre- and postmenopausal women. *Cancer Epidemiology, Biomarkers & Prevention,* Vol. 5, No. 10, (October 1996), pp. 785-794. ISSN 1055-9965.

Rochfort, S. & Panozzo, J. (2007). Phytochemicals for health, the role of pulses. *Journal of agricultural and food chemistry,* Vol. 55, No. 20, (October 2007), pp. 7981-7994. ISSN 0021-8561.

Ruiz-Larrea, M. B.; Mohan, A. R.; Paganga, G.; Miller, N. J.; Bolwell, G. P. & Rice-Evans, C. A. (1997). Antioxidant activity of phytoestrogenic isoflavones. *Free Radical Research,* Vol. 26, No. 1, (January 1997), pp. 63-70. ISSN 1071-5762.

Ryan, C. A. (1990). Protease inhibitors in plants: Genes for improving defenses against insects and pathogens. *Annual Review of Phytopathology,* Vol. 28, pp. 425–449.

Sakla, M. S.; Shenouda, N. S.; Ansell, P. J.; Macdonald, R. S. & Lubahn, D. B. (2007). Genistein affects HER2 protein concentration, activation, and promoter regulation in BT-474 human breast cancer cells. *Endocrine,* Vol. 32, No. 1, (August 2007), pp. 69-78. ISSN 1355-008X.

Shimizu, H.; Ross, R. K.; Bernstein, L.; Pike, M. C. & Henderson, B. E. (1990). Serum oestrogen levels in postmenopausal women: comparison of American whites and Japanese in Japan. *British journal of cancer,* Vol. 62, No. 3, (September 1990), pp. 451-453. ISSN 0007-0920.

Shu, X. O.; Jin, F.; Dai, Q.; Wen, W.; Potter, J. D.; Kushi, L. H.; Ruan, Z.; Gao, Y. T. & Zheng, W. (2001). Soyfood intake during adolescence and subsequent risk of breast cancer among Chinese women. *Cancer Epidemiology, Biomarkers & Prevention,* Vol. 10, No. 5, (May 2001), pp. 483-488. ISSN 1055-9965.

Shu, X. O.; Zheng, Y.; Cai, H.; Gu, K.; Chen, Z.; Zheng, W. & Lu, W. (2009). Soy food intake and breast cancer survival. *Jama,* Vol. 302, No. 22, (December 2009), pp. 2437-2443. ISSN 1538-3598.

Silva, L. P.; Leite, J. R. S. A.; Jr., C. B. & Freitas, S. M. (2001). Thermal stability of a black eyed pea trypsin/chymotrypsin inhibitor (BTCI). *Protein and Peptide Letters,* Vol. 7, No. 2001), pp. 397–401. ISSN

So, F. V.; Guthrie, N.; Chambers, A. F. & Carroll, K. K. (1997). Inhibition of proliferation of estrogen receptor-positive MCF-7 human breast cancer cells by flavonoids in the presence and absence of excess estrogen. *Cancer Letters,* Vol. 112, No. 2, (January 1997), pp. 127-133. ISSN 0304-3835.

Theil, C.; Briese, V.; Gerber, B. & Richter, D. U. (2010). The effects of different lignans and isoflavones, tested as aglycones and glycosides, on hormone receptor-positive and -negative breast carcinoma cells in vitro. *Archives of gynecology and obstetrics,* Vol. No. (September 2010), pp. ISSN 1432-0711.

Trock, B. J.; Hilakivi-Clarke, L. & Clarke, R. (2006). Meta-analysis of soy intake and breast cancer risk. *Journal of the National Cancer Institute,* Vol. 98, No. 7, (April 2006), pp. 459-471. ISSN 1460-2105.

Velie, E. M.; Schairer, C.; Flood, A.; He, J. P.; Khattree, R. & Schatzkin, A. (2005). Empirically derived dietary patterns and risk of postmenopausal breast cancer in a large prospective cohort study. *The American journal of clinical nutrition,* Vol. 82, No. 6, (December 2005), pp. 1308-1319. ISSN 0002-9165.

Ventura, M.M.; Xavier-Filho, J. (1966). A trypsin and chymotrypsin inhibitor from black-eyed pea (*Vigna sinensis*).I. Purification and partial characterization. *Anais da Academia Brasileira de Ciências,* Vol. 38 (1966), pp 553–566.

Verheus, M.; van Gils, C. H.; Keinan-Boker, L.; Grace, P. B.; Bingham, S. A. & Peeters, P. H. (2007). Plasma phytoestrogens and subsequent breast cancer risk. *Journal of Clinical Oncology,* Vol. 25, No. 6, (February 2007), pp. 648-655. ISSN 1527-7755.

Wan, X. S.; Hamilton, T. C.; Ware, J. H.; Donahue, J. J. & Kennedy, A. R. (1998). Growth inhibition and cytotoxicity induced by Bowman-Birk inhibitor concentrate in cisplatin-resistant human ovarian cancer cells. *Nutrition and cancer,* Vol. 31, No. 1, 1998), pp. 8-17. ISSN 0163-5581.

Wan, X. S.; Lu, L. J.; Anderson, K. E.; Ware, J. H. & Kennedy, A. R. (2000). Urinary excretion of Bowman-Birk inhibitor in humans after soy consumption as determined by a monoclonal antibody-based immunoassay. *Cancer Epidemiology, Biomarkers & Prevention,* Vol. 9, No. 7, (July 2000), pp. 741-747. ISSN 1055-9965.

Wang, J. & Shen, W. C. (2000). Gastric retention and stability of lipidized Bowman-Birk protease inhibitor in mice. *International journal of pharmaceutics,* Vol. 204, No. 1-2, (August 2000), pp. 111-116. ISSN 0378-5173.

Wang, T. T.; Sathyamoorthy, N. & Phang, J. M. (1996). Molecular effects of genistein on estrogen receptor mediated pathways. *Carcinogenesis,* Vol. 17, No. 2, (February 1996), pp. 271-275. ISSN 0143-3334.

Willett, W. C. (1995). Diet, nutrition, and avoidable cancer. *Environmental health perspectives,* Vol. 103, No. 8, (November 1995), pp. 165-170. ISSN 0091-6765.

Wu, A. H.; Ziegler, R. G.; Horn-Ross, P. L.; Nomura, A. M.; West, D. W.; Kolonel, L. N.; Rosenthal, J. F.; Hoover, R. N. & Pike, M. C. (1996). Tofu and risk of breast cancer in Asian-Americans. *Cancer Epidemiology, Biomarkers & Prevention,* Vol. 5, No. 11, (November 1996), pp. 901-906. ISSN 1055-9965.

Yan, L.; Li, D. & Yee, J. A. (2002). Dietary supplementation with isolated soy protein reduces metastasis of mammary carcinoma cells in mice. *Clinical & experimental metastasis,* Vol. 19, No. 6, 2002), pp. 535-540. ISSN 0262-0898.

Ye, X. & Ng, T. B. (2009). A trypsin-chymotrypsin inhibitor with antiproliferative activity from small glossy black soybeans. *Planta Medica,* Vol. 75, No. 5, (April 2009), pp. 550-556. ISSN 1439-0221.

Zhang, L.; Wan, X. S.; Donahue, J. J.; Ware, J. H. & Kennedy, A. R. (1999). Effects of the Bowman-Birk inhibitor on clonogenic survival and cisplatin- or radiation-induced cytotoxicity in human breast, cervical, and head and neck cancer cells. *Nutrition and cancer,* Vol. 33, No. 2, 1999), pp. 165-173. ISSN 0163-5581.

Zheng, W.; Dai, Q.; Custer, L. J.; Shu, X. O.; Wen, W. Q.; Jin, F. & Franke, A. A. (1999). Urinary excretion of isoflavonoids and the risk of breast cancer. *Cancer Epidemiology, Biomarkers & Prevention,* Vol. 8, No. 1, (January 1999), pp. 35-40. ISSN 1055-9965.

Zhou, J. R.; Yu, L.; Mai, Z. & Blackburn, G. L. (2004). Combined inhibition of estrogen-dependent human breast carcinoma by soy and tea bioactive components in mice. *International journal of cancer,* Vol. 108, No. 1, (January 2004), pp. 8-14. ISSN 0020-7136.

8

Experimental Therapeutics in Breast Cancer Cells

Weena Jiratchariyakul[1] and Tanawan Kummalue[2]
[1]*Department of Pharmacognosy, Faculty of Pharmacy, Mahidol University, Bangkok*
[2]*Department of Clinical Pathology, Faculty of Medicine Siriraj Hospital, Mahidol University, Bangkok*
Thailand

1. Introduction

Many cancer patients have medicated themselves with traditional herbal remedies, which are mostly composed of a single or combined medicinal plants. The effectiveness of the remedies can be explained by the presence of the phytochemicals and the bioactivity. The investigators select the traditional-used and evidence-based herbs for the research and development. The investigation of the following Thai herbs and their reasonable utilization are presented.

2. The selected medicinal plants

2.1 Single plant

2.1.1 *Trichosanthes cucumerina* L.

It is a cucurbitaceous vine, grooved stem with scattered hairs and tendrils. The leaf is simple, alternate, five-lobed margin and 8-12 cm blade width. It is dioecious, the male flower is white and the female yellow. The fruit is round with pointed ends and green striped lengthwise, usually 3-4 cm wide and 5-6 cm long (Fig. 1).

It is distributed wildly in the tropical Asia, climbs over the big trees along the riverside and mixed forest. The fruit is very bitter and inedible. It is used for shampooing to relieve itching, dandruff and lice. The fruit and the aerial plant parts are the ingredients in traditional Thai herbal medicine for dizziness. The dried fruit is ground, mixed with tobacco and smoked to alleviate the asthma. The seed (20-30 seeds) is an emetic, antidysentery, febrifuge, emenagogue and anthelmintic. The root decoction is laxative, febrifuge and used to relieve headach and bronchitis. The vine is decocted and used as febrifuge, laxative and tonic.

The bitterness of *T. cucumerina* fruit arises from the presence of cucurbitacins, the highly oxygenated C30-triterpenes, which are frequently found in the cucurbitaceous plants. The fruit juice was extracted with diethyl ether. The extract was concentrated and the crystalline solid was produced. The marc was continuously extracted with petroleum ether, chloroform and methanol in a Soxhlet apparatus. We tested the biological activities of the fruit juice, crystalline solid (TC compound) and the methanol extract. The fruit juice which was prepared as lyophilized (spray dried) solid, did not inhibit the standard strains of the microorganism (*E. coli, S. aureus, B. subtitis, M. smegmatis* and *C. albicans*), whereas the

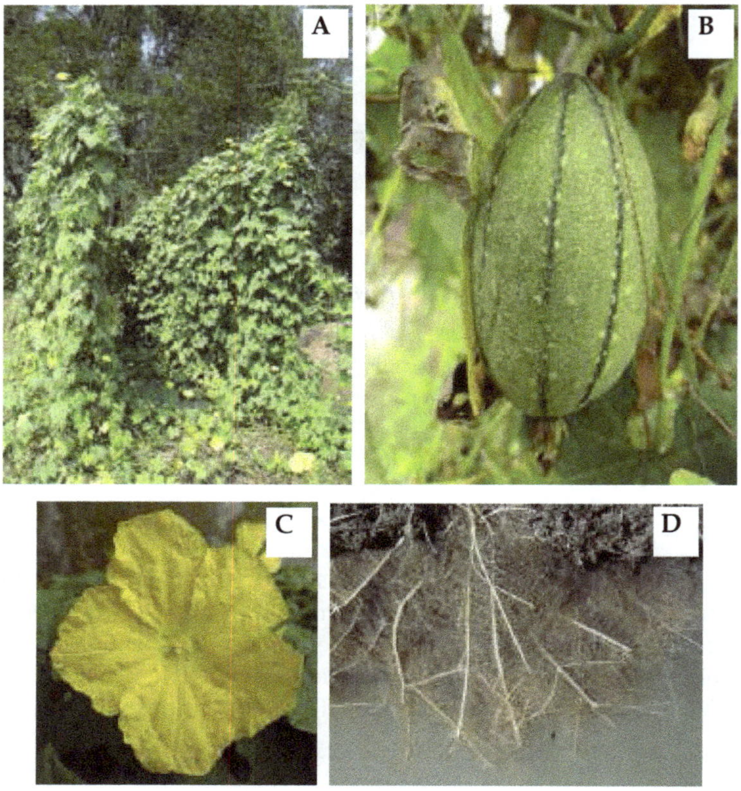

Fig. 1. *Trichosanthes cucumerina* L. : A whole plant; B fruit; C flower; D root.

methanol extract inhibited *S. aureus, M. smegmatis* and had a bactericidal action against *C. diptheriae* (Tiangda et al, 1986). TC compound comprised cucurbitacin B (Fig. 2) and dihydrocucurbitacin B, which had a strongly cytotoxic action, in vitro, against KB cell (human nasopharynx carcinoma cell) (Silapaarcha et al, 1981; Jiratchariyakul et al, 1992).

The MTT colorimetric assay for cytotoxicity against breast cancer cell line (SKBR3) of the TC compound, cucurbitacin B and dihydrocucurbitacin B resulted the ED_{50} of 0.48, 0.05 and 0.40 μg/mL, respectively (Jiratchariyakul et al, 1999). The lyophilized fruit juice of 5 mg/kg body weight was injected peritoneally to Swiss albino mice exhibited no sign of toxicity as in the control group. The LD_{50} of the juice was 13 mg/kg body weight, which was considered as moderate toxicity according to Casarett and Doull (Tiangda et al, 1986; Casarett & Doull, 1975).

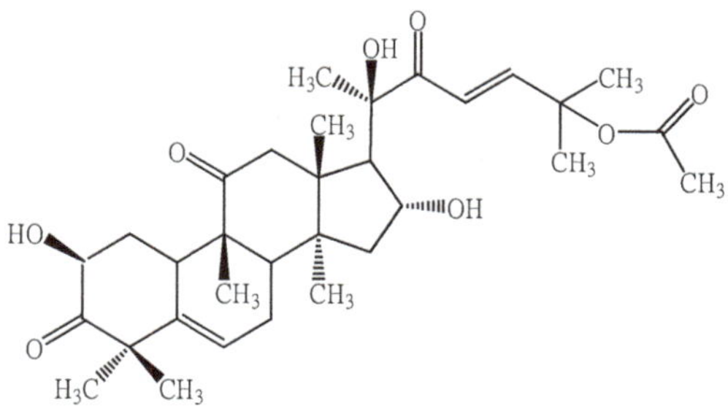

Fig. 2. Structure of cucurbitacin B.

The antiproriferative effect of the fruit juice and the isolated cucurbitacin against four breast cancer cell lines was further carried out. The cell lines included SKBR3, MCF7, T47D and MDA-MB435. SKBR3 is a human breast cancer cell line with overexpression of the HER2/neu receptor and absence of the ER receptor. In contrast, T47D and MCF7 are breast cancer cell lines that are ER receptor positive and HER2/neu negative, whereas the MDA-MB435 breast cancer cell line, both the ER receptor and HER2/neu expressions are absent (Table 1).

Breast cancer cell lines	ER receptor	HER2/neu	IC_{50} (μg/mL)		Doxorubicin (positive control)
			Lyophilized fruit juice	Cucurbitacin B	
MDA-MB435	Negative	Negative	155.77 ± 0.14	25.84 ± 0.83	0.48 ± 0.05
SKBR3	Negative	Overexpressed	130.52 ± 0.17	73.29 ± 0.88	0.65 ± 0.13
MCF7	Positive	Negative	374.77 ± 0.19	34.52 ± 0.11	0.62 ± 0.04
T47D	Positive	Negative	249.32 ± 0.40	60.26 ± 0.61	0.63 ± 0.04

Table 1. Cytotoxicity of the fruit juice of *T. cucumerina* (Kongtun et al., 2009).

The mechanism that cucurbitacin B inhibits the breast cancer cell can be explained through the increased telomerase expression, which is associated with the neoplastic growth. Over 90% of breast cancer has highly telomerase expression. We investigated the effect of cucurbitacin B on telomerase activity. Cucurbitacin B inhibited telomerase activity especially in the ER-negative breast cancer cell SKBR3 with IC_{50} of 3.29 μg/mL, wheras TC compound 4.6 μg/mL and the lyophilized fruit juice less than 10 μg/mL. The activity of human telomerase reverse transcriptase (hTERT) and the level of c-Myc protein were also decreased by cucurbitacin B. Thus cucurbitacin B possibly inhibited the breast cancer cell by reducing the telomerase activity via down regulating both hTERT and c-Myc expressions (Duangmano et al, 2010). Cucurbitacin B inhibited also lung and especially colon cancer cell lines (Kummalue et al, 2009). The recent research indicated the strong cancerostatic action of cucurbitacins B which worked through Jak/STAT-signal ways (Jak = Janus-kinase; STAT = signal transducer and activator of transcription). Cucurbitacin B specifically inhibited STAT 3 which involved in the formation of interleukin 6 (IL-6), an important mediator in immune system (Haensel & Sticher, 2007). Cucurbitacin B was possible to act as immunosuppressive agent according to its inhibition of PHA-activated PBMC (U-pratya et al, 2010).

2.1.2 *Murdannia loriformis* (Hassk.) Rolla Rao et Kammathy

M. loriformis is commelinaceous, and monocotyledonous, perennial herb, about 10 cm high. The leaves are simple, glabrous, and alternate. The leaf blade is linear about 1.5-2.0 cm wide, 15-20 cm long. The flowers are inflorescence, terminal and densely panicle. The pedicels slightly curved, translucent bracts about 4 mm, sepal ovate-elliptic, about 3 mm; petals blue or bluish violet (Fig.3). The plant is also used in traditional Chinese medicine as a remedy for detoxification and respiratory tract complaints (Book of traditional Chinese medicine in Sichuan, 1992).

For over 30 years pressed herb juice from *M. loriformis* has been used to support self-medication in Thailand by patients who suffer from different types of cancer. It is supposed to prolong the patient's life and reduce the side effects resulting from modern therapy (radiation and chemotherapy) (Report from the first seminar on herbs and cancer, 1988).

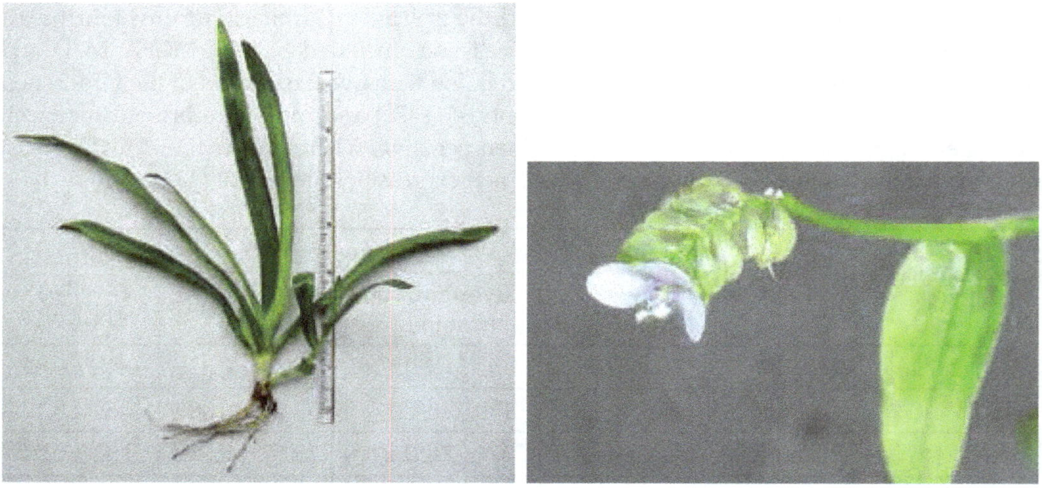

Fig. 3. *Murdannia loriformis* Rolla Rao et Kammathy.

The phytochemical work on this plant indicated the presence of cytotoxic glycosphingolipid namely 1β-*O*-D-glucopyranosyl-2-(2′-hydroxy-6′-ene-cosamide)-sphingosine (Fig. 4) which had moderate cytotoxicity with ED_{50} of 10.7, 15.6, 18.9 and 32.5 $\mu molL^{-1}$ against human breast, lung, colon and liver cancer cell lines, respectively, whereas the positive control (quercetin) had the ED_{50} of 23.2, 13.2, 24.8 and 59.6 $\mu molL^{-1}$, respectively (Jiratchariyakul et at., 1997, 1998, 2006).

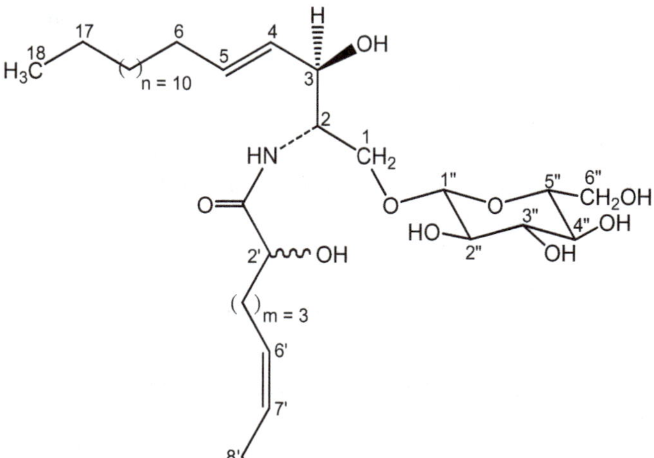

Fig. 4. Structure of 1β-*O*-D-glucopyranosyl-2-(2′-hydroxy-6′-ene-cosamide)-sphingosine, a glycosphingolipid from *M. loriformis.*

The investigation of the indirect (immune-mediated) cytotoxicity was also carried out. The pressed herb juice and the isolated cytotoxic glycosphingolipid were not toxic to the peripheral blood mononuclear cells (PBMCs) in vitro. Both increased PBMCs proliferation in the presence of the mitogen PHA (phytohaemagglutinin); the glycosphingolipid had the stronger effect. The pressed juice slightly increased the CD3, 4 : CD3, 8 ratio in the 3 day culture and the glycosphingolipid increased this ratio at both the 3 and 7 day cultures. They were the indicative of an in vitro immunomodulatory effect of the pressed juice and the glycosphingolipid (Jiratchariyakul et al., 2006).

The pressed juice had LD_{50}, orally in rats, more than 120 g/kg body weight, and did not damage the growth, the blood chemistry and the pathology of organs. It was safe according to World Health Organization (Tappayuthpijarn et al., 1991; Intayot et al., 2002). The sub-chronic toxicity study of *M. loriformis* in rats for 3 months did not damage the growth, the blood chemistry and the pathology of organs (Tappayuthpijarn et al., 1991). The ethanol extract of this plant induced in vitro DT-diaphorase, a detoxifying enzyme (Vinitketkumnuen, 1996), and decreased in vivo the formation of aberrant crypt foci (ACF), which was related to the colon cancer (Intayot et al., 2002).

2.1.3 *Ficus hispida* L. f.

F. hispida is a traditional Thai plant from family Moraceae. It is a moderate sized tree and grows well in damp and shady place (Fig. 5). Almost all parts of this plant can be used in traditional medicine for the treatment of various ailments, for example, an anti-diarrhea, emetic, astringent, hepatoprotective, antitussive, antipyretic, antiinflammatory, depurative, vulnerary, hemostatic, antiulcer as well as in the treatment of anemia (Wuttidhammaved, 1997; Mandal and Ashok Kumar, 2002; Peraza-Sanchez et al., 2002).

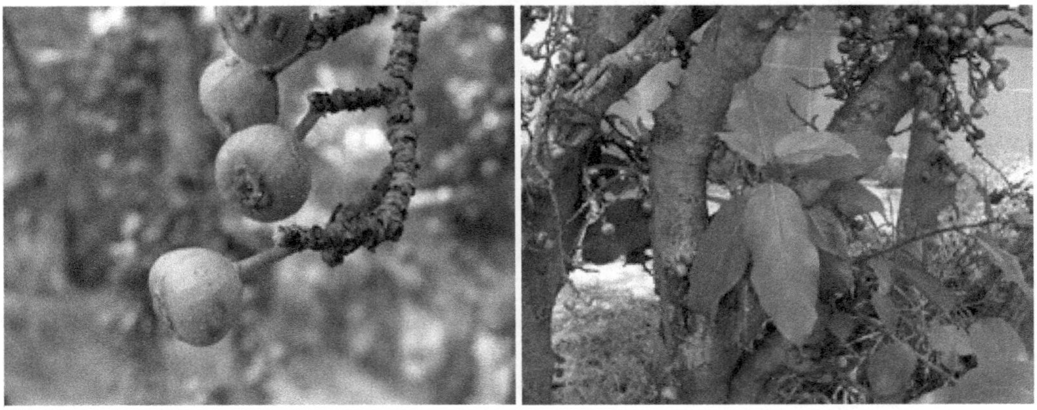

Fig. 5. *Ficus hispida* L. f.

F. hispida, was investigated for antiproliferative activity on human breast cancer cell lines: SKBR3, MDA-MB435, T47D, and MCF7. Based on the results, the methanolic extract exhibited the most powerful activity on T47D breast cancer cell line with ED_{50} of 110.3±9.63 μg/mL as compared to DMSO, the negative control. Confirmation of the result using colony-forming assay (clonogenic assay) yielded the effect in a dose - dependent manner. The cell cycle analysis of this plant extract revealed non-specificity with prominent in apoptosis. Therefore, *F. hispida* might provide some benefits in the treatment of breast cancer. (Pratumvinit et al., 2009)

2.1.4 *Erycibe elliptilimba* Merr. & Chun.

Erycibe elliptilimba, belonging to the Convolvulaceae family, is a Thai medicinal plant that has long been used for many decades to relieve symptoms from fever caused by infection, inflammation and prescribed in the mixture of traditional medicine for treating of various malignancies (Wuttidhammaved, 1997; Sintusarn, 2002).

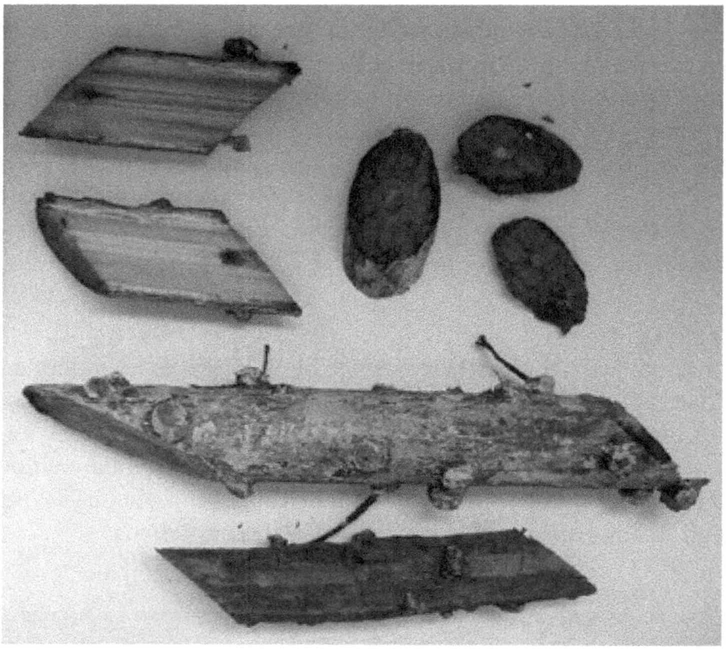

Fig. 6. *Erycibe elliptilimba* Merr. & Chun.

The ED_{50} values of the methanol fraction against SKBR3 and MDA-MB435 were 56.07 and 30.61 μg/mL, respectively. Doxorubicin as a positive control. This inhibitory growth activity of the treated cells acted in a dose-dependent manner which was also confirmed by the cell viability with the trypan blue exclusion assay. (Kummalue et al., 2007).

2.2 Herbal mixture

Two Thai remedies (TR1 and TR2) were tested for antiproliferative effect. TR1 was composed of following ingredients : *Albizia procera* (stem), *Diospyros mollis* (stem), *Ficus hispida* (stem), *Smilax glabra* (stem), *Smilax china* (stem) and cobra bone. TR2 was composed of *Gelonium multiflorum* (stem), *Erycibe elliptilimba* (stem), *Balanophora abbreviate* (stem), *Smilax glabra* (stem), *Smilax china* (stem) and *Millingtonia hortensis* (stem). TR1 and TR2 had no antiproliferative effect on breast, lung and colon cancer cell lines. However the combination of the remedies (either TR1 or TR2, 30 μg/mL) with doxorubicin (0.5 μg/mL) could significantly inhibit growth of lung cancer cell line (A549) at G2/M phase stronger than doxorubicin alone (Srisapoomi et al., 2008).

In addition two Thai medicinal plants, they were *P. indica and S. rarax*, were tested for antiproliferative effect. *P. indica* inhibited the leukemic cancer cells (NB4, HT93A) (U-pratya et al., 2008) and *S. rarax* inhibited the lung cancer cell (A549) (Kummalue et al., 2011). Both did not inhibit the breast cancer cell.

3. The herbal preparation

The usage of herbs nowadays has been developed according to the laboratory evidence. Herbs are prepared as drug materials, which are conformed to the following pattern (Dingermann, 2000).

- The nature (crude drug, tincture, pressed juice, fluidextract, dry extract, etc.) of the drug material (drug composition) must be specified.
- The quantity of the drug material in each dose of the solid dosage form (tablets) or in each package of the liquid dosage form must be specified.

  For example: 200 mg dry extract / tablet or
  100 mL fluidextract
- The drug extract ratio (DER), the amount (g) of crude drug to produce one g extract or drug material, and the extraction method must be specified.
- The solvent or solvent mixture used for the extraction must be specified.
- The indication must be conformed to the monograph established by the Ministry of the Public Health, or supported by the clinical evidence.
- The daily dose must be specified as the weight of the crude drug.

  For example :

labeled DER	=	4-6.7 : 1
recommended daily dose	=	500 mg extract
thus, the daily dose	=	2-3.35 g crude drug.

3.1 The preparation of *Trichosanthes cucumerina*

- Declaration

  The drug material comprises pressed juice from *T. cucumerina* fruit, which is standardized with cucurbitacin B, a specific marker compound.
- DER

  10.5:1

  One g pressed juice is prepared from 10.5 g fresh fruit.
- According to the preparation which is made from the pressed juice it is non-drug and can be considered as traditional remedy (Haensel & Hoelzl, 1996). The indication is supported by the laboratory evidence and the traditional use. It is supposed to be used as natural cytostatic agent.
- The daily dose

  10.5 g fresh fruit

3.2 The preparation of *Murdannia loriformis*

- Declaration

  The drug material comprises pressed juice from *M. loriformis* herb, which is standardized with glycosphingolipid namely 1β-*O*-D-glucopyranosyl-2-(2′-hydroxy-6′-ene-cosamide)-sphingosine, a specific marker compound.
- DER

  1.7:1

  One g pressed juice is prepared from 1.7 g fresh herb.

- According to the preparation made from the pressed juice it is non-drug and can be considered as traditional remedy (Haensel & Hoelzl, 1996). The indication can be supported by the traditional use over 30 years and the case reported by the physicians. To use as an adjunct to anticancer therapy in order to reduce the side effects and prevent the cancer metastasis.
- The daily dose

  100 g fresh herb (aerial plant parts)

4. Breast cancer cells and experimental procedure in antiproliferative activity background

Breast cancer is one of the leading causes of cancer death around the world. In Thailand, the incidence of breast cancer disease accounts for 20.5 per 100,000 female population (Chaiwerawatana, 2007). Though breast cancer treatment nowadays has dramatically improved due to new drug emerging such as monoclonal antibody, and tyrosine kinase inhibitor, the resistance to the drug itself, unfortunately, has significantly increased. Therefore, searching for the new drug to treat breast cancer is very essential. Based on this important issue, four specific breast cancer cell lines, i.e., SKBR3, MCF7, T47D, and MDA-MB435 have been used to evaluate the potential and promising chemotherapeutic agents from medicinal plants sources.

These four breast cancer cell lines, SKBR3, MCF7, T47D, and MDA-MB435, have different origins and properties which are considered as the very useful tools for investigating the medicinal plants effects. Actually, medicinal plants have long been prescribed for over centuries to treat various diseases including infections and malignancies such as breast cancer in many countries, for example, China, and Thailand. This traditional medicine nowadays plays an important role in healthcare system with approximately 80% of people around the world using it (Itharat and Ooraikul, 2007). Determination of the plants activities especially growth inhibition and their mechanisms for cancer therapy is, indeed, undergoing in much effort.

In this section, four breast cancer cell lines and their experiments on medicinal plants are demonstrated. These include antiproliferative activity and cytotoxicity, cell cycle study, apoptotic study, mechanisms of action in plants, and future direction for testing the drugs from plant sources. Most of the experiments are performed in the biosafety level 1 which is suitable enough for manipulating these breast cancer cell lines in vitro.

4.1 Breast cancer cell lines: Their origins and properties

Breast cancer cell lines can be categorized into three groups according to their phenotypes and invasiveness (Lacroix and Leclercq, 2004).

The first group is luminal epithelial-like cells. This group expresses high amount of typical luminal epithelial phenotype of breast cells such as estrogen receptor (ER), E-cadherin (gene CDH1), zonula occludens-1(TJP1), desmoplakin I/II (DSP), and desmosomal junctions. This group of breast cancer cells will grow as interconnected colonies of polygonal cells on plastic and as fused colonies in Matrigel, which is semisolid medium. This kind of cells are weakly invasive. BT-483, MCF7, T47D, and ZR-75 are all in this group.

The second group is called weakly luminal epithelial-like cells. This group of cells shows the expression closely to the first group with a reduced extent or at least some of those markers.

Cells are weakly invasive in vitro. In Matrigel, most of these cells grow as non-fused spheres. Moreover, on plastic, they will accumulate in clusters of loosely attached cells and rarely reach full confluency. Breast cancer cell lines in this group are BT-474, CAMA-1, MDA-MB134, MDA-MB361, MDA-MB453, MDA-MB468, and SKBR3.

The third group is mesenchymal-like or stromal-like cells. It does not express the markers found in the first and second group. In contrast, it exhibits a high level of vimentin (gene VIM) which is the marker of mesenchymal cells. These cells have fibroblastoid phenotype on plastic and grow as colonies with large stellate projections in Matrigel. They are highly invasive in vitro. MDA-MB435S, MDA-MB231, Hs578T, and BT-549 are classified in this group.

Herein, details of breast cancer cell lines which have been employed in our medicinal plant research are demonstrated.

4.1.1 SKBR3 breast cancer cell line

SKBR3 is a human breast carcinoma cell line established in late 1970s and derived from pleural effusion of Caucasian patient diagnosed as invasive ductal carcinoma (CLS, Germany). It is an adherent cell which is the usual character found in most breast cancer cell lines. Ultra structures of cells show microvilli and desmosomes, large lysosomes, and bundles of cytoplasmic fibrils. In nude mice, these cells can form poorly differentiated adenocarcinoma (http://www.cell-lines-service). In addition in nude mice, c-Jun, the ending molecule of signal transduction pathways, is demonstrated to have the critical role in the tumorigenesis and metastasis in SKBR3 breast cancer cells (Zhang et al, 2007).

Estrogen receptor (ER) is found to be absent or expressed at the very low level in SKBR3 cells and progesterone receptor is also absent in this type of cell (Lacroix and Leclercq, 2004). In contrast, Her2/neu receptor including leptin receptor are overexpressed in this cell line whereas insulin- like growth factor receptor- I is expressed at the lower level when compared with those in MCF7 cells (Ozbay and Nahta, 2008). Interestingly, recent report revealed that SKBR3 expressed NMDAR1 and NMDAR2 receptors, both of which are important calcium channels. These receptors are reported to be essential for the growth of human breast cancer xenografts in mice (North et al, 2010).

This SKBR3 cell line with high expression of HER2 protein has long been used in various research. Recently, it has been shown to be the suitable candidate for reference materials in quality control of HER2 testing together with MCF7 cell line. Based on this report, SKBR3 and MCF7 breast cancer cells provide valuable controls for quantitative measurement of HER2 amplification and production (Xiao et al, 2009). The photograph of SKRB3 cultured in the flask is shown in Figure 7.

4.1.2 MCF7 breast cancer cell line

MCF7 is a human breast carcinoma cell line derived from pleural effusion of Caucasian patient diagnosed with breast adenocarcinoma (CLS, Germany). It is a relatively resistant to cisplatin treatment (Westmose Yde and Issinger, 2006). Morphology of this cell line exhibits epithelial-like cell including the ability to process estradiol via cytoplasmic estrogen receptors and domes formation. This cell line has oncogene, wnt7h and can induce tumor in nude mice (http://www.cell-lines-service).

This MCF7 cell line expresses both estrogen and progesterone receptors whereas the expression of Her2/neu is absent (Lacroix and Leclercq, 2004). The cells can be suppressed by catechin hydrate, product from plant sources such as green tea, through TP53/caspase-

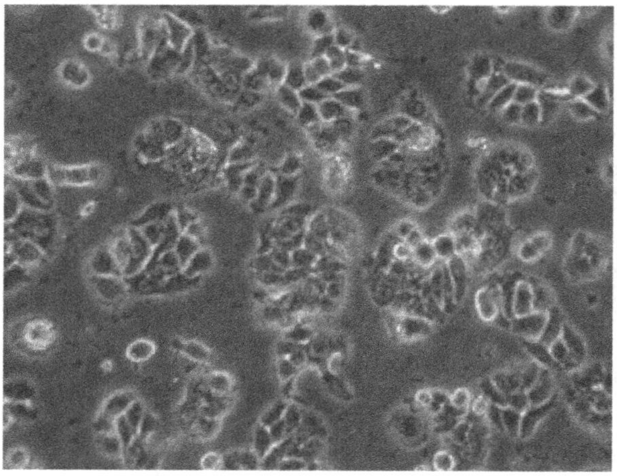

Fig. 7. SKBR3 cells grow in DMEM supplemented with 10% fetal bovine serum and 1% penicillin+ streptomycin. Cells show monolayer when grow in plastic with polygonal shaped. This cell line is categorized as weakly luminal epithelial-like cell.

mediated apoptosis (Alshatwi, 2010). Some vasoactive peptides such as endothelin 1 is found at low level in MCF7 while in SKBR3 is expressed at the higher level. This expression might correlate with high invasiveness phenotype in breast cancer (Hagemann et al, 2005). MCF7 has been extensively used as the model for breast cancer and breast cancer therapy. However, different sources of MCF7 show the differences in response to 17beta-estradiol resulting from activation or inhibition of insulin-like growth factor I (IGF-1) (Hamelers et al, 2003). Therefore, the different responses of MCF7 should be realized due to the expression of IGF-1. As mentioned above, MCF7 is suitable to be candidate of reference materials in quality control for HER2 testing (Xiao et al, 2009).

4.1.3 T47D breast cancer cell line

T47D is a human breast carcinoma cell line derived from pleural effusion of an infiltrating ductal carcinoma of the breast (CLS, Germany). It contains cytoplasmic junctions, receptors to 17 beta estradiol including steroids and calcitonin (Moseley et al, 1983). Receptors for estrogen and progesterone are also present (Hevir et al, 2011). This cell line has tumorigenicity in nude mice and has three oncogenes, i.e., wnt3, wnt7h, and wnt7b (http://www.cell-lines-service).

By activation Janus kinase2/signal transducer and transcription 5 pathway, this cell line expresses ample growth hormone receptor and prolactin receptor (Xu et al, 2011). Both receptors are structurally similar cytokine receptor superfamily members. Direct protein identification by MALDI post-source decay (PSD) or MALDI collision-induced dissociation (CID) in T47D cells showed only histone H2B (Pevsner et al, 2007). Chemokine CXCL12 and its promoter activity are found to be increase in human T47D breast cancer cells (Chen et al, 2010). Indeed, T47D cell line, as well as MCF7, represents the good model of estrogen-dependent breast cancer with capacity of 17beta-estradiol local production (Hevir et al, 2011).

4.1.4 MDA-MB435 breast cancer cell line

MDA-MB435 is derived from the pleural effusion of metastatic ductal adenocarcinoma of the breast. Recent data have pointed out that MDA-MB435 cells are from melanoma

(Lacroix, 2009; Rae et al, 2004). This cell line is found to express certain genes commonly transcribed in melanocyte which are not seen in breast cancer cell lines such as DCP gene. Moreover, expression of melanocyte proteins tyrosinase and melan-A has also been demonstrated in MDA-MB435. However, some evidences have been presented that MDA-MB435 might be breast cancer cell line expressing a poorly differentiated aggressive breast tumor together with epithelial and melanocyte markers (Chambers, 2009; http://www.cell-lines-service).

Investigation on protein identification in MDA-MB435 cells was performed and found 30 important proteins expressing in this cell line (Chandramouli et al, 2009). For example, caspase 14 precursor, heat shock protein 60, cell adhesion proteins, and some immune response proteins such as complement C3 were also demonstrated.

4.2 Breast cancer cells: Experimental procedures in antiproliferative activity

Antiproliferative and cytotoxic activity are the basic and very common investigations used for determination in the efficacy of plant extracts for searching the novel drugs. The measurement of herb treated mammalian cells either surviving or proliferating cells could be achieved by several techniques. Counting cells that include or exclude a dye such as trypan blue dye with the use of a hemocytometer under a microscope or in an automated cell counter is one assay. Quantitation of suspension cells could be performed by counting them directly whereas adherent cells which grow in monolayer culture require proteolytic agents such as trypsin prior to quantitation. This method is, therefore, not only time consuming, labor intensive, but also dependent upon individual skills.

A number of various indirect methods to quantitate living or dead cell number has been developed. Based on the fact that active or living cells will increase or decrease some specific proteins or even nucleic acids that can indicate cellular proliferation or cytotoxicity. Measuring released 51Cr-labeled protein after cell lysis, and measuring incorporation of 3H-thymidine during cell proliferation have been employed (Mosmann, 1983). These traceable radioactive moieties are very efficient and specific. However, the radioactive methods could handle very limited numbers of samples at each time and also require long sample preparation procedure with inherent dangers and high cost (Haslam et al, 2000). Therefore, several non-radioactive methods have been developed instead of an old traditional method, the cell counting.

In this section, breast cancer cells and experimental procedures in antiproliferative activity, three non-radioactive assays, i.e., MTT assay, Lactate dehydrogenase (LDH) cytotoxicity assay, and clonogenic assay, commonly used have been demonstrated in details.

4.2.1 MTT assay

Principle & mechanism of action

This colorimetric assay was first developed and reported by Mosmann (Mosmann, 1983). Tetrazolium salt MTT (3-(4, 5-dimethylthiazol-2-yl)-2, 5-diphenyl tetrazolium bromide) is tested and used in this assay. These tetrazolium salts can measure the activity of several dehydrogenase enzymes especially mitochondrial enzyme succinate-dehydrogenase (Slater et al., 1963). The reaction is known to be occurred in the living cells by cleaving the tetrazolium ring in the metabolically active mitochondria, not in dead cells or erythrocytes. From the MTT pale yellow substrate, the dark blue (purple) formazan products are generated in the direct proportion to the living cell numbers. Notably, this MTT assay cannot distinquish between the cytotoxic and cytostatic effect of the tested drug or herb (Plumb, 2004).

Interestingly, MTT solution at 1 mg/mL increases the formazan product whereas MTT solution at 1-2 mg/mL will slow down the production (Sylvester, 2011). This is the reason why MTT solution is usually used at the concentration of 1 mg/mL. From the kinetics of formazan production, incubation time over 4 hours will get the plateau production curve. Therefore, standard incubation time at 3-4 hours is usually enough for the production time (Denizot and Lang, 1986).

As reported, the blue formazan products are partially dissolved in the medium. To induce complete solubilization of these MTT formazan products, several organic solvents have been tested and used such as ethanol, dimethylsulfoxide (DMSO), and isopropanol which is reported to be the most suitable solvent. After getting the homogeneous solution, optical density (OD) will be measured by reading on a scanning multiwell spectrophotometer (ELISA reader). The absorption spectrum of MTT formazan crystal is pH dependent. At pH 10.5, the maximum absorption is 570 nm. whereas, at pH 7.0, the absorption peak will show at 500 and 570 nm. (Plumb, 2004). The use of flat-bottomed well will help in increasing the sensitivity due to the doubled light-path length in the final optical density reading (Denizot and Lang, 1986).

In general, the accurate and reliable results from the MTT assay depend upon various important parameters which need to be optimized first. The proper cell number for seeding should be characterized by using standard curve. Changing into fresh medium prior to adding MTT solution is also critical in getting the good yield because of reduction of MTT activity in nutrient-depleted medium. Time and dose of MTT solution in each experiment may be different for each cell or cell lines used (Sylvester, 2011). Importantly, chemotherapeutic agents and some drugs such as valproic acid can yield the lower results from the MTT assay (Ari et al, 2010; Ulukaya et al, 2008). The experimental procedure is as followed (Kummalue et al, 2005).

Experimental procedure:

- Breast cancer cells will be seeded at $1x10^4$ cells per well in 96 flat-bottomed well plate containing 100µl of the culture medium DMEM supplemented with 10% heat inactivated fetal bovine serum and 1% antibiotic.
- After 24 hours, the cells will be treated with herbal extract at final concentrations from 1, 10, 100, and 500 µg/mL for 48 hours. These serial concentrations are used for determining the activity in crude extracts only.
- After 48 hours incubation, medium will be changed into fresh medium, and MTT 50 µl (stock concentration at 1mg/mL in PBS) will be added to each well.
- After 4 hours incubation, the MTT solution will then be removed by rapid flick-off of the medium and 100 µl of 100% DMSO will be added to solubilize the formazan products. The dark purple solution from formazan products can be seen as shown in Figure 8.
- Plate will be rotated on the platform rotator for 10 minutes before further measurement the O.D. by a microplate Elisa reader at 595 nm.
- Calculation of ED_{50} (50% of inhibition of cancer cell growth) will be performed by using the formula:

$$\text{percentage of viability} = \text{OD sample}/\text{OD control} \times 100 \quad (1)$$

$$\text{percentage of inhibition} = 100 - \%\ \text{viability}$$

Special comments:

- For pure compounds, serial concentrations can be diluted to the final concentrations as low as 0.1 μg/mL. This is because pure compounds are active compounds which are purified from crude extracts.
- After adding MTT solution, remember to wrap plate with aluminium foil because MTT substrate is light sensitive.
- We usually perform the O.D. measurement at 595 nm. because of the limitation of our instrument.
- Rotate the cell culture plate at the rotator platform for 10 minutes is important to induce the homogeneous solution that will be easy for the O.D. measurement and to achieve the correct data.
- The rapid flick-off of the medium after the MTT incubation will be done only in adherent cell lines such as breast cancer cell lines. For suspension cells such as leukemic cell lines, K562, the 100 μl of the stop solution (10% SDS dissolved in 0.01 N HCl) will be added into each well and incubated overnight.
- If dilute the herbal extract with DMSO, it is better to keep the percentage of DMSO in the final concentration not more than 0.5% to avoid cell damage and false positive result. In our experience, 1% DMSO still can cause some effect on cell viability.
- Please remember to set the control wells (both positive and negative control). We usually use doxorubicin or vinca alkaloid for positive control. Only cells in the medium will be used as negative control.
- The number of the seeding cells used in our experiment is from the standard curve at the O.D 0.7-1.2.
- We always perform the MTT assay with three independent experiments.

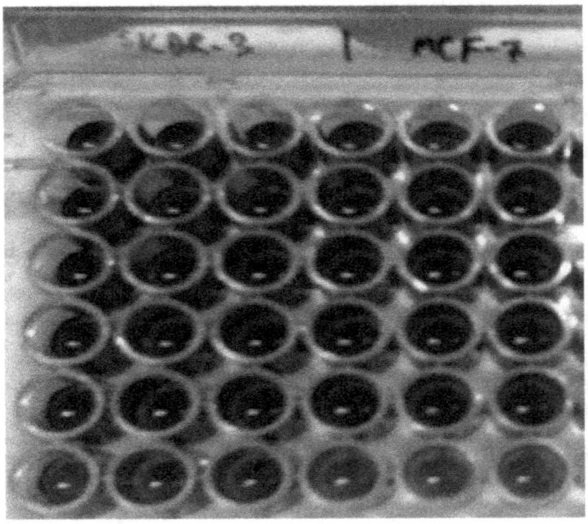

Fig. 8. The MTT assay showed the dark purple formazan products in the wells after dissolving the crystal with 100 μl of 100% DMSO.

4.2.2 Lactate dehydrogenase (LDH) cytotoxicity assay

Principle & mechanism of action

For MTT tetrazolium salt assay, the method measures the surviving cells after treatment with chemical substances. However, for the very low toxic reagents, calculation from the data of control cells and treated cells from MTT assay results in low sensitivity. In this case, direct measurement of dead cells will give more accurate information (Sasaki et al, 1992). Therefore, development of assay using cytolytic enzymes releasing from dead cells has been initiated which can represent proportionally to the dead cell number (Sasaki et al, 1992). Detection of lactate dehydrogenase enzyme, one of the stable cytolytic enzyme found in animal cells, has been established for this purpose (Decker and Lohmann-Matthes, 1988).

Lactate dehydrogenase (LDH) enzyme has the function to catalyze lactate to pyruvate under anaerobic condition. It is a soluble enzyme in the cytoplasm. This enzyme will be released to the culture medium when the cell is ruptured or dead. Usually the assay will contain two steps. First, LDH releasing from the cells will oxidize lactate to generate NADH and H+. The second step, diaphorase in the reaction will use NADH and H+ to catalyze the tetrazolium salt such as WST-8, or INT to generate colored formazan which will absorbs strongly at wavelength 490-520 nm. The amount of the formazan production will correlate in the proportion to the damaged cells in the reaction (Haslam et al, 2000; Rodney et al, 1966). The experimental procedure is shown belowed (Kummalue et al, 2009; LDH-cytotoxicity assay kit with WST-8, MBL international corporation).

Experimental procedure:

- Breast cancer cells will be seeded at a density of 1×10^4 cells per well in 96 well plates flat-bottom in 100 µl of culture medium DMEM supplemented with 10% heat inactivated fetal bovine serum and 1% antibiotic.
- The next morning, cells will be treated with the herbal extract at various final concentrations from 1 to 500 µg/mL for 48 hours in the incubator. These concentrations are used to evaluate the ED50 for crude extracts only.
- Centrifuge the cells at 1500 rpm or 250 g for 10 minutes.
- Transfer 10 µl of culture medium into the new 96 well plate with corresponding well.
- Add 100 µl of LDH reaction mix (containing LDH and WST-8) to 10 µl of tested culture medium and incubated at 37 °C with a 5% CO_2 incubator for an additional 30 minutes.
- The absorbance at 450 nm of the dissolved solution will be measured by using an Elisa plate reader.

Special comments:

All MTT, WST-8, XTT, and INT are commonly used tetrazolium salts. They have different chemical structures and properties such as solubility. These properties depend on the substituents on the tetrazole rings in the compounds (Zhivich et al, 1990).

4.2.3 Clonogenic assay

Principle & mechanism of action

This method for cell sensitivity assay is considered as the gold standard technique and has been used for a long time (Plumb, 2004). It is a well known method for testing the effects of drugs on the proliferation of treated cell lines. This assay can measure the ability of cells to proliferate and form colonies after treating cells with chemical substances or herbal extracts (cytostatic effect of drug) whereas cells that are killed by the drugs cannot grow and form colonies (cytotoxic effect of drug). In addition, clonogenic assay is reported to be able to detect cell survival as low as 1% (Plumb, 2004).

Staining technique is a very important step because the accuracy of counting colonies depends on the good visualization. Colony staining has been performed with several dye solutions such as methylene blue, ethidium bromide, and crystal violet (Guda et al, 2007). Counting colony can be done by using manual counting with microscope or using the specific software (Niyazi et al, 2007). The experimental procedure is demonstrated belowed (Pratumvinit et al, 2009).

Experimental procedure:

- Breast cancer cell lines will be plated in 12 well plate at a density of $7x10^2$ cells per well.
- The next morning, cells will be treated with the herbal extract at the concentrations of 0, 50, 100, and 150 μg/mL.
- After 48 hours incubation, culture medium will be changed into fresh medium.
- Cells will be further cultured for 7-14 days until colonies are observed.
- Plates will be stained with 1 gm of crystal violet in 50% methanol for 30 minutes.
- Pour off the stain, carefully rinse with running water.
- Colonies will be counted by using ChemiDocXRS with specific software. Figure 9 showed the colonies detected in our experiment.

Special comments:

- The number of cells seeded in each well will be vary depending on the area of the well.
- The concentrations used in the experiment depend upon the ED_{50} value of each medicinal plant.
- Changing into fresh medium (after treated cells) before continue keeping cells in culture is very important for cell growth and colony formation.
- The time for culturing after exposure to the herbal extract depend upon the cell growth curve. For breast cancer cell lines, small colony can be detected after culturing cells for at least 7 days.
- Counting the colonies can be achieved by using only light microscope, no software use (but may be too difficult to count in some cases).
- We always perform the clonogenic assay with three independent experiments.

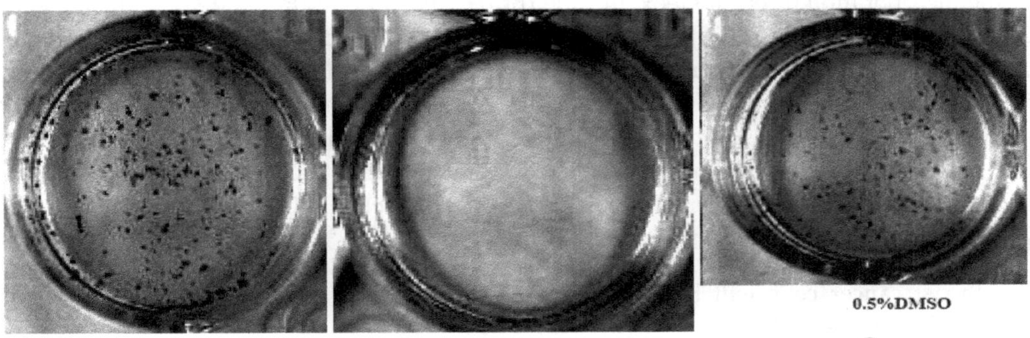

A B C

Fig. 9. Demonstration of colonies detected in the well. A. T47D breast cancer cells as a negative control. B. T47D treated with plant extract at 0.5 times ED_{50}. No colony was detected which was due to the cytotoxicity of the extract. C. T47D treated with 0.5% DMSO as a control because the extract was diluted with 0.5% DMSO. Colonies could be seen as dots at the bottom of the wells after staining with crystal violet in this experiment and counted by using the software.

4.3 Breast cancer cells and experimental procedures in mechanism of actions

This is usually the next step of investigation in searching for the new drug from plant sources. Plant extracts that exhibit the promising ED_{50} values, i.e., the plant extracts show some antiproliferative or cytotoxic activities on specific breast cancer cell lines, the extracts will be further studied to find the mechanism of actions in view of inhibition of cancer cells growth or even killing cells. Cell cycle analysis and apoptotic study are the most two common methods used in the field for searching the mechanism of actions in plants.

4.3.1 Breast cancer cells and experimental procedure in cell cycle study

Based on the knowledge of normal cell cycle, breast cancer cells actively synthesize DNA in the same process (Ross et al, 2003). Normally, the cell cycle phase contains G0, G1, S, G2, and M phase in order. Cells in the G0 phase or resting state contain diploid DNA which will enter the second step G1 (Gap 1). After this step, cells increase their DNA content to two folds with twice the diploid DNA content at the end. This accumulation state of DNA is S phase. Cells then enter the G2 phase (Gap 2) and finally go into the M phase, while M means the mitotic state. Finally, each mitotic cell will end up with 2 daughter cells.

In breast cancer cells, DNA ploidy has been reported to correlate with the prognosis in patients. The first retrospective report using flow cytometry to study DNA content as a predictor in breast cancer was done by Auer et al with pure diploid showing an excellent prognosis (Auer et al, 1980). However, the use of DNA ploidy as an prognostic indicator in clinical practice still remains in controversy (Ross et al, 2003). Estrogen has also been reported to induce breast cancer which might due to the inappropriate activation of cyclin dependent kinase and consequently abnormal transition through G1 phase (Foster et al, 2001).

The most popular technique used for demonstration DNA content in the cells is by flow cytometry (Nunez, 2001). Four distinct phases could be categorized, i.e., G1, G2, S, and M phases with G2 and M phase will represent at the same DNA content (so called G2/M phase). The staining techniques to distinquish these cell cycle phases are the measurement of the incorporation of bromodeoxyuridine (BrdU) and propidium iodide (Kummalue et al, 2002; Pratumvinit et al, 2009). Interference from RNA may result in misinterpretation as false positive. Therefore, the use of RNase should be added in the protocol. The experiment in breast cancer demonstrated here will share the experience in using the cell cycle kit which is much easier than the traditional technique. (The details of cell cycle study using BrdU incorporation and propidium iodide can be found in the references as mentioned in the text.) Belowed is the experimental procedure (Kummalue et al, 2007).

Experimental procedure:

- Breast cancer cells will be seeded at $1x10^6$ cells in 100 mm tissue culture dish and incubated overnight.
- The next morning, cells will be treated with the plant extract at the dosage ranging from 0.5 times ED_{50} to 2 times ED_{50}.
- After 48 hours incubation, cells will be harvested and incubated with reagents as described in the protocol of the CycleTEST™PLUS DNA reagent kit (Becton Dickinson, USA).
- Measurement of DNA content of cells will be performed within 3 hours by flow cytometry and analysed by CellQuest Software.

Special comments:

- The incubation time for cell cycle study depends on the time that is used for cell sensitivity assay.
- Dosage used in the experiment to investigate the effect of plant on cell cycle depends upon the ED_{50} of the plant extract.

4.3.2 Breast cancer cells and experimental procedure in apoptotic study

Apoptosis or programmed cell death is a very interesting investigation in drug discovery and development especially for cancer therapies. Searching for the anticancer agents that can induce apoptosis is necessary and needed for the effective treatment. For example, tamoxifen, which is prescribed as an adjuvant therapy in breast cancer, has been shown to induce apoptosis by down regulation of bcl-2 (Zhang et al, 1999). Therefore, most of medicinal plant researchers keep looking on finding these properties of plants. By the way, high cost and time consumption are unavoidable to face.

Apoptosis is a process that organisms, including human beings, use to tightly regulate the cell numbers and tissue size (Hengartner, 2000). It is caused by a group of cysteine proteases known as caspases. There are 2 major apoptotic pathways. One is via death receptor pathway which is triggered by death receptor superfamily such as CD95 and also tumor necrosis factor receptor I. This results in activation of caspase 8. The other pathway is mitochondrial pathway. This activates pro-apoptotic member of the Bcl-2 family and then pro caspase 9. Both pathways converge at the caspase 3 activation (Hengartner, 2000). To evaluate the apoptotic activity of plant extracts, caspase activity is usually investigated either by detection at the level of the enzyme caspase itself or by the level of its cleavage product, poly (ADP-ribose) polymerase-1 (PARP-1) (Los et al, 2002; Kummalue et al, 2011).

In summary, characterization of apoptosis is chromatin condensation, fragmentation of DNA (seen as ladder pattern in gel electrophoresis), and reduction of cell volume. Externalization of phosphatidylserine at the cell surface also plays an important role in macrophages recognition and consequently eradication of these apoptotic cells (Koopman et al, 1994). With these specific expression of phosphatidylserine, the new method was developed for detection of apoptotic cells by flow cytometry and has been frequently used nowadays. (Koopman et al, 1994). The experimental procedure is shown belowed. (Kummalue et al, 2011)

Experimental procedure:

- Cells will be seeded on 100 cm tissue culture dish at the density of $1x10^6$ cells.
- After 24 hours, cells will be treated with plant extracts at the various final concentrations ranging from 0.5 times ED_{50}, to 2 times ED_{50}.
- After incubating cells for various time points, cells will be harvested. The time points used to treat cells depend on the efficacy of the plant extract itself.
- Cells will be labeled with Annexin V-PI following the protocol of Annexin V-FITC Apoptosis Detection Kit from the manufacture and analysis by flow cytometry.

Special comments:

Detection of early and late apoptosis using annexin V depends upon the doses and time that treating the cells.

4.3.3 Breast cancer cells and specific mechanism of action of the plant extracts

Elucidation of the mechanism of action will greatly help in understanding the activity from plant sources on these breast cancer cell lines. Following the cell cycle and apoptotic studies as the basis, the mechanisms of these activities such as telomerase activity, antioxidant activity, and details of special signaling pathways are always considered for studying.

Telomerase is a eukaryotic ribonucleoprotein complex that helps in stabilizing telomere length in human stem cells, reproductive cells, and cancer cells (Shay and Bacchetti, 1997; Shay et al, 2001). The activity of telomerase increases in almost all human cancers except for the normal cells (Shay et al, 2001;Kim et al, 1994). Based on several studies, there are correlations between telomere shortening and growth failure of human cells (Harley et al, 1990; Shay et al, 2001). Therefore, human cancer cells show to have short telomeres with high telomerase, which is in contrast to normal human cells. Notably, cancer cells need to maintain telomeres for their immortalization. Based on this correlation, investigations of human cancer on telomerase activity have been done for over decades due to the potential development in drug targeting cancers.

Human telomerase consists of a catalytic protein component (hTERT) and integral RNA which are essential for the function of telomerase (Shay et al, 2001). hTERT is reported to be the critical for the production of telomerase (Nakamura et al, 1997). Investigation on telomerase activity can usually perform by detection the hTERT expression using RT-PCR. RNA extraction from treated breast cancer cells will be done before further processing to quantitate the level of transcripts. The method can be undertaken by real time RT-PCR and specific software for interpretation (Duangmano et al, 2010).

5. Breast cancer cells in medicinal plants research: Future direction in drug testing

Generating of induced pluripotent stem cells (iPS) for the first time in the world by Professor Dr. Shinya Yamanaka in Year 2006 has very high impact on several fields such as stem cell therapies, regenerative medicine, replacement therapy, and also drug screening and toxicity (Inoue and Yamanaka, 2011). Researchers worldwide are very interested in this iPS technology because of the high possibility in its usefulness and application to human diseases.

Induced pluripotent stem cells or iPS has first been generated from mouse tip tail fibroblasts which were somatic cells (Takahashi and Yamanaka, 2006). The process involved in transduction of fibroblasts with retrovirus carrying 4 transcription factors, i.e., Sox2, Klf4, c-Myc, and Oct3/4. These four factors are now known as Yamanaka's four factors. iPS cells exhibit several features characteristics of embryonic stem cells such as positive for alkaline phosphatase, forming teratoma in mice, and expression of specific embryonic antigen (Park et al, 2008). Nowadays, iPSs have been generated from various kinds of animals cells such as monkey, mouse, etc., including normal human cells, human cancer cell lines, and patients' cells to generate the patient-specific iPSs (Chun et al, 2010; Raya et al, 2009).

In drug screening and toxicity testing, human iPSs offer the high values in this field. For example, breast cancer patients' fibroblasts can be induced with transcription factors either 2 or 4 factors to create patient-specific iPS. Based on the fact that the iPS cells are generated from patients' own somatic cells, therefore, these specific iPS cells can be used to identify and test with the novel drug developing for cancer patients including the toxic effects of the drugs themselves (Chun et al, 2010). Interestingly, the advantage of iPS is the generation of the library for human cancer that will represent the genetic and epigenetic variation of the population (Chun et al, 2010). In addition, since iPSs grow in culture like cell lines, therefore, this technology can provide the unlimited sources of cells for desired situation.

6. Discussion and conclusion

The investigation of the traditional used and evidence-based medicinal plants provides the chance to discover natural anticancer agents. The breast cancer cell lines with specific properties and the progress in antiproliferative and cytotoxic experiments are the important tools for the investigation of the medicinal plants. Clear differences in specific properties including receptors of these 4 breast cancer cell lines have been demonstrated so far. Comparing specific receptors, i.e., estrogen receptor, progesterone receptor, and Her2/neu in these 4 breast cancer cell lines: SKBR3, MCF7, T47D, and MDA-MB435 are demonstrated in Table 2. These 4 breast cancer cell lines are classified in different groups and express different receptors. Therefore, treatment of plant extracts on these 4 breast cancer cell lines can help, at least, in the decision whether or not the extracts will exert activities in breast cancer with different subtypes. However, the established cell lines from patients do not always represent the genotypes of parental tumor tissues (Tsuji et al, 2010). Therefore, testing in cell lines may not yield the same results when performing in vivo though most of these cells deregulate in signaling along the EgfR-MAPK pathway (Heiser et al, 2009).

Characters	**SKBR3**	**MCF7**	**T47D**	**MDA-MB435**
Category	Second group	First group	First group	Third group
Estrogen receptor	-	+	+	-
Progesterone receptor	-	+	+	-
Her-2/neu	overexpression	-	-	-

(-) = not expressed; (+) = expressed

Table 2. Characters of receptors on four breast cancer cell lines: SKBR3, MCF7, T47D, and MDA-MB435 (http://www.cell-lines-service; Lacroix and Leclercq, 2004; Hevir et al, 2011).

Searching for the novel chemotherapeutic agents from plant sources usually involves with the initial process of antiproliferative activity. These three non-radioactive assays are commonly used nowadays in the determination of antiproliferative and cytotoxic activities. Several aspects from them are summarized in Table 3, i.e., sensitivity, cost and time consuming for each assay. Notably, each assay has its own advantages and disadvantages which should be carefully considered.

Prediction of toxicology and therapeutic responses induced by the novel drugs can be approached by iPS technology as mentioned aboved. Lots of current disease specific based patients iPS have been reported since then (Chun et al, 2010). This application as a personalized approach leads to the specialized model in vitro. However, the safety and risk in applying to the clinical trials should be aggressively considered because of the techniques in generation of iPS with viral gene transfer.

The elucidation of the action mechanism provides the concrete evidence of the study plant. The utilization of herbs as natural anticancer agents can solve the problem of the

	MTT assay	LDH assay with WST-8	Clonogenic assay
Sensitivity	++ (high sensitivity for antiproliferative activity)	+++ (high sensitivity for cytotoxic activity)	+ (low sensitivity and high false negative result due to small colony formation)
Cost consuming	++ (high cost reagent)	++ (high cost reagent)	+ (low cost staining)
Time consuming	++ (moderate term culture)	+ (short term culture)	+++ (long term culture and time spending in counting)

+++ represent the highest scores
+ represent the lowest scores

Table 3. Comparison of three non-radioactive methods for assaying the antiproliferative activities (Kosaka et al, 1996; Kawada et al, 2002; Fotakis and Timbrell, 2006; Miyamoto et al, 2002).

unaccessible anticancer drugs. We investigated thoroughly two Thai herbs and discovered the possible benefit to the breast cancer patients. *T. cucumerina* fruit juice exerted strongly antiproliferative effect. The juice itself can be considered as a natural cytostatic agent because of its potent effect. According to the presence of cucurbitacins, the juice irritates the mucous membrane of the gastrointestinal tract. The juice produced toxicity to the central nervous system and the respiratory tract, the usage of the herbal juice should be under the supervision of the physician.

For the part of *M. loriformis* herb juice, it can be used as an adjunct to the modern therapy according to the moderate cytotoxicity, immunomodulatory effect and safety. The patient cases, which were reported by the physicians, have supported the use of herbal juice to reduce the side effects from the modern therapy. Several active compounds in the pressed juice worked together to exert the activities, which were expected to have broad spectrum and lowered toxicity. The appropriate daily doses of cytotoxic effect from *T. cucumerina* and immunomodulatory effect from *M. loriformis* require further clinical investigation.

F. hispida and *E. elliptilimba* are interesting herbs for further investigation. It was also noticeable that herbal remedy could potentiate the effect of anticancer drug.

7. References

Alshatwi AA. (2010) Catechin hydrate suppresses MCF7 proliferation through TP53/caspase-mediated apoptosis. J Exp Clin Cancer Res Vol. 29 pp. 167-75.

Ari F, Ikitimur E, Ulukaya E. (2010) The ATP assay, but not the MTT assay, detects further cytotoxicity of the combination of anthracycline-based therapy with histone deacetylase inhibitor (valproic acid) in breast cancer cells. Turk J Biochem Vol. 35 pp. 293-9.

Auer GU, Capersson TO, Wallgren AS. (1980) DNA content and survival in mammary carcinoma. Vol. 2 pp. 161-5.

Book of traditional Chinese Medicine in Sichuan. (1992) pp. 181. (chinese).

Casarett LJ and Doull J. (1975) Toxicology: The basic science of poisons. New York: MacMillan Publishing Co., pp. 24.

Chaiwerawatana A. (2007) Chapter 13. Cancer in Thailand Vol. IV, 1998-2000. Edited by Khuhaprema T, Srivatanakul P, Sriplung H, Wiangnon S, Sumitsawan Y, Attasara P. Bangkok Medical Publisher, Bangkok, Thailand. pp. 48-50.

Chambers A. (2009) MDA-MB435 and M14 cell line: Identical but not M14 melanoma Cancer Res Vol. 69 pp. 5292-3.

Chandramouli KH, Agrawal P, Thimmaiah KH. (2009) Protein identification in sub proteome fractions of breast cancer cells by OFFGEL-IEF and iTRAQ labeling. Current Proteomic Vol. 6 pp. 43-50.

Chen L, Xu S, Zeng X, Li J, Yin W, Chen Y, et al. (2010) c-myb activated CXCL12 transcription in T47D and MCF7 breast cancer cells. Acta Biochem Biophys Sin Vol. 42, pp. 1-7.

Chun YS, Chaudhari P, Jang YY. (2010) Application of patient-specific induced pluripotent stem cells; focused on disease modeling, drug screening and therapeutic potential for liver disease. Int J Biol Sci Vol.6, No.7, pp. 96-805.

Decker T, Lohmann-Matthes ML. (1988) A quick and simple method for the quantitation of lactate dehydrogenase release in measurements of cellular cytotoxicity and tumor necrosis factor (TNF) activity. J Immunolo Methods Vol. 15 pp. 61-9.

Denizot F, Lang R. (1986) Rapid colorimetric assay for cell growth and survival modifications to the tetrazolium dye procedure giving improved sensitivity and reliability. J Immunol Methods Vol. 89 pp. 271-7.

Dingermann T. (2000) (unter Mitarbeit der Expertenkommission BARMER/BPI). Transporenzkriterien fuer pflanzliche, homoeopathische und anthroposophische Arzueimittch Skarger. Freiburg. pp 3-4.

Duangmano S, Dakeng S, Jiratchariyakul W, Suksamrarn A, Smith DR and Patmasiriwat P. (2010) Antiproliferative effects of cucurbitacin B in breast cancer cells: down-regulate c-Myc/hTERT/telomerase pathway and obstruct the cell cycle. Int. J. Mol. Sci. Vol. 11 No. 12 pp. 5323-5338.

Foster JS, Henley DC, Ahamed S, Wimalasena J. (2001) Estrogens and cell cycle regulation in breast cancer. Trends Endocrinol Metabol Vol.12 pp. 320-7.

Fotakis G, Timbrell JA. (2006) In vitro cytotoxicity assays: Comparison of LDH, neutral red, MTT and protein assay in hepatoma cell lines following exposure to cadmium chloride. Toxicology Vol.160. pp. 171-7.

Guda K, Natale L, Markowitz S. (2007) An improved method for staining cell colonies in clonogenic assays. Cytotechnology Vol.54 pp. 85-8.

Haensel R, Hoelzl J. (1996) Lehrbuch der pharmazeutischen biologie. Spinger-Verlag. Heidelberg. pp. 516-7.

Haensel R, Sticher O. (2007) Pharmakognosie - Phytopharmazie. 8th rev.ed. Springer, Heidelberg : Springer-Medizin Verlag pp. 928-30.

Hagemann T, Binder C, Binder L, Pukrop T, Trumper L, Grimshaw M. (2005) Expression of endothelins and their receptors promotes an invasive phenotype of breast tumor cells but is insufficient to induce invasion on benigh cells. DNA Cell Biol Vol.24 pp.766-76.

Hamelers I, van Schaik R, Sussenbach J, Steenbergh P. (2003) 17 beta-estradiol responsiveness of MCF7 laboratory strains is dependent on an autocrine signal activating the IGF type I receptor. Cancer Cell Inter 3:10. Published online 2003 July 11. doi:10.1186/1475-2867-3-10.

Harley CB, Fletcher AB, Greider CW. (1990) Telomeres shorten during aging. Nature Vol. 345 pp. 458-60.

Haslam G, Wyatt G, Kitos PA. (2000) Estimating the number of viable animal cells in multi-well cultures based on their lactate dehydrogenase activities. Cytotechnology Vol. 32 pp. 63-75.

Heiser LM, Wang NJ, Talcott CL, Laderoute KR, Knapp M, Guan Y, et al. (2009) Integrated analysis of breast cancer cell lines reveals unique signaling pathway. Genome Biol Vol. 10 No. 3: R31. Published online 2009 March 25. doi:10.1186/gb-2009-10-3-r31.

Hengartner M. (2000) The biochemistry of apoptosis. Nature Vol.407 pp.770-6.

Hevir N, Trost N, Debeljak N, Rizner L. (2011) Expression of estrogen and progesterone receptors and estrogen metabolizing enzymes in different breast cancer cell lines. Chemico biological Interaction 2011 online doi:10.1016/j.cbi.2010.12.013.

Inoue H, Yamanaka S. (2011) The use of induced pluripotent stem cells in drug development. Nature 23 March, 2011. Doi:10.1038/clpt.2011.38.

Intayot Y, Kinouchi T, Kataoka K, et al. (2002) Antimutagenicity of *Murdannia loriformis* in the Salmonella mutation assay and its inhibitory effects on azoxymethane-induced DNA methylation and aberrant crypt focus formation in male F344 rats. J Med Invest Vol. 49 pp. 25-34.

Itharat A, Ooraiku B. (2007). Chapter 13 Research on Thai medicinal plants for cancer treatment, In: Advance Medicinal Plant Research Acharaya SN, Thomas JE, Trivandrum, pp.287-317,

Jiratchariyakul W and Frahm AW. (1992) Cucurbitacin B and dihydrocucurbitacin B from *Trichosanthes cucumerina* L. Mahidol Univ J Pharm Sci Vol. 19 pp, 5-12.

Jiratchariyakul W, Moogkarndi P, Theppeang K, Sethjintanin D, Jarikasem S and Frahm AW. (1999) Cytotoxic principles from *Trichosanthes cucumerina* L. Thai J Phytopharmacy Vol. 6, No. 2 pp. 1-9.

Jiratchariyakul W, Moongkarndi P, Okabe H, Frahm AW. (1997) Investigation of anticancer components from *Murdannia loriformis* (Hassk.) Rolla Rao et Kammathy. In : Proceeding of the first Pharma Indochina conference on Pharmaceutical Sciences. Pharmacy in Harmony. Faculty of Pharmacy, Mahidol Univ. Bangkok, Thailand, 20-23 May 1pp. 171-92.

Jiratchariyakul W, Okabe H, Moongkarndi P, et al. (1998) Cytotoxic glycosphingolipid from *Murdannia loriformis* (Hassk.) Rolla Rao et Kammathy. Thai Journal of Phytopharmacy Vol. 5 No. 1 pp. 10-20.,

Jiratchariyakul W, Vongsakul M, Sunthornsuk L, Moongkarndi P, Narintorn A, Somanabandhu A, Okabe H, Frahm A.W. (2006) Immunomodulatory Effect and Quantitation of a Cytotoxic Glycosphingolipid from *Murdannia loriformis.* J Nat Med Vol. 60 pp. 210-216.

Kawada K, Yonei T, Ueoka H, Kiura K, Tabata M, Takigawa N, et al. (2002) Comparison of hemosensitivity tests: Clonogenic assay versus MTT assay. Acta Med Okayama Vol. 56 pp. 129-34.

Kim NW, Piatyszek MA, Prowse KR, Harley CB, West MD, Ho PL, et al. (1994) Specific association of human telomerase activity with immortal cells and cancer. Science Vol. 266 pp. 2011-15.

Kongtun S, Jiratchariyakul W, Kummalue T, Tan-ariya P, Kunnachak S, Frahm AW. (2009) Cytotoxic properties of root extract and fruit juice of *Trichosanthes cucumerina*. Planta Med Vol. 75 pp. 839-842.

Koopman G, Reutelingsperger CPM, Kuijten GAM, Keehnen RMJ, Pals ST, Oers V. (1994) Annexin V for flow cytometric detection of phosphatidylserine expression on B cells undergoing apoptosis. Blood Vol. 84 pp. 1415-20.

Kosaka T, Fukaya K, Tsuboi S, Pu H, Ohno T, Tsuji T, et al. (1996) Comparison of various methods of assaying the cytotoxic effects of ethanol on human hepatoblastoma cells (HUH-6 line). Acta Med Okayama Vol. 50 pp.151-6.

Kummalue T, Jiratchariyakul W, Srisapoomi T, Sukpanichnant S, Hara T, Tani K. (2009) Antiproliferative effect of cucurbitacin B extracted from *Trichosanthes cucumerina* L. on human cancer cell Lines. Siriraj Med J Vol. 61 No. 2 pp. 75-7.

Kummalue T, Lou J, Friedman A.D. (2002) Multimerization via Its Myosin domain facilitates nuclear localization and Inhibition of CBF activities by the CBFbeta- SMMHC myeloid leukemia oncoprotein. Mol. Cell. Biol. Vol. 22 No.23 pp. 8278-91.

Kummalue T, O-charoenrat P, Jiratchariyakul W, Chanchai M, Iemsri S. (2005) Antiproliferative activities of three Thai medicinal plants on human cancer cells. Siriraj Med J Vol. 57 pp. 491-5.

Kummalue T, O-charoenrat P, Jiratchariyakul W, Chanchai M, Pattanapanyasat K, Sukapirom K, Iemsri S. (2007) Antiproliferative effect of *Erycibe elliptilimba* on human breast cancer cell lines. J Ethnopharmacol Vol. 110 No. 3 pp. 439-43.

Kummalue T, Sujiwattanarat P, Jiratchariyakul W. (2011) Apoptotic inducibility of *Sapindus rarax* water extract on A549 human lung cancer cell line. J Med Plants Res Vol. 5(7), pp. 1087-94.

Lacroix M, Leclercq G. (2004) Relevance of breast cancer cell lines as models for breast tumours: an update. Breast Cancer Res Treat Vol. 83 pp. 249-89.

Lacroix M. (2009) MDA-MB435 cells are from melanoma, not from breast cancer. Cancer Chemother Pharmacol Vol. 63 pp. 567.

Los M, Mozoluk M, Ferrari D, Stepczynska A, Stroh C, Renz A, et al. (2002) Activation and caspase-mediated inhibition of PARP a molecular switch between fibroblast necrosis and apoptosis in death receptor signaling. Molecular biol Cell 13:978-8.

Mandal SC, Ashok CK (2002). Studies on anti-diarrhoeal activity of *Ficus hispida*. Leaf extract in rats. Fitoterapia Vol. 73 pp. 663-7.

Miyamoto T, Min W, Lillehoj HS. (2002) Lymphocyte proliferation response during Eimeria tenella infection assessed by a new, reliable, nonradioactive colorimetric assay. Avian Dis vol.46 pp. 10-6.

Moseley JM, Findlay DM, Gorman JJ, Michelangeli VP, Martin TJ. (1983) The calcitonin receptor on T47D breast cancer cells. Biochem Vol. 212 pp.609-16.

Mosmann T. (1983) Rapid colorimetric assay for cellular growth and survival: Application to proliferation and cytotoxicity assays. J Immunol Methods Vol. 65 pp.55-63.

Nakamura TM, Morin GB, Chapman KB, Weinrich SL, Andrews WH, Linger J, et al. (1997) Telomerase catalytic subunit homologs from fission yeast and humans. Science Vol.277 pp. 955-9.

Niyazi M, Niyazi I, Belka C. (2007) Counting colonies of clonogenic assays by using densitometric software. Rad Oncol 2:4 Published online 2007 January 9. doi:10.1186/1748-717x-2-4.

North WG, Gao G, Memoli VA, Pang RH, Lynch L. (2010) Breast cancer expresses functional NMDA receptors. Breast Cancer Res Treat Vol. 122 pp. 307-14.

Nunez R. (2001) DNA measurement and cell cycle analysis by flow cytometry. Curr Issues Mol Biol Vol.3 pp.67-70.

Ozbay T, Nahta R. (2008) A novel unidirectional cross-talk from the insulin-like growth actor -I receptor to leptin receptor in human breast cancer cells. Mol Cancer Res Vol. 6 pp. 1052-8.

Park I, Zhao R, West J, Yabuuchi A, Huo H, Ince T, et al. (2008) Reprogramming of human somatic cells to pluripotency with defined factors. Nature Vol. 451 pp. 141-7.

Peraza-Sanchez, SR, Chai HB, Shin YG, Santisuk T, Reutrakul V, Farnsworth NR, Cordell GA, Pezzuto JM, Kinghorn AD (2002). Constituents of the leaves and twigs of *Ficus hispida*. Planta Med. Vol. 68 pp. 186-8.

Pevsner P, Naftolin F, Hillman D, Miller D, Fadiel A, Kogus A, et al. (2007) Direct identification of proteins from T47D cells and murine brain tissue by matrix-assisted laser desorption/ionization post-source decay/collision-induced dissociation. Rapid Commun Mass Spectrom Vol. 21 pp. 429-36.

Plumb Jane A. (2004) Cell sensitivity assays: The MTT assay. Methods Mol Med 88:165-9.

Pratumvinit B, Srisapoomi T, Worawattananon P, Opartkiattikul N, Jiratchariyakul W and Kummalue T. (2009) In vitro antineoplastic effect of *Ficus hispida* L. plant against breast cancer cell lines. Journal of Medicinal Plants Research Vol. 3 No. 4 pp. 255-261.

Rae JM, Ramus SJ, Waltham M, Armes JE, Campbell IG, Clarke R, et al. (2004) Common origins of MDA-MB435 cells from various sources with those shown to have melanoma properties. Clin Exp Met Vol. 21 pp. 543-52.

Raya A, Rodriguez-Piza I, Guenechea G, Vassena R, Navarro S, Barrero MJ, et al. (2009) Disease-corrected haematopoietic progenitors from Fanconi anemia induced pluripotent stem cells. Nature Vol. 460 pp. 53-60.

Report from the first seminar on herbs and cancer : *Murdannia loroformis*, held by National Cancer Institute of Thailand (1988) RamaVI Rd., Bangkok, June.

Rodney D, Capps II, Batsakis J, Briere RO, Calam R. (1966) An automated colorimetric (Tetrazolium salt) assay for serum lactate dehydrogenase. Clin Chem Vol. 12 pp. 406-13.

Ross JS, Linette GP, Stec J, Ross M, Anwar S, boguniewicz A. (2003) DNA ploidy and cell cycle analysis in breast cancer. Am J Clin Pathol 120 (Suppl 1): S72-S84.

Sasaki T, Kawai K, Saijo-Kurita K, Ohno T. (1992) Detergent cytotoxicity: Simplified assay of cytolysis by measuring LDH activity. Toxic In Vitro Vol. 6 pp. 451-7.

Shay JW, Bacchetti S. (1997) A survey of telomerase activity in human cancer. Eur J Cancer Vol. 33 pp. 787-91.

Shay JW, Zou Y, Hiyama E, Wright W. (2001) Telomerase and cancer. Hum Mol Gen Vol. 10 pp. 677-85.

Silapaarcha W, Picha P, Lurwongrattana O, Kittiwongsunthorn W, Ungsunthornsarit P. (1981) Investigation of the triterpenes in cucurbitaceae prevalent in Thailand. Mahidol University journal Pharmaceutical Science Vol. 8, No. 1 pp. 5-8.

Sintusarn, U. (2002) Natural Product of Chao-Krom-Po, 2nd ed. Thammasarn Printing, Bangkok, p. 190.

Slater TF, Sawyer B., Strauli UD. (1963) Studies on succinate tetrazolium reductase systems. III points of coupling of four different tetrazolium salts. Biochem Biophys Acta Vol. 77 pp. 383-93.

Srisapoomi T, Jiratchariyakul W, O-partkiattikul N, Kummalue T. (2008) Effects of two Thai herbal remedies on the sensitivity of chemotherapeutic agents in human cancer cells. Asian Journal of Traditional Medicine Vol. 3 No. 4 pp. 144-152.

Sylvester PW. (2011) Optimization of tetrazolium dye (MTT) colorimetric assay for cellular growth and viability. Methods Mol Biol Vol. 716 pp. 157-68.

Takahashi K, Yamanaka S. (2006) Induction of pluripotent stem cells from mouse embryonic and adult fibroblast cultures by defined factors. Cell Vol. 126 pp. 663-76.

Tappayuthpijarn P, Sattaboos P, Pidetcha P. (1991) Subchronic toxicity of *Murdannia loriformis*. Siriraj Hosp Gaz Vol. 43 pp. 529-533.

Tappayuthpijarn P, Wamanutajinda V, Pidetcha P. (1991) Acute toxicity of *Murdannia loriformis*. Siriraj Hosp Gaz Vol. 43 pp. 458-462.

Tiangda C, Silapaarcha W, wiwat C, Picha P. (1986) Chemical composition, acute toxicity and pharmacological screening of *Trichosanthes cucumerina* L., *Proceeding of the 11th Asian Congress of Pharmaceutical Sciences* pp. 320-324, Bangkok, Thailand,

Tsuji K, Kawauchi S, Saito S, Furuya T, Ikemoto K, Nakao M, et al. (2010) Breast cancer cell lines carry cell line-specific genomic alterations that are distinct from aberrations in breast cancer tissues: Comparison of the CGH profiles between cancer cell lines and primary cancer tissues. BMC Cancer 10:15 Published online 2010 January 14. doi:10.1186/1471-2407-10-15.

Ulukaya E, Ozdikicioglu F, Oral AY, Demirci M. (2008) The MTT assay yields a relatively lower result of growth inhibition than the ATP assay depending on the chemotherapeutic drugs tested. Toxicol In Vitro Vol. 22 No.1 pp. 232-9.

U-pratya Y, Jiratchariyakul W, Kummalue T. (2008) Anti-proliferative effects of *Pouzolzia indica* on acute promyelocytic cell lines: NB4 and HT93A. Asian Journal of Traditional Medicines Vol. 3 No. 4 pp. 124-133.

U-pratya Y, Lueangamornnara U, Jiratchariyakul W and Kummalue T. (2010) Immunosuppressive effects of Cucurbitacin B on human peripheral blood lymphocytes. Journal of Medicinal Plants Research Vol. 4 No. 22 pp. 2340–2347.

Vinitketkumnuen U, Charoenkunathum W, Kongtawelert P, Lertprasertsuk R, Picha P, Matsushima T. (1996) DT-diaphorase inducer activity of antimutagenic Thai medicinal plant, *Murdannia loriformis*. J. Herbs & Spices and Medicinal Plants. Vol. 4 pp. 45-51.

Westmose Yde C, Issinger OG. (2006) Enhancing cisplatin sensitivity in MCF7 human breast cancer cells by down regulation of Bcl-2 and cyclin D1. Inter J Oncol 29:1397-1404.

Wuttidhammaved,W. (1997) Thai Traditional Medicine, revised ed. O-dien Store Printing, Bangkok, p. 339.

Xiao Y, Gao X, Maragh S, Telford WG, Tona A. (2009) Cell lines as candidate reference materials for quality control of ERBB2 amplification and expression assays in breast cancer. Clin Chem Vol. 55 pp.7.

Xu J, Zhang Y, Berry PA, Jiang J, Lobie PE, Langenheim JF, et al. (2011) Growth hormone signaling in human T47D breast cancer cells: Potential role for a growth hormone receptor-prolactin receptor complex. Mol Endocrinol Vol. 25 pp. 597-610.

Zhang GJ, Kimijima I, Onda M, Kanno M, Sato H, Watanabe T, et al. (1999) Tamoxifen-induced apoptosis in breast cancer cells relates to down-regulation of bcl-2, but not bax and bcl-XL, without alteration of p53 protein levels. Clin Cancer Res Vol. 5 pp. 2971-7.

Zhang Y, Pu X, Shi M, Chen L, Qian L, Song Y, et al. (2007) c-Jun, a crucial molecule in metastasis of breast cancer and potential target for biotherapy. Oncology Reports Vol. 18 pp. 1207-12.

Zhivich AB, Koldobskii GI, Ostrovskii VA. (1990) Tetrazolium salts (Review) Chemistry of Heterocyclic compounds Vol. 26 pp. 1319-28.

9

Novel Therapeutic Strategies and Combinations for HER2-Overexpressing Breast Cancer

Sylvia Shabaya and Rita Nahta
Emory University,
USA

1. Introduction

Approximately 20-30% of breast cancers show increased expression of the HER2 receptor tyrosine kinase. Elevated levels of HER2 are associated with aggressive disease, high metastatic potential, and reduced survival versus other breast cancer subtypes (Slamon, 1987). Trastuzumab (Herceptin) is a monoclonal antibody targeted against an extracellular region of HER2 (Carter, 1992). Clinical trials have shown that 15-30% of patients with HER2-overexpressing metastatic breast cancer respond to single-agent trastuzumab for a median duration of approximately 10 months (Baselga, 1996; Cobleigh, 1999). Response rates improve when trastuzumab is combined with chemotherapy in patients with HER2-overexpressing metastatic breast cancer (Esteva, 2002; Slamon, 2001). A subset of trastuzumab-resistant breast cancers respond to the dual EGFR/HER2 kinase inhibitor lapatinib, although the majority (70% or more) show primary resistance (Geyer, 2006). Similar to trastuzumab treatment, clinical trials with lapatinib indicated that the median duration of response to lapatinib in a heavily pre-treated, trastuzumab-refractory population was less than one year (Geyer, 2006). Hence, resistance to clinically available HER2-targeted agents is a major concern in the treatment of patients with HER2-overexpressing metastatic breast cancer.

2. HER2 and breast cancer

The human epidermal growth factor receptor 2 (HER2) is overexpressed in approximately 25% of invasive breast carcinomas. HER2 is a member of the epidermal growth factor receptor (EGFR) family, which also contains two other receptors, HER3 and HER4 (Fig. 1). Each of these cell surface receptors has an extracellular ligand-binding domain and a transmembrane-spanning domain (Nielsen, 2008). All HER family receptors except HER2 bind specific ligands that induce conformational changes and receptor homo- or hetero-dimerization. Several HER family ligands have been identified including transforming growth factor alpha (TGFa), epidermal growth factor (EGF), and the heregulins (Nielsen, 2008). In addition, all except HER3 contain an intracellular tyrosine kinase domain. Receptor dimerization activates the kinase function of receptors, leading to receptor auto- or trans-phosphorylation. The phosphorylated tyrosine residues serve as docking sites for SH2 and PTB-domain containing proteins, which links the receptors to multiple cell survival and proliferation pathways including the phosphatidylinositol-3 kinase (PI3K) and mitogen-activated protein kinase (MAPK) cascades (Spector, 2009; Graus-Porta, 1997). HER2 is the preferred dimerization partner for the other HER family members, as HER2 heterodimers have increased ligand binding affinity and increased catalytic activity relative to other heterodimer complexes (Spector, 2009; Graus-Porta, 1997). In particular, the HER2-HER3 heterodimer has the strongest kinase activity and transforming ability, as HER3 possesses multiple PI3K docking sites in its cytoplasmic tail.

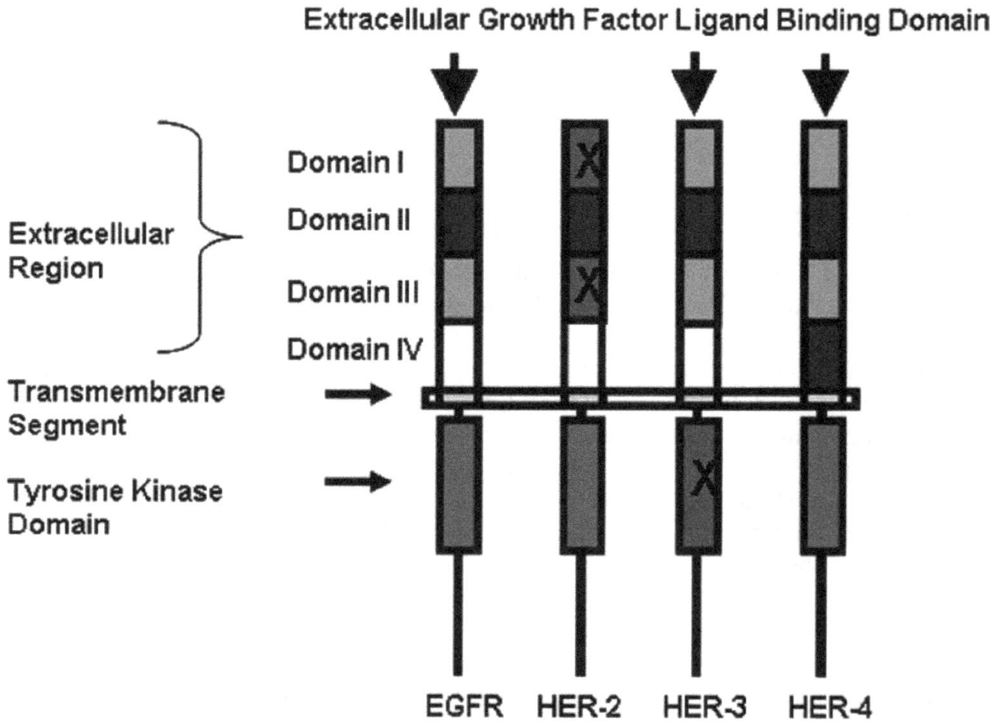

Fig. 1. HER/erbB family of growth factor receptors. The four members of the EGFR family are illustrated. The inactive ligand-binding domains of HER2 and the inactive kinase domain of HER3 are denoted with an X. Trastuzumab binds to domain IV of the extracellular region of HER2.

2.1 Targeting HER2 in breast cancer

Patients who are diagnosed with HER2-overexpressing breast cancer have a poor prognosis, and shorter progression-free and overall survival compared to patients with other subtypes of breast cancer (Eccles, 2001). HER2-overexpressing tumors have been found to be larger in size, and higher in nuclear grade, S phase fraction, and aneuploidy (Nielsen, 2008). Traditional cancer treatments have targeted DNA replication or cell division, leading to nonspecific cytotoxicity (Oakman, 2010). The identification of abnormal signaling from HER2 led to the development of trastuzumab (Herceptin) (Genentech, San Francisco, CA, USA), which is the first drug to target the genetic lesion or oncogenic addiction found in patients with HER2-overexpressing breast cancer. Clinically, trastuzumab was found to significantly enhance the effectiveness of conventional chemotherapies. However, the median duration of response was less than one year, indicating rapid development of resistance. The precise mechanism of action of trastuzumab is unclear, but it is thought to involve HER2 downregulation (Cuello, 2001; Gajria, 2011), selective inhibition of HER2-HER3 heterodimerization (Junttila, 2009; Gajria, 2011), prevention of HER2 extracellular domain proteolytic cleavage (Molina, 2001; Gajria, 2011), and activation of an immune response including antibody-dependent cellular cytotoxicity (Sliwkowski, 1999). As a single agent, trastuzumab achieved an overall response rate for a median duration of about nine months (Baselga, 1996; Cobleigh, 1999; Nielsen, 2008; Slamon, 2001). The low response rate indicates that many patients with HER2-overexpressing breast cancer have primary resistance to trastuzumab, while the short duration of response indicates rapid development of acquired resistance. Multiple mechanisms contributing to trastuzumab resistance have been proposed, resulting in multiple approaches to potentially treat resistant cancers (Table 1).

Target	Role in trastuzumab resistance
PI3K	Increased PI3K signaling due to *PIK3CA* mutations or PTEN loss was reported in trastuzumab-resistant cancers
mTOR	As a downstream molecule of PI3K, mTOR has become a target of inhibition in resistant cancers; multiple mTOR inhibitors are in advanced phases of clinical development
IGF-IR	Increased expression of IGF-IR has been shown to reduce response to trastuzumab; increased IGF-IR overexpression was associated with lower response to neoadjuvant trastuzumab; IGF-IR/HER2 interaction and crosstalk were associated with acquired resistance
Src	Trastuzumab-mediated inhibition of Src activity appears to be important to its anti-cancer activity; resistance to trastuzumab was associated with PTEN loss and increased Src activity; targeting Src with dasatinib or genetic knockdown blocked growth of resistant cancers
Cdk2	Reduced p27kip1 levels or amplification of *cyclin E* gene have been reported to result in increased cdk2 activity in trastuzumab-resistant cancers

Table 1. Potential pharmacologic targets in trastuzumab-resistant HER2-positive breast cancers.

3. Targeting PI3K/mTOR signaling in HER2-overexpressing breast cancer

HER2 signaling is initiated upon receptor dimerization, which induces phosphorylation of tyrosine residues within the receptor cytoplasmic domain. The phosphorylated residues serve as docking sites for adaptor proteins and link the receptor to downstream survival pathways including the PI3K/Akt/mTOR axis (Spector, 2009). The PI3K pathway is frequently hyper-activated in many cancers. An association between oncogenic PI3K mutations and trastuzumab resistance was found in a study examining HER2-overexpressing tumors from patients with trastuzumab-refractory disease (Berns, 2007). About 25% of tumors analyzed had PIK3CA mutations, and reduced phosphatase and tensin homolog (PTEN) expression was present in 22% of the tumors. Immunohistochemistry studies performed in a retrospective analysis of *HER2*-amplified breast tumors treated with trastuzumab plus taxanes showed a postive correlation between PTEN down-regulation and tumor response (Nagata, 2004). To evaluate the role of PI3K post-trastuzumab exposure, tumors that had progressed on trastuzumab were analyzed for changes in PI3K signaling. The findings demonstrated that PI3K mutations and PTEN loss were identified in patients who had initially responded to trastuzumab; reduced PTEN expression was identified in tumors that had developed trastuzumab resistance, but had not been identified before trastuzumab treatment. This finding indicates that PI3K mutations can occur as a result of trastuzumab treatment in some tumors (Kalinsky, 2009; Sakr, 2010; Gajria, 2011). Thus, there is ample rationale for co-targeting PI3K and HER2 in breast cancer. Activated Akt regulates several downstream signaling molecules including mTOR, a highly conserved 289-kDa serine/threonine kinase that plays roles in cell proliferation, survival, and motility (Lang, 2010). mTOR activation is initiated when phosphorylated PI3K/Akt inhibits the TSC1/TSC2 complexes, thereby preventing Rheb from inhibiting mTOR. mTORC1 (mTOR, Raptor, mLST8/GBL and PRAS40) and mTORC2 (mTOR, RICTOR, mLST8/GBL, SIN1, and PROTOR/PRR5) are the two distinct complexes through which mTOR exerts cellular effects. The complexes have different functional roles, with mTORC1 having been implicated in cell cycle progression, motility, and protein biosynthesis, while mTORC2 regulates cytoskeleton organization, and regulates cell growth and survival (Wullschleger, 2005; Van der Heijen, 2011).

Preclinical *in vivo* studies in which mice were treated with single agent trastuzumab, the mTOR inhibitor rapamycin, or a combination of trastuzumab plus rapamycin showed that the combination was more effective at inducing tumor regression than either of the single agent treatments (Miller, 2009). In cell culture experiments using the rapamycin analogue RAD001, a greater amount of growth inhibition was observed with combination mTOR inhibition plus HER2-targeting than with either drug alone. Trastuzumab partially decreased PI3K activity, but not mTOR activity (Miller, 2009). Increased PI3K signaling is a validated mechanism of trastuzumab resistance, but its association with lapatinib resistance is yet to be determined due to conflicting data (Eichhorn, 2008; O'Brien, 2010). Patients with HER2-overexpressing breast cancer who have developed resistance to trastuzumab may be given the dual EGFR/HER2 tyrosine kinase inhibitor lapatinib. Response to single agent lapatinib is less than 25%, indicating cross-resistance between trastuzumab and lapatinib (Blackwell, 2010; Eichhorn, 2008). As with trastuzumab treatment, the small subset of patients who initially responded to lapatinib eventually developed resistance, at which point there is no standard therapeutic approach available. Phase I trials have indicated that in patients with trastuzumab-resistant, heavily pretreated breast cancer, combined everolimus plus trastuzumab could be a promising treatment (Jerusalem, 2011). It is thought that the inability of trastuzumab to completely inhibit PI3K/Akt/mTOR signaling may permit escape from growth inhibition; mTOR inhibitors would thus synergize with trastuzumab to prevent the continued growth of HER2-dependent cancer cells.

In contrast to PI3K, very little has been published regarding the role of MAPK signaling in trastuzumab resistance. Our data suggests that phosphorylation of Erk1/2, which is a marker of MAPK activity, is not increased in resistant cells (Fig. 2A). Inhibition of MEK (upstream of Erk1/2) using a small molecule MEK kinase inhibitor called PD0325901 reduces p-Erk1/2 levels in parental HER2-overexpressing breast cancer cells and in acquired trastuzumab-resistant and primary trastuzumab-resistant cells (Fig. 2B). However, trastuzumab-naïve and trastuzumab-resistant cells are relatively resistant to PD0325901, in that doses up to 10 uM do not block proliferation of HER2-overexpressing trastuzumab-naïve or resistant cells (Fig. 2C). Thus, our data indicate that MAPK signaling may not be a major mechanism of trastuzumab resistance.

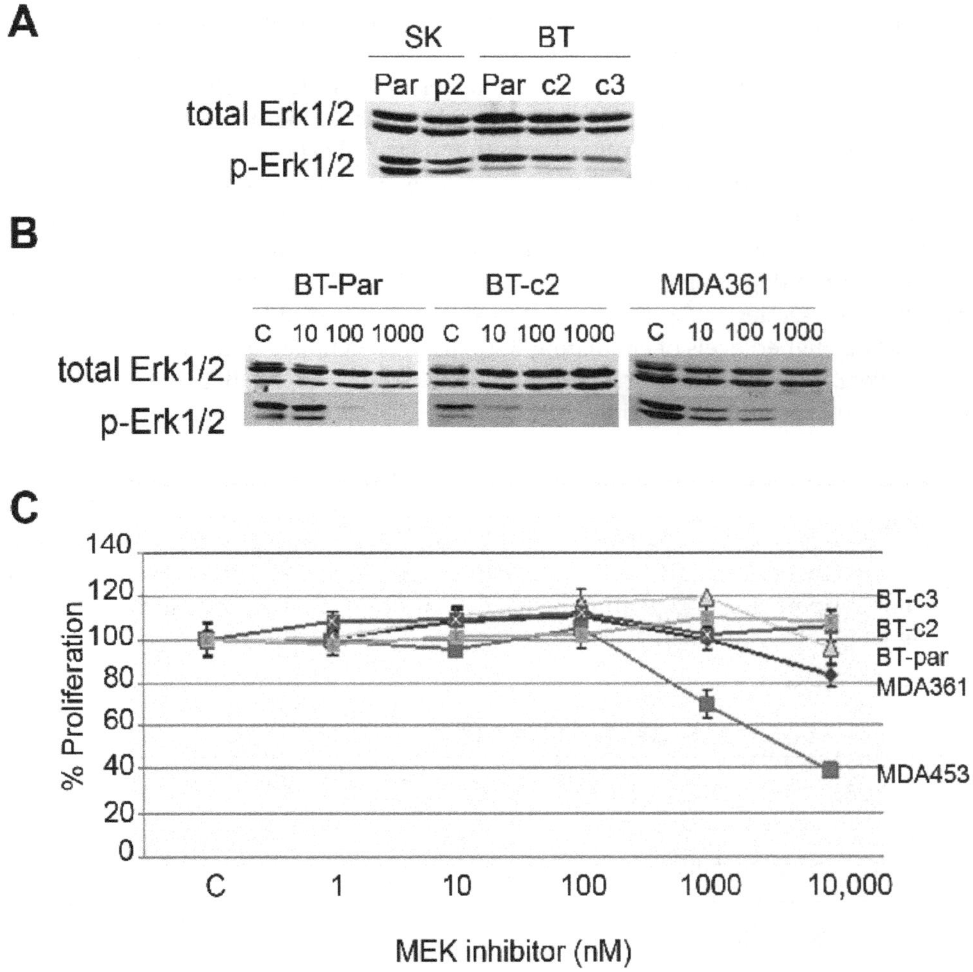

Fig. 2. Role of MAPK signaling in trastuzumab-resistant cells. (A) SKBR3 parental, trastuzumab-resistant pool 2, and BT474 parental, and trastuzumab-resistant clone 2 and clone 3 cells were Western blotted for phosphorylated and total Erk1/2. (B) BT-parental, BT-c2 (resistant clone 2), and MDA-MB-361 primary trastuzumab-resistant cells were treated with MEK inhibitor PD0325901 at 10, 100, or 1000nM for 6 hours or with DMSO control (C) corresponding to the volume found in the highest dose of PD0325901. Total protein lysates were Western blotted for phosphorylated and total Erk1/2. (C) BT-parental, resistant clone 2 and 3, MDA361, and MDA453 cells were treated with MEK inhibitor PD0325901 at 1, 10, 100, 1000, or 10, 000nM for 48 hours with six replicates per treatment group. Control cells were treated with DMSO corresponding to the volume found in the highest dose of PD0325901. Proliferation was assessed by MTS assay, and is shown as a percentage of control group per line.

4. Targeting IGF-IR signaling in HER2-overexpressing breast cancer

The insulin-like growth factor receptor I (IGF-IR) is a heterotrimeric transmembrane tyrosine kinase receptor that regulates cell metabolism and growth (Chaves, 2010), and has been associated with increased risk and maintenance of multiple cancers including HER2-overexpressing breast cancer (Esparis-Ogando, 2008; Hankinson, 1998; Surmacz, 2000). Circulating ligands of the insulin-like growth factor (IGF) system include IGF-I and IGF-II, with IGF-I having the highest affinity for IGF-IR. Upon binding to IGF-IR, a receptor conformational change is induced that leads to tyrosine phosphorylation and activation of several downstream survival signaling pathways such as the Ras/Raf/mitogen activated protein kinase pathway (MAPK), and the PI3K/Akt/mTOR pathway. Activation of these pathways results in cell cycle progression and resistance to apoptosis (Chaves, 2011; Adams, 2000). The IGF binding proteins (IGFBPs) modulate IGF-IR activity by binding to the IGF ligands thereby sequestering them and preventing ligand-induced receptor activation (Adams, 2000). Higher levels of circulating IGF-I have been linked to trastuzumab resistance in HER2-overexpressing breast cancer, with the addition of IGFBP3 decreasing IGF-IR activity, and subsequently resulting in an increased response to trastuzumab (Lu, 2001; Jerome, 2006).

We found by gene microarray analysis that IGFBP3 and IGFBP5 were down-regulated in resistant versus sensitive cells (Table 2). However, ELISA of secreted IGFBP3 (Fig. 3A) or real-time PCR analysis of endogenous IGFBP3 or IGFBP5 transcript level (Fig. 3B) failed to show any differences in IGFBP3 or IGFBP5 level in resistant versus parental cells. Thus, our data do not support down-regulation of IGFBP3 or IGFBP5 as a mechanism of increased IGF-IR signaling in trastuzumab resistance.

Gene Name	Fold Change	ILMN_GENE	DEFINITION
IGFBP5	-20. 55848937	IGFBP5	Homo sapiens insulin-like growth factor binding protein 5 (IGFBP5), mRNA.
IGFBP5	-20. 0185274	IGFBP5	Homo sapiens insulin-like growth factor binding protein 5 (IGFBP5), mRNA.
IGFBP3	-7. 77282369	IGFBP3	Homo sapiens insulin-like growth factor binding protein 3 (IGFBP3), transcript variant 2, mRNA.
PKIA	-6. 484521044	PKIA	Homo sapiens protein kinase (cAMP-dependent, catalytic) inhibitor alpha (PKIA), transcript variant 7, mRNA.
IGFBP3	-6. 193624741	IGFBP3	Homo sapiens insulin-like growth factor binding protein 3 (IGFBP3), transcript variant 1, mRNA.
PKIA	-5. 371909749	PKIA	Homo sapiens protein kinase (cAMP-dependent, catalytic) inhibitor alpha (PKIA), transcript variant 6, mRNA.
BASP1	-4. 444496135	BASP1	Homo sapiens brain abundant, membrane attached signal protein 1 (BASP1), mRNA.
HERC6	-4. 048474978	HERC6	Homo sapiens hect domain and RLD 6 (HERC6), mRNA.
FRAS1	-3. 988854857	FRAS1	Homo sapiens Fraser syndrome 1 (FRAS1), mRNA.
THBS1	-3. 966312615	THBS1	Homo sapiens thrombospondin 1 (THBS1), mRNA.

Table 2. Genes that are down-regulated in SKBR3- and BT474-derived acquired trastuzumab-resistant cells versus parental SKBR3 and BT474 cells by 4-fold or more.

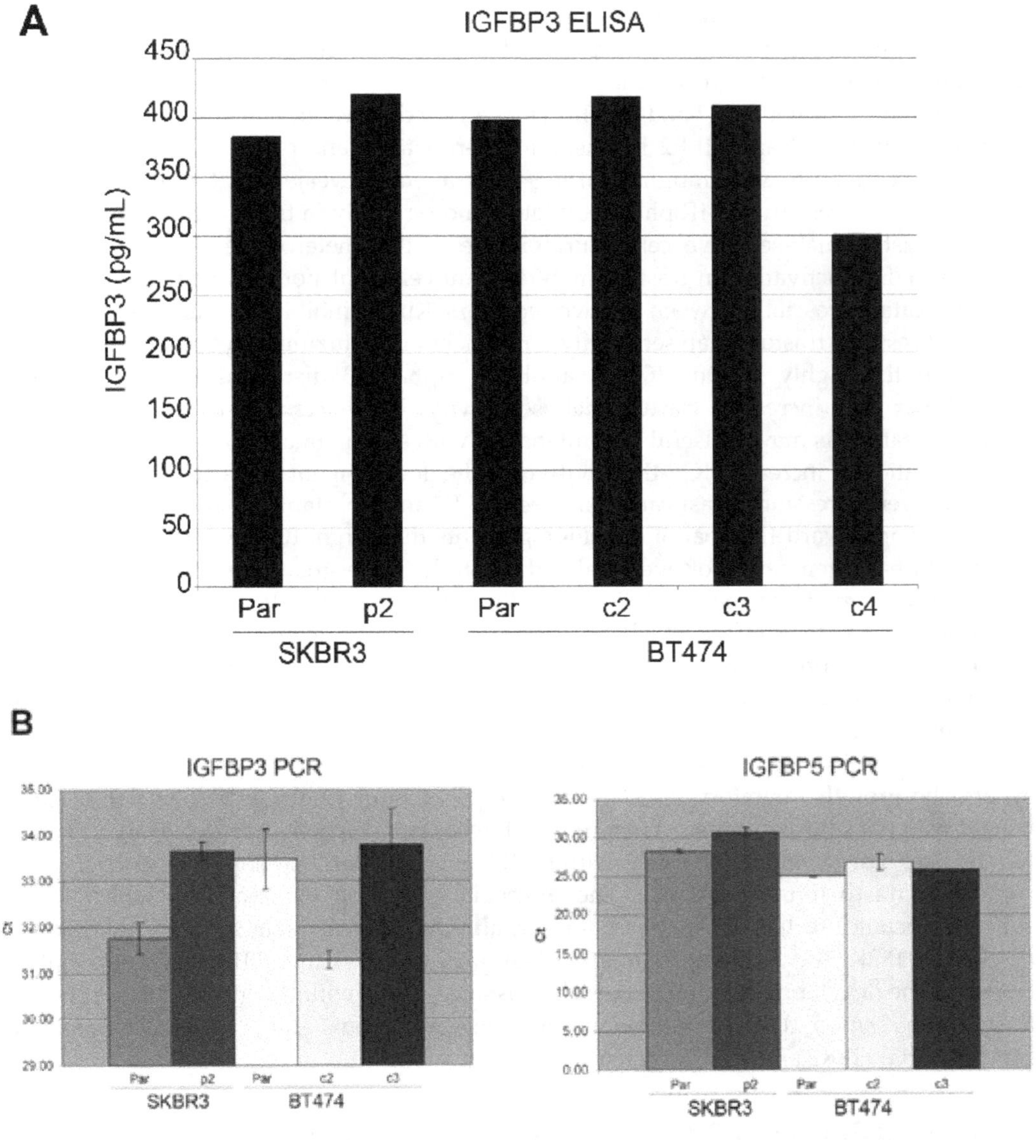

Fig. 3. IGFBP3 and IGFBP5 in resistant and sensitive cells. (A) Secreted IGFBP3 was assessed by ELISA in SKBR3 parental, resistant pool 2, BT474 parental, resistant clone 2 and clone 3 cells. IGFBP3 is shown in pg/mL and was measured in triplicate with reproducible results per line. (B) Real-time PCR analysis of IGFBP3 and IGFBP5 was examined in triplicate per line, with error bars representing standard deviation between replicates. Housekeeping gene RPLPO was measured as an internal control; IGFBP3 and IGFBP5 values are normalized to RPLPO.

A subset of HER2-/ IGF-IR-overexpressing cells were found to be less sensitive to the growth inhibitory effects of trastuzumab when compared to HER2-overexpressing cells that do not overexpress IGF-IR (Lu, 2001). Flow cytometry revealed that after trastuzumab treatment, HER2 overexpressing cells were less likely to progress through the cell cycle and stopped at the G1 phase, while a greater number of HER2/IGF-IR overexpressing cells passed the restriction point and completed the cell cycle. These results demonstrate that IGF-IR interferes with the growth inhibitory actions of trastuzumab, supporting therapeutic strategies that co-target HER2 and IGF-IR. Further, we discovered that signaling interactions exist between IGF-IR and HER2 in trastuzumab-resistant cancers (Nahta, 2005; Jin, 2008). Immunoprecipitation and immunoblotting experiments revealed that IGF-I stimulation results in an increase in IGF-IR phosphorylation more rapidly in trastuzumab-resistant cells than in trastuzumab-sensitive cells. Furthermore, IGF-IR heterodimerization with HER2 results in HER2 activation in trastuzumab-resistant cells, but not in trastuzumab-sensitive cells, indicating crosstalk between the two receptors. Kinase inhibition or antibody blockade of IGF-IR restores trastuzumab sensitivity. Treatment of trastuzumab-resistant breast cancer cells with the highly specific IGF-IR antibody alpha IR3 disrupted the IGF-IR/HER2 heterodimer and increased trastuzumab sensitivity. These results suggest that IGF-IR-targeted treatments may be useful in combination with trastuzumab.

The association of increased IGF-IR activity with the development of trastuzumab resistance in HER2-overexpressing breast cancer makes IGF-IR an important target. Researchers have been working toward the goal of developing agents that target IGF-IR for the past several years with each generation of agents aimed at producing a greater benefit for the patient while decreasing adverse effects. IGF-IR and the insulin receptor (IR) are 60% homologous, with one of the adverse effects of IGF-IR antibody treatment being downregulation of the IR, leading to hyperglycemia (Sachdev, 2006). In an effort to remedy this problem, pharmacological agents like the small molecule tyrosine kinase inhibitor NVP-AEW541 (Novartis Pharma, Basel Switzerland) are specific for IGF-IR and less likely to interfere with glucose metabolism. Combination treatment with NVP-AEW541 and trastuzumab showed synergistic growth inhibitory effects, indicating that inhibiting IGF-IR plus HER2 could benefit patients whose tumors overexpress both receptors (Esparis-Ogando, 2008).

IGF-IR overexpression and crosstalk with HER2 suggests that IGF-IR plays a crucial role in conferring trastuzumab resistance. The molecular signaling pathways by which IGF-IR confers resistance to trastuzumab is not clear, although downstream focal adhesion kinase (FAK) and PI3K/Akt pathway signaling likely play a role (Yang, 2010). This data linking IGF-IR to the development of trastuzumab resistance, along with the increased sensitivity to trastuzumab upon IGF-IR inhibition provides a rational for the development of combinatorial HER2 and IGF-IR targeting.

5. Targeting Src in HER2-overexpressing breast cancer

Trastuzumab treatment of HER2-overexpressing breast cancer cells results in inhibition of Src non-receptor tyrosine kinase (Nagata, 2004). Src inhibition appears to be important to trastuzumab-mediated anti-cancer activity, as increased Src signaling is associated with trastuzumab resistance (Mitra, 2009; Liang, 2010; Zhang, 2011). One mechanism leading to increased Src activity appears to be a variant of HER2 called HER2 delta 16 (Mitra, 2009), which shows increased oncogenic activity. Local disease progression involved HER2Delta16 in 89% of breast cancer patients with HER2-positive tumors (Mitra, 2009). Transfection of MCF7 or NIH3T3 cells with HER2 delta 16 promoted receptor dimerization, invasion, and trastuzumab resistance (Mitra, 2009). The oncogenic properties of HER2Delta16 were mediated through direct interaction of HER2Delta16 with Src kinase. Activated Src kinase was found in 44% of HER2Delta16-positive breast carcinomas (Mitra, 2009). Dual targeting of HER2Delta16 plus Src with dasatinib resulted in Src inactivation, destabilization of HER2Delta16, and decreased tumorigenicity (Mitra, 2009). In addition, Src activation via Jak2 has been shown to reduce trastuzumab activity (Liang, 2010). Recombinant human erythropoietin activated Jak2-Src signaling and inactivated PTEN in HER2-positive cells (Liang, 2010). Combined treatment with recombinant human erythropoietin plus trastuzumab reduced response to trastuzumab in cell culture and *in vivo* models. Further, shorter progression-free and overall survival was found in patients with HER2-positive breast cancer treated concurrently with erythropoietin and trastuzumab (Liang, 2010). Src was also shown to be activated in primary and acquired trastuzumab resistance as a consequence of PTEN loss (Zhang, 2011). Src-targeted therapy blocked growth of trastuzumab-resistant tumors *in vivo* (Zhang, 2011). Thus, Src activation may occur via multiple mechanisms, ultimately abrogating sensitivity to trastuzumab. Combining Src-targeted therapy with trastuzumab may offer benefit to patients with HER2-overexpressing breast cancer.

6. Role of p27 and cdk2 in HER2-overexpressing breast cancer

Trastuzumab induces G1 arrest by several mechanisms including increased expression of cyclin-dependent kinase inhibitor p27kip1, which inhibits cyclin E/cdk2 and cyclin A/cdk2 complexes and blocks cell cycle progression through S phase (Lane, 2001; Le, 2003). Trastuzumab induces p27kip1expression by suppressing expression of proteins that sequester p27kip1, which also results in increased interaction between p27kip1 and cdk2 leading to cdk2 inactivation (Lane, 2001). We previously reported (Nahta, 2004b) that cells with acquired trastuzumab resistance showed increased proliferation, reduced p27kip1 expression, reduced p27kip1-cdk2 interaction, and increased cdk2 activity relative to parental, trastuzumab-sensitive cells. Transfection of wild-type p27kip1 increased trastuzumab sensitivity in cells with acquired resistance (Nahta, 2004b). Yakes et al. (Yakes, 2002) showed that knockdown of p27kip1 reduced trastuzumab sensitivity in HER2-overexpressing breast cancer cell lines, further supporting a requirement of p27kip1 expression for optimal response to trastuzumab. Post-translational modification of p27kip1 occurs primarily by phosphorylation, with subsequent protein ubiquitination and degradation. Preliminary data supporting ubiquitin-proteasome degradation of p27kip1 as a mechanism of p27kip1 down-regulation in trastuzumab resistance includes our finding that proteasome inhibitor MG132 induced p27 expression and reduced viability of resistant cells (Nahta, 2004b). Further, Cardoso et al. (Cardoso, 2006) showed that proteasome inhibitor bortezomib induced p27kip1 and increased the efficacy of trastuzumab in HER2-overexpressing breast cancer cells. PI3K inhibition has been shown to induce p27kip1 expression, and is believed to contribute to p27kip1 down-regulation and acquired trastuzumab resistance. In addition to observing reduced p27kip1 levels in models of acquired resistance, our data indicates that p27kip1 expression is down-regulated post-transcriptionally in cells with primary trastuzumab resistance (Fig. 4). Cyclin E expression has been shown to be regulated by HER2 expression status, in that HER2 knockdown resulted in reduced cyclin E level and reduced cyclin E-associated kinase activity (Mittendorf, 2010). In addition, HER2-overexpressing breast cancers that also show increased cyclin E expression have lower 5 year disease-free survival versus those that have lower cyclin E levels (Mittendorf, 2010). Recently, cyclin E overexpression in HER2-overexpressing breast cancer cells that have acquired trastuzumab resistance was shown to be due to amplification of the *cyclin E* gene (Scaltriti, 2011). Amongst 34 patients with HER2-overexpressing breast cancer, cyclin E amplification was associated with worse response to trastuzumab (Scaltriti, 2011). Knockdown of cyclin E or cdk2 inhibition reduced proliferation and induced apoptosis of trastuzumab-resistant tumors (Scaltriti, 2011). Thus, cdk2 inhibition is a potential pharmacologic strategy for treating trastuzumab-resistant HER2-overexpressing breast cancers that show reduced p27kip1 or increased cyclin E levels.

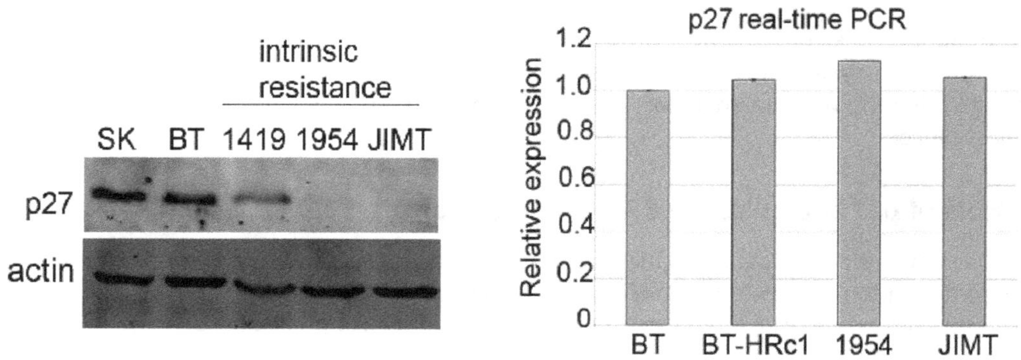

Fig. 4. p27 down-regulation in models of intrinsic (primary resistance). (A) SKBR3 and BT474 trastuzumab-sensitive cells and trastuzumab-resistant HCC1419, HCC1954, and JIMT-1 cells were examined by Western blotting for p27 and actin internal control. (B) BT474 and acquired resistant clone BT-HRc1 and primary resistant HCC1954 and JIMT-1 cells were examined by real-time PCR for p27 transcript which was normalized to RPLPO housekeeping gene.

7. Combining multiple HER2-targeted agents in HER2-overexpressing breast cancer

Two HER2-targeted agents are currently approved for use in the setting of metastatic HER2-positive breast cancer, trastuzumab and lapatinib. These agents target HER2 via distinct mechanisms (Fig. 5). Trastuzumab is a monoclonal antibody that specifically recognizes and binds to an extracellular part of HER2. Since antibodies are large, bulky molecules, trastuzumab is unable to cross the blood-brain barrier and thus cannot combat brain metastases. In contrast, lapatinib is a small molecule kinase inhibitor targeted against the EGFR and HER2 active sites. Since it is a small molecule, it is believed that lapatinib has the potential to enter the brain and target metastatic cells that overexpress HER2. A phase II trial of lapatinib in patients with trastuzumab-refractory disease and CNS metastases showed some volumetric changes in brain lesions and improved neurologic symptoms (Lin, 2008; Lin, 2009). Amongst 50 patients who were terated with lapatinib plus capecitabine, 20% showed a CNS objective response and 40% experienced 20% or greater volumetric reduction in their CNS lesions (Lin, 2009), suggesting that lapatinib may have some utility in limiting CNS metastases of primary HER2-overexpressing breast cancers.

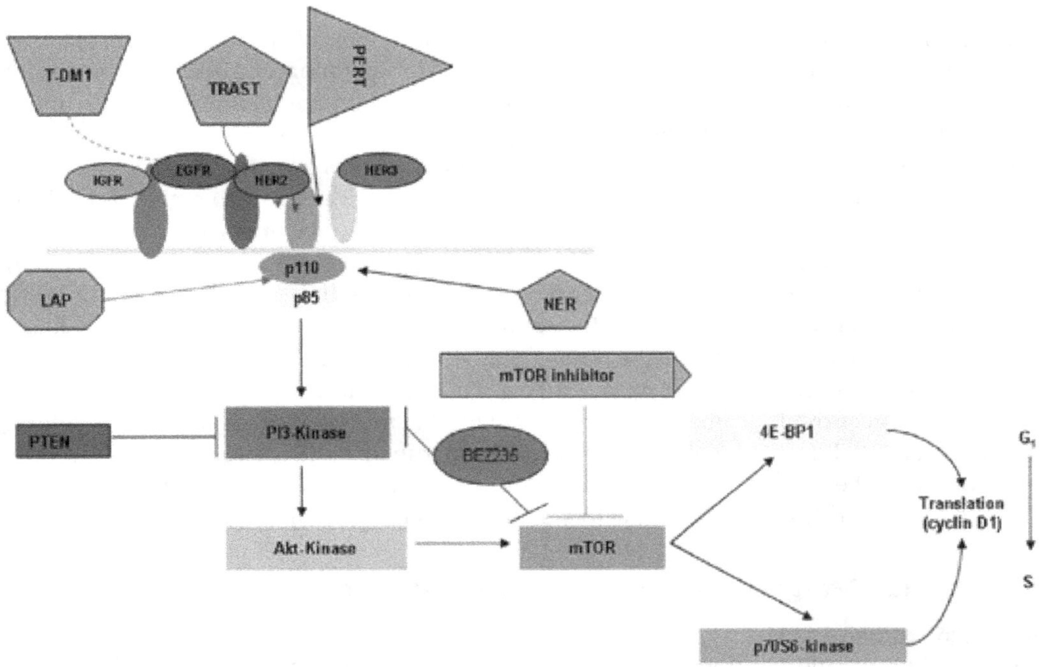

Fig. 5. Novel targeted agents in trastuzumab-resistant HER2-positive breast cancer. T-DM1, Trastuzumab-DM1; TRAST, Trastuzumab; PERT, Pertuzumab; IGFR, insulin growth factor receptor; EGFR, epidermal growth factor receptor; LAP, lapatinib; NER, neratinib.

7.1 Combining trastuzumab with lapatinib

Combination of trastuzumab plus lapatinib has been shown to induce apoptosis in part via down-regulation of survivin in cell culture and animal models (Xia, 2005). Initial phase I data suggested that the combination is well-tolerated and elicits partial or complete responses in a subset of patients who have progressed on prior trastuzumab therapy (Storniolo, 2008). The combination has been tested clinically in advanced phase trials in patients who have progressed on trastuzumab-based regimens. Progression-free survival and quality of life were improved in patients treated with the combination versus lapatinib alone (Wu, 2011). EGF104900 showed that the combination was superior to lapatinib alone in the trastuzumab-resistant setting, with a clonical benefit rate of 24. 7% versus 12. 4% (Blackwell, 2010). A potentially important mechanism of action of this drug combination is that lapatinib has been shown to induce accumulation of inactive HER2 dimers via reduced receptor ubiquitination, providing increased pharmacologic target for trastuzumab-mediated antibody-dependent cellular cytotoxicity (Scaltriti, 2009). Combining trastuzumab with lapatinib offers a chemotherapy-free option for treating HER2-positive trastuzumab-resistant disease.

7.2 Combining trastuzumab with pertuzumab

Pertuzumab is an anti-HER2 monoclonal antibody that targets an extracellular epitope distinct from what is targeted by trastuzumab. Pertuzumab binds to HER2 near the center of domain II, sterically blocking a binding pocket necessary for receptor dimerization and signaling (Franklin, 2004). In contrast, trastuzumab does not significantly inhibit HER2 interaction with other erbB receptors. We were the first to show that combining pertuzumab with trastuzumab results in synergistic inhibition of proliferation of HER2-overexpressing breast cancer cells (Nahta, 2004a). Trastuzumab increased pertuzumab-mediated disruption of HER2 dimerization with EGFR and HER3, and further reduced pertuzumab-mediated inhibition of PI3K signaling (Nahta, 2004a). Phase II data shows that combining trastuzumab with pertuzumab in patients who have progressed on prior trastuzumab regimens achieves clinical benefit rate of 50%, objective response rates of 24%, and median progression-free survival of 5. 5 months (Baselga, 2010a). A potential mechanism of synergy is non-overlapping mechanisms by single agents, trastuzumab-mediated inhibition of p95HER2 cleavage and pertuzumab-mediated disruption of dimerization (Scheuer, 2009). Clinical evaluation of pertuzumab and trastuzumab (CLEOPATRA) is an international, randomized, double-blind, placebo-controlled phase III trial. Patients with HER2-positive breast cancer with locally recurrent or metastatic disease will be randomized to receive docetaxel, trastuzumab, and pertuzumab or docetaxel, trastuzumab, and placebo. Progresion-free survival will be assessed to determine efficacy of combination pertuzumab plus trastuzumab in the trastuzumab-refractory setting (Baselga, 2010b).

8. Novel HER2-targeted agents in clinical development

8.1 Trastuzumab-DM1

One novel preparation of trastuzumab is a drug conjugate called trastuzumab-DM1, which is trastuzumab conjugated to a microtubule-depolymerizing drug called maytansinoid (Lewis Phillips, 2008). Trastuzumab-DM1 blocks growth of trastuzumab-naive and trastuzumab-refractory HER2-overexpressing breast tumors *in vivo* (Lewis Phillips, 2008), and retains the mechanistic activity of unconjugated trastuzumab (Junttila, 2010). Antibody-dependent cellular cytotoxicity was induced by trastuzumab-DM1, and tumor growth of trastuzumab-resistant cells was blocked by trastuzumab-DM1 due to induction of apoptosis and mitotic catastrophe (Barok, 2011). A phase I dose-escalation study in patients who had progressed on trastuzumab showed clinical benefit of 73% in 15 of 24 patients, including objective responses in 5 patients (Krop, 2010). A phase II study of trastuzumab-DM1 in patients with trastuzumab-refractory HER2-positive breast cancer showed objective response of 25. 9% and median progression-free survival of 4. 6 months (Burris, 2011). Thus, trastuzumab-DM1 HER2 antibody-chemotherapy conjugate is a promising treatment for HER2-positive breast cancer that has progressed on prior HER2-directed therapies.

8.2 Irreversible pan-HER kinase inhibitors

In contrast to lapatinib, which is a reversible EGFR/HER2 kinase inhibitor, irreversible pan-HER inhibitors are being developed for use against HER2-dependent breast cancers (Ocana, 2009). Neratinib, an irreversible EGFR/HER2 inhibitor, achieved a response rate of 26% in trastuzumab-pretreated patients and 55% in trastuzumab-naïve patients (Burstein, 2009). Progression-free survival at 16 weeks was 60% and 77%, respectively, for trastuzumab-pretreated and naïve patients (Burstein, 2009). Finally, the median time to progression was 23 weeks and 40 weeks, respectively, for trastuzumab-pretreated and naïve patients (Burstein, 2009). Canertinib (CI-1033) is an irreversible inhibitor of all HER proteins. Response to canertinib was higher in patients with HER2-positive breast cancer, although toxicity at the most effective dose was limiting and unacceptable (Rixe, 2009).

9. Conclusion

In conclusion, several major mechanisms of trastuzumab resistance have been proposed, including increased signaling from PI3K/mTOR, Src, and IGF-IR, as well as reduced p27kip1 and increased cdk2 activity. These mechanisms have uncovered new therapeutic targets for which multiple pharmacologic agents have been developed. Some of the most promising include mTOR-targeted agents derived from rapamycin and trastuzumab-DM1. Combining multiple HER2-targeted agents appears to be beneficial due to different mechanisms of action. Future studies should more clearly address the role of IGF-IR in acquired versus primary resistance, and test IGF-IR-targeted agents in combination with trastuzumab and/or lapatinib in a trastuzumab-refractory setting. In addition, studies examining the role of estrogen receptor (ER) signaling in trastuzumab resistant HER2-positive ER-positive disease should be performed. Finally, biological predictors of response or resistance need to be developed to determine which patients are most likely to benefit from trastuzumab therapy, thus allowing for more specific individualization of targeted therapy in patients with HER2-overexpressing breast cancer.

10. References

Adams TE, Epa VC, Garrett TP, & Ward CW. (2000). Structure and function of the type 1 insulin-like growth factor receptor. *Cell Mol Life Sci*, Vol. 57, No. 7, (July 2000), pp. 1050-93

Barok M, Tanner M, Koninki K, & Isola J. (2011). Trastuzumab-DM1 causes tumor growth inhibition by mitotic catastrophe in trastuzumab-resistant breast cancer cells in vivo. Breast *Cancer Res* Vol. 13, No. 2, (2011 Apr 21), pp. R46

Baselga J, Tripathy D, Mendelsohn J, Baughman S, Benz CC, Dantis L, Sklarin NT, Seidman AD, Hudis CA, Moore J, Rosen PP, Twaddell T, Henderson IC, & Norton L. (1996). Phase II study of weekly intravenous recombinant humanized anti-p185HER2 monoclonal antibody in patients with HER2/neu-overexpressing metastatic breast cancer. *J Clin Oncol*, Vol. 14, No. 3, (March 1996), pp. 737-44

Baselga J, Gelmon KA, Verma S, Wardley A, Conte P, Miles D, Bianchi G, Cortes J, McNally VA, Ross GA, Fumoleau P, & Gianni L. (2010a). Phase II trial of pertuzumab and trastuzumab in patients with human epidermal growth factor receptor 2-positive metastatic breast cancer that progressed during prior trastuzumab therapy. *J Clin Oncol* Vol. 28, No. 7, (2010 Mar 1), pp. 1138-44

Baselga J & Swain SM. (2010b). CLEOPATRA: a phase III evaluation of pertuzumab and trastuzumab for HER2-positive metastatic breast cancer. *Clin Breast Cancer* Vol. 10, No. 6, (2010 Dec 1), pp. 489-91

Berns K, Horlings HM, Hennessy BT, Madiredjo M, Hijmans EM, Beelen K, Linn SC, Gonzalez-Angulo AM, Stemke-Hale K, Hauptmann M, Beijersbergen RL, Mills GB, van de Vijver MJ, & Bernards R. (2007). A functional genetic approach identifies the PI3K pathway as a major determinant of trastuzumab resistance in breast cancer. *Cancer Cell* Vol. 12, No. 4, (2007 Oct), pp. 395-402

Blackwell KL, Burstein HJ, Storniolo AM, Rugo H, Sledge G, Koehler M, Ellis C, Casey M, Vukelja S, Bischoff J, Baselga J, O'Shaughnessy J. (2010). Randomized study of Lapatinib alone or in combination with trastuzumab in women with ErbB2-

positive, trastuzumab-refractory metastatic breast cancer. *J Clin Oncol*, Vol. 28, No. 7, (March 2010), pp. 1124-30

Burris HA 3rd, Rugo HS, Vukelja SJ, Vogel CL, Borson RA, Limentani S, Tan-Chiu E, Krop IE, Michaelson RA, Girish S, Amler L, Zheng M, Chu YW, Klencke B, & O'Shaughnessy JA. (2011). Phase II study of the antibody drug conjugate trastuzumab-DM1 for the treatment of human epidermal growth factor receptor 2 (HER2)-positive breast cancer after prior HER2-directed therapy. *J Clin Oncol* Vol. 29, No. 4, (2011 Feb 1), pp. 398-405

Burstein HJ, Sun Y, Dirix LY, Jiang Z, Paridaens R, Tan AR, Awada A, Ranade A, Jiao S, Schwartz G, Abbas R, Powell C, Turnbull K, Vermette J, Zacharchuk C, & Badwe R. (2010). Neratinib, an irreversible ErbB receptor tyrosine kinase inhibitor, in patients with advanced ErbB2-positive breast cancer. *J Clin Oncol* Vol. 28, No. 8, (2010 Mar 10), pp. 1301-7

Cardoso F, Durbecq V, Laes JF, Badran B, Lagneaux L, Bex F, Desmedt C, Willard-Gallo K, Ross JS, Burny A, Piccart M, & Sotiriou C. (2006). Bortezomib (PS-341, Velcade) increases the efficacy of trastuzumab (Herceptin) in HER-2-positive breast cancer cells in a synergistic manner. *Mol Cancer Ther* Vol. 5, No. 12, (2006 Dec), pp. 3042-51

Carter P, Presta L, Gorman CM, Ridgway JB, Henner D, Wong WL, Rowland AM, Kotts C, Carver ME, & Shepard HM. (1992). Humanization of an anti-p185HER2 antibody for human cancer therapy. *Proc Natl Acad Sci U S A* Vol. 89, No. 10, (1992 May 15), pp. 4285-9

Casalini P, Iorio MV, Berno V, Bergamaschi A, Børresen Dale AL, Gasparini P, Orlandi R, Casati B, Tagliabue E, & Ménard S. (2007). Relationship between p53 and p2 7 expression following HER2 signaling. *Breast*, Vol. 16, No. 6, (December 2007), pp. 597-605

Chaves J, Saif MW. IGF system in cancer: from bench to clinic. (2011). *Anticancer Drugs*, Vol. 22, No. 3, (March 2011), pp. 206-12

Cobleigh MA, Vogel CL, Tripathy D, Robert NJ, Scholl S, Fehrenbacher L, Wolter JM, Paton V, Shak S, Lieberman G, & Slamon DJ. (1999). Multinational study of the efficacy and safety of humanized anti-HER2 monoclonal antibody in women who have HER2-overexpressing metastatic breast cancer that has progressed after chemotherapy for metastatic disease. *J Clin Oncol*, Vol. 17, No. 9, pp. 2639-48

Cuello M, Ettenberg SA, Clark AS, Keane MM, Posner RH, Nau MM, Dennis PA, & Lipkowitz S. (2001). Down-regulation of the erbB-2 receptor by trastuzumab (herceptin) enhances tumor necrosis factor-related apoptosis-inducing ligand-mediated apoptosis in breast and ovarian cancer cell lines that overexpress erbB-2. *Cancer Res*, Vol. 61, No. 12, (June 2001), pp. 4892-4900

Eccles SA. (2001). The role of c-erbB-2/HER2/neu in breast cancer progression and metastasis. *J Mammary Gland Biol Neoplasia* Vol. 6, No. 4, (2001 Oct), pp. 393-406

Eichhorn PJ, Gili M, Scaltriti M, Serra V, Guzman M, Nijkamp W, Beijersbergen RL, Valero V, Seoane J, Bernards R, Baselga J. Phosphatidylinositol 3-kinase hyperactivation results in lapatinib resistance that is reversed by the mTOR/phosphatidylinositol 3-kinase inhibitor NVP-BEZ235. *Cancer Res* Vol. 68, No. 22, (2008 Nov 15), pp. 9221-30

Esparís-Ogando A, Ocaña A, Rodríguez-Barrueco R, Ferreira L, Borges J & Pandiella A. (2008). Synergic antitumoral effect of an IGF-IR inhibitor and trastuzumab on HER2-overexpressing breast cancer cells. *Ann Oncol*, Vol. 19, No. 11, (November 2008) pp. 1860-9

Esteva FJ, Valero V, Booser D, Guerra LT, Murray JL, Pusztai L, Cristofanilli M, Arun B, Esmaeli B, Fritsche HA, Sneige N, Smith TL, & Hortobagyi GN. (2002). Phase II study of weekly docetaxel and trastuzumab for patients with HER-2-overexpressing metastatic breast cancer. *J Clin Oncol*, Vol. 20, No. 7 (2002 Apr 1), pp. 1800-8

Franklin MC, Carey KD, Vajdos FF, Leahy DJ, de Vos AM, & Sliwkowski MX. (2004). Insights into ErbB signaling from the structure of the ErbB2-pertuzumab complex. *Cancer Cell* Vol. 5, No. 4, (2004 Apr), pp. 317-28

Gajria D, & Chandarlapaty S. (2011). HER2-amplified breast cancer: mechanisms of trastuzumab resistance and novel targeted therapies. *Expert Rev Anticancer Ther,* Vol. 11, No. 2, (February 2011), pp. 263-75

Geyer CE, Forster J, Lindquist D, Chan S, Romieu CG, Pienkowski T, Jagiello-Gruszfeld A, Crown J, Chan A, Kaufman B, Skarlos D, Campone M, Davidson N, Berger M, Oliva C, Rubin SD, Stein S, & Cameron D. (2006). Lapatinib plus capecitabine for HER2-positive advanced breast cancer. *N Engl J Med*, Vol. 355, No. 26 (2006 Dec 28), pp. 2733-43.

Graus-Porta D, Beerli RR, Daly JM, & Hynes NE. (1997). ErbB-2, the preferred heterodimerization partner of all ErbB receptors, is a mediator of lateral signaling. *EMBO J*, Vol. 16, No. 7, (April 1997), pp. 1647-55

Hankinson SE, Willett WC, Colditz GA, Hunter DJ, Michaud DS, Deroo B, Rosner B, Speizer FE, & Pollak M. Circulating concentrations of insulin-like growth factor-I and risk of breast cancer. *Lancet* Vol. 351, No. 9113, (1998 May 9), pp. 1393-6.

Huang X, Qian X, Cheng C, He S, Sun L, Ke Q, Zhang L, Pan X, He F, Wang Q, Meng J, Ni R, & Shen A. (2011). Expression of Pirh2, a p27(Kip1) ubiquitin ligase, in hepatocellular carcinoma: correlation with p27(Kip1) and cell proliferation. *Hum Pathol*, Vol. 42, No. 4, (April 2011), pp. 507-15

Jerome L, Alami N, Belanger S, Page V, Yu Q, Paterson J, Shiry L, Pegram M, & Leyland-Jones B. (2006). Recombinant human insulin-like growth factor binding protein 3 inhibits growth of human epidermal growth factor receptor-2-overexpressing breast tumors and potentiates herceptin activity in vivo. *Cancer Res* Vol. 66, No. 14, (2006 Jul 15), pp. 7245-52

Jerusalem G, Fasolo A, Dieras V, Cardoso F, Bergh J, Vittori L, Zhang Y, Massacesi C, Sahmoud T, & Gianni L. (2011). Phase I trial of oral mTOR inhibitor everolimus in combination with trastuzumab and vinorelbine in pre-treated patients with HER2-overexpressing metastatic breast cancer. *Breast Cancer Res Treat*, Vol. 125, No. 2, (January 2011), pp. 447-55

Jin Q & Esteva FJ. (2008). Cross-talk between the ErbB/HER family and the type I insulin-like growth factor receptor signaling pathway in breast cancer. *J Mammary Gland Biol Neoplasia*, Vol. 13, No. 4, (December 2008), pp. 485-98

Junttila TT, Akita RW, Parsons K, Fields C, Lewis Phillips GD, Friedman LS, Sampath D, & Sliwkowski MX. (2009). Ligand-independent HER2/HER3/PI3K complex is disrupted by trastuzumab and is effectively inhibited by the PI3K inhibitor GDC-0941. *Cancer Cell*, Vol. 15, No. 5, (May 2009), pp. 429-40

Junttila TT, Li G, Parsons K, Phillips GL, & Sliwkowski MX. (2010). Trastuzumab-DM1 (T-DM1) retains all the mechanisms of action of trastuzumab and efficiently inhibits growth of lapatinib insensitive breast cancer. *Breast Cancer Res Treat* (2010 Aug 21. [Epub ahead of print])

Kalinsky K, Jacks LM, Heguy A, Patil S, Drobnjak M, Bhanot UK, Hedvat CV, Traina TA, Solit D, Gerald W, & Moynahan ME. (2009). PIK3CA mutation associates with improved outcome in breast cancer. *Clin Cancer Res*, Vol. 15, No. 16, (August 2009), pp. 5049-59

Kotoshiba S, Kamura T, Hara T, Ishida N, & Nakayama KI. (2005). Molecular dissection of the interaction between p27 and Kip1 ubiquitylation-promoting complex, the ubiquitin ligase that regulates proteolysis of p27 in G1 phase. *J Biol Chem*, Vol. 280, No. 18, (May 2005), pp. 17694-700

Krop IE, Beeram M, Modi S, Jones SF, Holden SN, Yu W, Girish S, Tibbitts J, Yi JH, Sliwkowski MX, Jacobson F, Lutzker SG, & Burris HA. (2010). Phase I study of trastuzumab-DM1, an HER2 antibody-drug conjugate, given every 3 weeks to patients with HER2-positive metastatic breast cancer. *J Clin Oncol* Vol. 28, No. 16, (2010 Jun 1), pp. 2698-704

Lane HA, Motoyama AB, Beuvink I, & Hynes NE. (2001). Modulation of p27/Cdk2 complex formation through 4D5-mediated inhibition of HER2 receptor signaling. *Ann Oncol* Vol. 12, Suppl 1, (2001), pp. S21-2.

Lang SA, Hackl C, Moser C, Fichtner-Feigl S, Koehl GE, Schlitt HJ, Geissler EK, & Stoeltzing O. (2010). Implication of RICTOR in the mTOR inhibitor-mediated induction of insulin-like growth factor-I receptor (IGF-IR) and human epidermal growth factor receptor-2 (Her2) expression in gastrointestinal cancer cells. *Biochim Biophys Acta*, Vol. 4, (April 2010), pp. 435-42

Le XF, Claret FX, Lammayot A, Tian L, Deshpande D, LaPushin R, Tari AM, & Bast RC Jr. (2003). The role of cyclin-dependent kinase inhibitor p27Kip1 in anti-HER2 antibody-induced G1 cell cycle arrest and tumor growth inhibition. *J Biol Chem*, Vol. 278, No. 26, (June 2003), pp. 23441-50

Lewis Phillips GD, Li G, Dugger DL, Crocker LM, Parsons KL, Mai E, Blättler WA, Lambert JM, Chari RV, Lutz RJ, Wong WL, Jacobson FS, Koeppen H, Schwall RH, Kenkare-Mitra SR, Spencer SD, & Sliwkowski MX. (2008). Targeting HER2-positive breast cancer with trastuzumab-DM1, an antibody-cytotoxic drug conjugate. Cancer Res Vol. 68, No. 22, (2008 Nov 15), pp. 9280-90

Liang K, Esteva FJ, Albarracin C, Stemke-Hale K, Lu Y, Bianchini G, Yang CY, Li Y, Li X, Chen CT, Mills GB, Hortobagyi GN, Mendelsohn J, Hung MC, & Fan Z. (2010). Recombinant human erythropoietin antagonizes trastuzumab treatment of breast cancer cells via Jak2-mediated Src activation and PTEN inactivation. *Cancer Cell* Vol. 18, No. 5, (2010 Nov 16), pp. 423-35

Lin NU, Carey LA, Liu MC, Younger J, Come SE, Ewend M, Harris GJ, Bullitt E, Van den Abbeele AD, Henson JW, Li X, Gelman R, Burstein HJ, Kasparian E, Kirsch DG, Crawford A, Hochberg F, & Winer EP. (2008). Phase II trial of lapatinib for brain metastases in patients with human epidermal growth factor receptor 2-positive breast cancer. *J Clin Oncol* Vol. 26, No. 12, (2008 Apr 20), pp. 1993-9

Lin NU, Diéras V, Paul D, Lossignol D, Christodoulou C, Stemmler HJ, Roché H, Liu MC, Greil R, Ciruelos E, Loibl S, Gori S, Wardley A, Yardley D, Brufsky A, Blum JL, Rubin SD, Dharan B, Steplewski K, Zembryki D, Oliva C, Roychowdhury D, Paoletti P, & Winer EP. (2009). Multicenter phase II study of lapatinib in patients with brain metastases from HER2-positive breast cancer. *Clin Cancer Res* Vol. 15, No. 4, (2009 Feb 15), pp. 1452-9

Lu Y, Zi X, Zhao Y, Mascarenhas D, & Pollak M. (2001). Insulin-like growth factor-I receptor signaling and resistance to trastuzumab (Herceptin). *J Natl Cancer Inst,* Vol. 93, No. 24, (December 2001), pp. 1852-7

Marches R, & Uhr JW. (2004). Enhancement of the p27Kip1-mediated antiproliferative effect of trastuzumab (Herceptin) on HER2-overexpressing tumor cells. *Int J Cancer,* Vol. 112, No. 3, (November 2004), pp. 492-501

Miller TW, Forbes JT, Shah C, Wyatt SK, Manning HC, Olivares MG, Sanchez V, Dugger TC, de Matos Granja N, Narasanna A, Cook RS, Kennedy JP, Lindsley CW, & Arteaga CL. (2009). Inhibition of mammalian target of rapamycin is required for optimal antitumor effect of HER2 inhibitors against HER2-overexpressing cancer cells. *Clin Cancer Res,* Vol. 15, No. 23, (December 2009), pp. 7266-76

Mitra D, Brumlik MJ, Okamgba SU, Zhu Y, Duplessis TT, Parvani JG, Lesko SM, Brogi E, & Jones FE. (2009). An oncogenic isoform of HER2 associated with locally disseminated breast cancer and trastuzumab resistance. *Mol Cancer Ther* Vol. 8, No. 8, (2009 Aug), pp. 2152-62

Mittendorf EA, Liu Y, Tucker SL, McKenzie T, Qiao N, Akli S, Biernacka A, Liu Y, Meijer L, Keyomarsi K, & Hunt KK. (2010). A novel interaction between HER2/neu and cyclin E in breast cancer. *Oncogene* Vol. 29, No. 27, (2010 Jul 8), pp. 3896-907

Molina MA, Codony-Servat J, Albanell J, Rojo F, Arribas J, & Baselga J. (2001). Trastuzumab (herceptin), a humanized anti-Her2 receptor monoclonal antibody, inhibits basal and activated Her2 ectodomain cleavage in breast cancer cells. *Cancer Res,* Vol. 61, No. 12, (June 2001), pp. 4744-9

Nagata Y, Lan KH, Zhou X, Tan M, Esteva FJ, Sahin AA, Klos KS, Li P, Monia BP, Nguyen NT, Hortobagyi GN, Hung MC, & Yu D. (2004). PTEN activation contributes to tumor inhibition by trastuzumab, and loss of PTEN predicts trastuzumab resistance in patients. *Cancer Cell,* Vol. 6, No. 2, (2004 Aug), pp. 117-27

Nahta R, Hung MC, & Esteva FJ. (2004a). The HER-2-targeting antibodies trastuzumab and pertuzumab synergistically inhibit the survival of breast cancer cells. *Cancer Res* Vol. 64, No. 7, (2004 Apr 1), pp. 2343-6

Nahta R, Takahashi T, Ueno NT, Hung MC, & Esteva FJ. (2004b). P27(kip1) down-regulation is associated with trastuzumab resistance in breast cancer cells. *Cancer Res,* Vol. 64, No. 11, (June 2004), pp. 3981-6

Nahta, R, Yuan, L X, Zhang, Kobayashi, R, & Esteva FJ. (2005). Insulin-like growth factor-i receptor/human epidermal growth factor receptor 2 heterodimerization contributes to trastuzumab resistance of breast cancer cells. *Cancer Res,* Vol. 65, No. 23, (Nov 2008), pp. 11118-28

Nielsen DL, Andersson M, & Kamby C. (2008). HER2-targeted therapy in breast cancer. Monoclonal antibodies and tyrosine kinase inhibitors. *Cancer Treat Rev,* Vol. 35, No. 2, (April 2009), pp. 121-36

O'Brien NA, Browne BC, Chow L, Wang Y, Ginther C, Arboleda J, Duffy MJ, Crown J, O'Donovan N, & Slamon DJ. (2010). Activated phosphoinositide 3-kinase/AKT signaling confers resistance to trastuzumab but not lapatinib. *Mol Cancer Ther* Vol. 9, No. 6, (June 2010), pp. 1489-502

Oakman C, Pestrin M, Zafarana E, Cantisani E, & Di Leo A. (2010). Role of lapatinib in the first-line treatment of patients with metastatic breast cancer. *Cancer Manag Res,* Vol. 2, (January 2010), pp. 13-25

Ocaña A & Amir E. (2009). Irreversible pan-ErbB tyrosine kinase inhibitors and breast cancer: current status and future directions. *Cancer Treat Rev* Vol. 35, No. 8, (2009 Dec), pp. 685-91

Rixe O, Franco SX, Yardley DA, Johnston SR, Martin M, Arun BK, Letrent SP, & Rugo HS. (2009). A randomized, phase II, dose-finding study of the pan-ErbB receptor tyrosine-kinase inhibitor CI-1033 in patients with pretreated metastatic breast cancer. *Cancer Chemother Pharmacol* Vol. 64, No. 6, (2009 Nov), pp. 1139-48

Sachdev D, Singh R, Fujita-Yamaguchi Y, & Yee D. (2006). Down-regulation of insulin receptor by antibodies against the type I insulin-like growth factor receptor: implications for anti-insulin-like growth factor therapy in breast cancer. *Cancer,* Vol. 66, No. 4, (February 2006), pp. 2391-402

Sakr RA, Barbashina V, Morrogh M, Chandarlapaty S, Andrade VP, Arroyo CD, Olvera N, & King TA. (2010). Protocol for PTEN expression by immunohistochemistry in formalin-fixed paraffin-embedded human breast carcinoma. *Appl Immunohistochem Mol Morphol* Vol. 18, No. 4, (July 2010), pp. 371-4

Scaltriti M, Verma C, Guzman M, Jimenez J, Parra JL, Pedersen K, Smith DJ, Landolfi S, Ramon y Cajal S, Arribas J, & Baselga J. (2009). Lapatinib, a HER2 tyrosine kinase inhibitor, induces stabilization and accumulation of HER2 and potentiates trastuzumab-dependent cell cytotoxicity. *Oncogene* Vol. 28, No. 6, (2009 Feb 12), pp. 803-14

Scaltriti M, Eichhorn PJ, Cortés J, Prudkin L, Aura C, Jiménez J, Chandarlapaty S, Serra V, Prat A, Ibrahim YH, Guzmán M, Gili M, Rodríguez O, Rodríguez S, Pérez J, Green SR, Mai S, Rosen N, Hudis C, & Baselga J. (2011). Cyclin E amplification/overexpression is a mechanism of trastuzumab resistance in HER2+ breast cancer patients. *Proc Natl Acad Sci U S A* Vol. 108, No. 9, (2011 Mar 1), pp. 3761-6

Scheuer W, Friess T, Burtscher H, Bossenmaier B, Endl J, & Hasmann M. (2009). Strongly enhanced antitumor activity of trastuzumab and pertuzumab combination treatment on HER2-positive human xenograft tumor models. *Cancer Res* Vol. 69, No. 24, (2009 Dec 15), pp. 9330-6

Slamon DJ, Clark GM, Wong SG, Levin WJ, Ullrich A, & McGuire WL. (1987). Human breast cancer: correlation of relapse and survival with amplification of the HER-2/neu oncogene. *Science* Vol. 235, No. 4785 (1987 Jan 9), pp. 177-82

Slamon DJ, Leyland-Jones B, Shak S, Fuchs H, Paton V, Bajamonde A, Fleming T, Eiermann W, Wolter J, Pegram M, Baselga J, & Norton L. (2001) Use of chemotherapy plus a monoclonal antibody against HER2 for metastatic breast cancer that overexpresses HER2. *N Engl J Med* Vol. 15, No. 344, (March 2001), pp. 783-92

Sliwkowski MX, Lofgren JA, Lewis GD, Hotaling TE, Fendly BM, & Fox JA. (1999). Nonclinical studies addressing the mechanism of action of trastuzumab (Herceptin). *Semin Oncol* Vol. 26, No. 4 Suppl 12, (1999 Aug), pp. 60-70

Spector NL & Blackwell KL. (2009). Understanding the mechanisms behind trastuzumab therapy for human epidermal growth factor receptor 2-positive breast cancer. *J Clin Oncol*, Vol. 27. No. 34 (December 2009), pp. 5838-47

Storniolo AM, Pegram MD, Overmoyer B, Silverman P, Peacock NW, Jones SF, Loftiss J, Arya N, Koch KM, Paul E, Pandite L, Fleming RA, Lebowitz PF, Ho PT, & Burris HA 3rd. (2008). Phase I dose escalation and pharmacokinetic study of lapatinib in combination with trastuzumab in patients with advanced ErbB2-positive breast cancer. *J Clin Oncol* Vol. 26, No. 20, (2008 Jul 10), pp. 3317-23

Surmacz E. (2000). Function of the IGF-I receptor in breast cancer. *J Mammary Gland Biol Neoplasia*, Vol. 5, No. 1 (January 2000), pp. 95-105

Van der Heijden, M S, & Bernards, R. (2010). Inhibition of the PI3K pathway: Hope we can believe in? *Clin Cancer Res*, Vol. 16, No. 12 (June 2010), pp. 3094-9

Vermeulen K, Van Bockstaele DR, & Berneman ZN. (2003). The cell cycle: a review of regulation, deregulation and therapeutic targets in cancer. *Cell Prolif.* Vol. 36, No. 3, (June 2003), pp. 131-49

Wu Y, Amonkar MM, Sherrill BH, O'Shaughnessy J, Ellis C, Baselga J, Blackwell KL, & Burstein HJ. (2011). Impact of lapatinib plus trastuzumab versus single-agent lapatinib on quality of life of patients with trastuzumab-refractory HER2+ metastatic breast cancer. *Ann Oncol* (2011 Mar 15 [Epub ahead of print])

Wullschleger S, Loewith R, Oppliger W, & Hall MN. (2005). Molecular organization of target of rapamycin complex 2. *J Biol Chem*, Vol. 280, No. 235, (September 2005), pp. 30697-704

Xia W, Gerard CM, Liu L, Baudson NM, Ory TL, & Spector NL. (2005). Combining lapatinib (GW572016), a small molecule inhibitor of ErbB1 and ErbB2 tyrosine kinases, with therapeutic anti-ErbB2 antibodies enhances apoptosis of ErbB2-overexpressing breast cancer cells. *Oncogene* Vol. 24, No. 41, (2005 Sep 15), pp. 6213-21

Yakes FM, Chinratanalab W, Ritter CA, King W, Seelig S, & Arteaga CL. (2002). Herceptin-induced inhibition of phosphatidylinositol-3 kinase and Akt Is required for antibody-mediated effects on p27, cyclin D1, and antitumor action. *Cancer Res* Vol. 62, No. 14, (2002 Jul 15), pp. 4132-41

Yang XH, Flores LM, Li Q, Zhou P, Xu F, Krop IE, & Hemler ME. (2010). Disruption of laminin-integrin-CD151-focal adhesion kinase axis sensitizes breast cancer cells to ErbB2 antagonists. *Cancer Res* Vol. 70, No. 6, (2010 Mar 15), pp. 2256-63

Zhang S, Huang WC, Li P, Guo H, Poh SB, Brady SW, Xiong Y, Tseng LM, Li SH, Ding Z, Sahin AA, Esteva FJ, Hortobagyi GN, & Yu D. (2011). Combating trastuzumab resistance by targeting SRC, a common node downstream of multiple resistance pathways. *Nat Med* Vol. 17, No. 4, (2011 Apr), pp. 461-9

10

Fractionation and Characterization of Bioactive Components in Kefir Mother Culture that Inhibit Proliferation of Cultured MCF-7 Human Breast-Cancer Cells

Chujian Chen[1,2], Hing Man Chan[3] and Stan Kubow[1]
[1]*School of Dietetics and Human Nutrition, Macdonald Campus of McGill University, Ste-Anne-de-Bellevue, Quebec*
[2]*School of Public Health, Nantong University, Nantong, Jiangsu*
[3]*Community Health Program, University of Northern British Columbia, Prince George, British Columbia*
[1,3]*Canada*
[2]*People's Republic of China*

1. Introduction

Breast cancer is the most commonly diagnosed cancer in women. Resistance to therapy is the major reason for failure of cancer treatment (Mesner *et al.*, 1997). There is a critical need to identify new chemotherapeutic agents that can increase susceptibility to anti-breast cancer drugs or overcome resistance mechanisms, which would improve patient outcomes, prevent relapse, and prolong patient survival. Kefir is an acidic and mildly alcoholic fermented milk that originated in the Caucasian mountains of former Soviet Union, and enjoys a rich tradition of health benefits. Consumption of fermented dairy foods has been associated with lower incidence of breast cancer (Ronco *et al.*, 2002). Research on the putative health benefits of fermented milks suggested that by-products of bacterial fermentation of proteins, lipids and carbohydrates present in fermented milks exert health benefits beyond basic nutrition including anti-tumor action, immune system enhancement and antioxidant effects (Parvez *et al.*, 2006). Conjugated linoleic acid (Schonberg *et al.*, 1995), sphingolipids (Dillehay *et al.*, 1994), polysaccharides (Shiomi *et al.*, 1982), organic acids (Garrote *et al.*, 2000) and some proteins and peptides (Svensson *et al.*, 1999) have been shown to have antimutagenic and antitumor effects. Promising results regarding anti-tumor activity of yogurt extracts in cell culture (Biffi *et al.*, 1997) and kefir extracts in animal feeding studies (Cervikbas *et al.*, 1994; Furukawa *et al.*, 2000; Shiomi *et al.*, 1982) have been reported. However, the bioactive components in kefir and the mechanisms involved in the various biofunctional effects of kefir are still not well characterized, particularly in terms of anti-cancer activities. In our recent studies, kefir extracts exerted potent anti-proliferative effects on cultured human mammary tumor cells as compared to extracts of yogurt or milk (Chen *et al.*, 2007). The aim of the present study was to fractionate and characterize bioactive components in kefir mother culture that exert antiproliferative effects in MCF-7 cells.

2. Materials and methods

Kefir samples were provided by Liberte Inc. (Brossard, Canada). The large-scale production of kefir involves a two-step fermentation process. The first fermentation is achieved by directly adding kefir grains (2-10%) to milk that has been pasteurized and cooled to 20-25°C. After a period of fermentation lasting around 24 h, the grains are removed by filtration. The filtrate (kefir mother culture) is added to milk (1-3%), which is further fermented for 24 h and packaged for the consumer market (final kefir commercial product). Samples from three different batches were used. Upon receipt of the samples, they were immediately well stirred, and centrifuged at 4°C, 32,000 x g, for 60 min (Sorvall RC 5C Centrifuge, rotor ss-34, Sorvall Instruments, Wilmington, USA). The supernatant was filtered with a 0.45 μm membrane filter followed by a 0.2 μm filter. The filtrates were stored at −80°C for future use.

2.1 Macronutrients and minerals

A Flexi-Dry MP lyophilizer (FTS Systems Inc., Stone Ridge, USA) was used for triplicate determination of moisture. Ten grams of homogenized sample was transferred into pre-weighed aluminium weigh boat, frozen at -80°C for approximately 1 h and then freeze dried for 48 h. The boat was weighed again and the moisture was calculated. A LECO FP-428 Nitrogen Determination System (LECO Corporation, St. Joseph, USA) was used to determine nitrogen content in triplicate for freeze-dried samples. Crude protein content was calculated using a conversion factor of 6.25. Protein in solution was determined by using Bio-Rad protein assay kit according to the instruction with the kit (Bio-Rad Laboratories, Hercules, USA). Peptide concentrations were analyzed by the method of Church *et al.* (1983) (opthialdehyde; OPA). Crude fat was analyzed in triplicate with an automatic Soxtec extraction system (Soxtec HT6 Tecator AB, Hoganas, Sweden). Three grams of freeze-dried, well-mixed sample was loaded and analyzed. Proper amount of freeze-dried samples were digested in 70% (w/v) nitric acid (Fisher Scientific, trace metal grade) and minerals (i.e., Ca, Mg, Zn, Fe, Na and K) were determined by using Hitachi Z-8200 Zeeman polarized atomic absorption spectrophotometer (Nissei Sango Ltd., Mississauga, ON, Canada).

2.2 Organic acids

Lactic acid content was analyzed using a Sigma lactate kit assay (Sigma Diagnostics, Cat. No. 735-10, St. Louis, USA). Organic acids were determined by HPLC according to the method of Guzel-Seydim *et al.* (2000). Five mL of each sample was diluted with 25 mL 0.01 M H_2SO_4, vortexed for 1 min followed by centrifugation at 2000 x g for 10 min. Supernatants were collected and filtered through 0.2 μm filter. Volumes of 20 μl of samples and standards were injected into a Beckman Gold HPLC system (Beckman Coulter, Fullerton, USA) equipped with an Aminex HPX-87H (300 mm x 7.8 mm) organic acid column (Bio-Rad Laboratories, Hercules, USA). Degassed 8 mM sulfuric acid (H_2SO_4) was used as the mobile phase. The organic acids oxalate, citrate, malate, succinate, formate and acetate were detected at 215 nm. Organic acids were quantified using external standards (organic acid analysis standard, Bio-Rad Laboratories, Hercules, USA).

2.3 Molecular weight cut-off fractionation (MWCO)

Centriplus centrifugal filter devices were used to get MWCO fractions at 3000 Da (Millipore, Bedford, USA). Ten milliliters whole extract were loaded to the sample reservoir and the assembled device was centrifuged at 4°C, 3000 x g for 290 min. The filtrates were collected for further analysis.

2.4 Size exclusion HPLC (SEC) separation

One hundred microliters of kefir mother culture extract was injected into a TSK G2000SWXL column (78 mm x 30 mm, SUPELCO, Bellefonte, USA) and separated with a Shimadzu LC-6AD Liquid Chromatograph system (Shimadzu Scientific Instruments, Inc. Columbia, USA) with UV detection at 210 nm. The separation buffer used was a mixture of 45% acetonitrile in 0.1% trifluoroacetic acid (TFA) with a flow rate of 0.4 ml/min for 40 min. Nine fractions were collected for each HPLC run, and fractions from five to ten runs were pooled. The above nine fractions were evaporated with N_2 and then freeze dried, stored at −80°C for cell culture incubations and for further analytical analyses.

2.5 Reverse phase HPLC (RP-HPLC) fractionation

The fraction(s) collected with SEC HPLC that showed antiproliferative effects on MCF-7 cells were further analyzed with a Prosphere 300 C4 column (5μm, 250 mm x 4.6 mm) (Alltech Associate, Inc. Deerfield, USA) using a Beckman Gold HPLC System (Beckman Coulter, Fullerton, USA). After the column was equilibrated with buffer A (0.1% TFA in water) at a flow rate of 1 ml per min, the fractions were eluted with a linear gradient of buffer A (0.1% TFA in water) and buffer B (60% of acetonitrile in 0.1% TFA: 40% of 0.1% TFA in water) as follows: 0 to 60 min, 0 to 90% B; and 61 to 65 min, 90 to 0% B. Dual channel absorbance was monitored at 210 nm (channel A) and 280 nm (channel B).

2.6 Preparative HPLC fractionation

Three batches of extracts of kefir mother culture were pooled and fractionated using the Centriplus centrifugal filter devices to obtain fractions of compounds with molecular weights less than 3000 Da. The fractions of MWCO less than 3000 Da were freeze-dried using a FLEXI-DRY MP Freeze Dryer (FTS Systems, Inc. Stone Ridge, U SA). Five g of the lyophilized MWCO fractions were dissolved in 20 ml of water. Ten milliliters of reconstituted solution were loaded on a C4 preparative column (300 Å, 5 μm, 300 mm x 50 mm) (Vydac Company, Herperia, CA) and separated with a Water Delta Prep 4000 HPLC system (Waters Corporation, Milford, USA). After the column was equilibrated with buffer A (0.6% acetic acid in water) at a flow rate of 13 ml and the fractions were eluted with a linear gradient of buffer A and buffer B (0.6% acetic acid in acetonitrile) as follows: 0 to 70 min, 0 to 60% B; 70 to 80 min, 60 to 70% B; 80 to 100 min, 70 to 80% B; 100 to 105 min, 80 to 0% B. A total of 100 fractions were collected between 0 and 100 min, with samples taken at 1-min intervals. The fractions were then lyophilized and kept at −80°C for further cell culture and analysis. The fractions were reconstituted by adding water and peptide and protein concentrations were determined before cell culture assays.

2.7 Capillary electrophoresis

Capillary zone electrophoresis (CE) was performed using a P/ACE ™ 2200 HPAC instrument controlled by System Gold software (Beckman, Fullerton, CA, USA) coupled to an IBM PC 486 computer (IBM Corp., Portmouth, England) for data acquisition and analysis. A neutral uncoated fused silica capillary column (57 cm × 50 μm, the length from intake to detector was 50 cm) was assembled in the P/ACE cartridge (Polymicro

Technologies, Phoenix, Arizona USA) for capillary separations. Injection volume, buffer concentration and running voltage were optimized to achieve the best resolution with the shortest running time. The capillary was flushed with 1 M sodium hydroxide, followed by nanopure water, 0.1 M sodium hydroxide, nanopure water, 1 M hydrochloric acid, and again water, each for 5 min at a pressure of 40 psi. A solution of 5% polybrene and 2% ethylene glycol was then passed for 10 min at 40 psi. Excessive coating was then removed by flushing with water for 2 min. Further capillary flushing was then performed for additional 10 min using 200 mM formic acid buffer. Before each sample application, the capillary was rinsed with 1 min water, 1 min 0.1 M sodium hydroxide, 1 min water and 3 min separation buffer (200 mM formic acid in water, pH 2.0). After the completion of each run, the capillary was rinsed with nanopure water for 1 min, 0.1 M sodium hydroxide for 1 min and nanopure water for 1 min. Peptide standard and sample injections were carried out at the anode end of the capillary using N_2 pressure (0.5 psi) for 5 sec and was separated at a constant temperature of 20°C with a 200 mM formic acid (pH 2.0) as separation buffer. On-line detection was performed using an UV detector at 200 nm. Twenty kilovolts was applied across the run buffers for best separation. The capillary was re-coated after every 5 runs.

2.8 MALDI-TOF for estimation of molecular weight

Reconstituted SEC-HPLC and RP-HPLC fractions were analyzed using a MALDI-TOF mass spectrometer (Voyager DE-STR; Applied Biosystems, Palo-Alto, CA, USA) with a laser at 337 nm and an acceleration voltage of 20.000 V.

2.9 Mass spectrometry

Mass spectrometric analysis in the positive ion mode was performed on a triple quadupole mass spectrometer (SCIEX API III Biomolecular mass analyzer, Thornhill, Ontario, Canada). Lyophilized reversed phase HPLC fractions having antiproliferative effect on MCF-7 cells were reconstituted in 0.5 mM ammonium acetate in methanol or in 10% acetic acid in 20% aqueous methanol. The resulting solution was then infused into the electrospray ion-source by a syringe pump (Harvard Apparatus Model 22, South Natick, MA) at a flow rate of 1.5 ml/min. The ion-spray voltage was set at 5.5 kV and the orifice potential was set at 50 V. Argon was used as the collision gas at a collision gas thickness (CGT) of 1.5 x 10^{14} for collision-induced fragmentation MS-MS analysis.

2.10 Cell Culture screening for antiproliferative effects

MCF-7 cells were purchased from ATCC (ATCC, Manassas, USA). Cells were routinely propagated as a monolayer culture in Dulbcco's Modified Eagle Medium (DMEM) (Gibco, Grand Island, NY, USA) supplemented with 10% heat-inactivated fetal bovine serum (FBS) (Gibco, Grand Island, NY, USA), in a 75-cm^2 plastic dish at 37°C in a humidified atmosphere with 5% CO_2, and passaged every 3-4 days. Normal human mammary epithelial cell lines (HMEC) were graciously provided by Dr. M.R. Stampfer (Lawrence Berkeley National Laboratory, Berkeley, USA). Cells were routinely propagated as a monolayer culture in Mammary Epithelial Growth Media (MEGM, Clonetics, San Diego, USA) supplemented with 10% heat-inactivated fetal bovine serum (FBS) in 75-cm^2 plastic dish at 37°C in a humidified atmosphere with 5% CO_2, and passaged every week. For the experiments, both

MCF-7 and HMEC cells were harvest from the dish using 0.25% trypsin-EDTA solution (Sigma, St Louis, MO, USA).

2.11 Cell proliferation experiments in 24-well plates

Cells previously harvested were seeded in 24-well plates, i.e., 10,000 cells for MCF-7 per well in DMEM supplemented with 10% FBS and 5,000 cells for HMEC per well in MEGM supplemented with 10% FBS. The cells were allowed to attach for 24 h. After that period, old media were removed and fresh media and extracts were added to each well. To study the dose response, a serial dilution of each the extract using the culture media was made to achieve final concentrations of extracts at 5%, 2.5%, 1.3%, 0.6%, and 0.3% (vol./vol.), respectively. Because the kefir extracts were acidic (approximately pH 4.5), Dulbecco's Phosphate Buffered Saline (PBS) buffer (Gibco BRL, Grand Island, NY) was added to the culture media to adjust the pH between 7.0 and 7.4. Cells were incubated at 37°C in a humidified atmosphere with 5% CO_2 for 6 d. Cell nuclei were counted in order to eliminate the difficulty in counting whole cells due to clumping. Furthermore, a more uniform distribution of nuclei over the grids of a hemacytometer was seen compared with whole cells. Media was aspirated from wells and cells were rinsed with 500 μl of PBS. 250 μl of hypotonic buffer (0.01 M HEPES, 1.5 M $MgCl_2$, pH 7.5) was added to each well. After 2 min, 250 μl of cell lysing solution (10% ethyl hexadecyl dimethyl ammonium bromide, 3% glacial acetic acid, in water) was added. The plate was shaken lightly every minute for 5 min. Cell lysis was confirmed microscopically as indicated by a suspension of clean nuclei. The suspension was mixed and the nuclei were counted using a Coulter Counter (Coulter Counter Corporation, Fullerton USA). Each sample was run in quadruplicate. Control cells were incubated with the culture medium with the dosing vehicle (PBS). To standardize results, each plate had its own control wells with cells treated with PBS and cell proliferation of different treatment was expressed as a percent of control.

2.12 Cell proliferation experiments in 96-well plates

Cells previously harvested were seeded in 96-well plates at 1,000 cells per well for MCF-7 in DMEM supplemented with 10% FBS and for HMEC in MEGM supplemented with 10% FBS. The cells were allowed to attach for 24 h. After that period, old media were removed and fresh media and extracts were added to each well. A serial dilution of each test fraction was made to study the dose-response. PBS buffer was added to the culture media to keep the final pH between 7.0 and 7.4. Cells were incubated at 37°C in a humidified atmosphere with 5% CO_2 for 6 d and the cell numbers in each well were determined by using a CellTiter 96® Aqueous One Solution Cell Proliferation Assay kit (Promega, Madison, USA). Each sample was run in quadruplicate. Control cells were incubated with the culture medium with the dosing vehicle (PBS). To standardize results, each plate had its own control wells with cells treated with PBS and cell proliferation of different treatments was expressed as a percent of control.

2.13 Statistics

All statistics test were performed using SAS 8.2 for PC (SAS, Cary, NC USA). Means were compared with Student's t test. Two-way ANOVA was used to analyze the effects of treatments and doses for the cell culture experiments. The differences among doses and treatments were determined by the Student-Newman-Keuls (SNK) multiple comparison test. Statistical significance was considered at $P < 0.05$.

3. Results

Moisture, macronutrients and some minerals in kefir mother culture and final kefir described in Table 1.

Component	Batch 1		Batch 2		Batch 3	
	Mother culture	Kefir	Mother culture	Kefir	Mother culture	Kefir
Moisture (g)	[1]89.78±0.09	90.40±0.06	91.22±0.19	90.03±0.02	89.56±0.07	90.17±0.08
Ash (g)	0.68±0.005	0.67±0.004	0.66±0.006	0.70±0.003	0.68±0.002	0.67±0.003
Protein (g)	3.05±0.16	2.81±0.03	2.78±0.03	3.14±0.04	3.28±0.01	2.77±0.02
Fat (g)	2.32±0.06	1.77±0.04	2.46±0.06	1.46±0.02	2.36±0.04	1.48±0.01
Calcium (mg)	78.20±0.66	77.70±0.71	78.93±0.58	77.40±0.64	81.53±0.73	80.40±0.56
Iron (mg)	0.02±0.001	0.02±0.001	0.02±0.001	0.02±0.001	0.02±0.001	0.02±0.001
Zinc (mg)	0.28±0.02	0.29±0.02	0.28±0.02	0.30±0.02	0.31±0.03	0.29±0.03
Magnesium (mg)	8.42±0.55	8.65±0.35	8.88±0.56	8.40±0.71	8.97±0.48	8.70±0.42
Sodium (mg)	28.51±1.86	29.0±0.71	28.60±2.03	30.05±2.05	30.99±1.08	31.05±0.72
Potassium (mg)	60.28±0.89	60.60±0.42	59.36±1.16	61.30±1.34	60.40±1.08	60.95±0.78

Table 1. Nutrient composition from three different batches of kefir mother culture and final commercial kefir product (per 100 g wet weight) ([1]Mean±SD, n=3).

No significant differences among nutrients and organic acids were found, except that lactic acid in the kefir commercial product was higher than that of kefir mother culture (Table 2).

Component	Mother culture	Kefir
Lactic acid[1]	[3]77.86±8.94	106.87±9.36*
Uric acid [2]	0.014±0.003	0.012±0.002
Pyruvic acid[2]	0.54±0.15	0.52±0.10
Oxalic acid[2]	[4]ND	ND
Citric acid[2]	3.27±0.17	3.22±0.28
Malic acid[2]	54.79±9.25	57.62±11.01
Succinic acid [2]	1.61±0.24	1.71±0.08
Formic acid[2]	Not detectable	Not detectable
Acetic acid[2]	3.81±0.74	3.46±0.47

Table 2. Organic acid concentrations (mmol/l) in mother culture and final kefir commercial product ([1]Determined by lactic acid kit assay method; [2]Determined by HPLC method of Guzel-Seydim *et al.* (2000); [3]Mean±SD, n=3; [4]ND = Not detectable; $^{*}P < 0.05$).

Capillary electrophoresis analyses showed that the profiles of extracts of mother culture and kefir were similar (data not shown). In our earlier study, the extract of kefir mother culture showed a tendency of having stronger antiproliferative effect on MCF-7 cells than other extracts (Chen *et al.*, 2007). Hence, mother culture was chosen for further fractionation and cell culture tests to identify the bioactive component(s). Extracts of kefir mother culture that were fractionated via the 3000 Da MWCO were analyzed for protein and peptide content (Table 3).

Samples	Moisture (g/100g)	Crude protein[1] (g/100g)	Protein[2] (μg/ml)	Peptides[3] (mmol/l)
Whole extract	[4]96.39±0.24	0.27±0.03	152.91±11.53	5.53±0.26
MWCO<3000	[5]ND	ND	5.10±0.07*	4.21±0.32*
MWCO>3000	ND	ND	195.94±4.11*	7.16±0.36*

Table 3. Protein and peptide concentrations in different MWCO fractions of extracts of kefir mother culture ([1]Determined by using Nitrogen Determinator; [2]Determined by Bradford method (1976); [3]Determined by OPA method of Church *et al.* (1983); [4]Mean±SD, n=3; [5]ND: No data is available; *Significant different at $P < 0.05$ when compared to protein or peptide concentration in whole extract).

Both protein and peptide concentrations were significantly lower in the fraction of MWCO less than 3000 Da ($P < 0.05$) relative to the whole kefir mother culture extract. Both the whole extract and the fraction with the MWCO less than 3000 Da were screened by MCF-7 cell culture using 24-well plates. As shown in Figure 1, the filtrate of MWCO less than 3000 Da had a dose dependent antiproliferative effect on MCF-7 cells comparable to that of the whole mother culture extract.

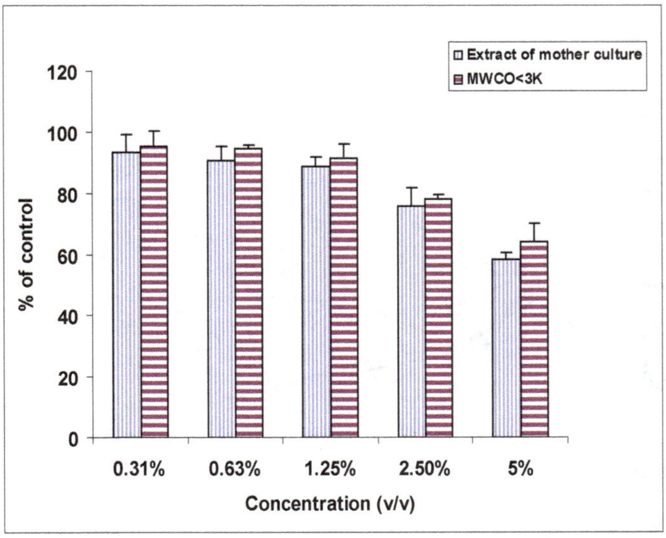

Fig. 1. Antiproliferative effects on MCF-7 cells induced by extracts of: (A) whole kefir mother culture; and (B) fraction of kefir mother culture obtained with MWCO less than 3000 Da. Cell proliferation was analyzed in 24-well plate. Values were graphed as Mean±SD, n=4.

The kefir mother culture filtrate that contained the MWCO less than 3000 Da was further separated with SEC-HPLC. Nine fractions were collected with each run with retention times of 14.6 to 17.0, 17.1 to 19.0, 19.1 to 21.0, 21.1 to 23.7, 23.8 to 25.6, 25.7 to 27.3, 27.4 to 29.1, 29.2 to 31.6, 31.7 to 33.7 min, respectively. Ten runs of SEC-HPLC fractions were pooled, freeze-dried and reconstituted in 2 ml water. The estimated molecular weight, protein and peptide concentrations are shown in Table 4. All the nine fractions were tested with MCF-7 cells in 96-well plates for their antiproliferative effects.

Fraction	Retention time (min)	Molecular Weight (Dalton)	Protein (µg/ml)	Peptides (µM/l)
1	14.4-17.0	13116-29507	145.7±5.12	274.53±2.19
2	17.1-19	7618-12745	118.56±4.89	284.70±5.31
3	19.1-21	4672-7425	43.62±2.84	208.33±2.26
4	21.1-23.7	2588-4565	16.80±1.56	491.14±6.67
5	23.8-25.6	1776-2535	3.23±0.26	422.01±5.17
6	25.7-27.3	1297-1742	2.92±0.2	655.11±4.58
7	27.4-29.1	949-1274	1.38±0.12	1168.33±8.22
8	29.2-31.6	635-934	4.77±0.16	1053.71±5.17
9	31.7-33.7	470-625	3.84±0.22	224.59±1.93

Table 4. Estimated molecular weight, protein and peptide concentration of the nine SEC HPLC fractions, Mean±SD, n=3.

Fractions 7 and 8 were the only fractions to demonstrate a dose-dependent antiproliferative effects on MCF-7 cells with the most potent effect exhibited with fraction 7 (Figure 2).

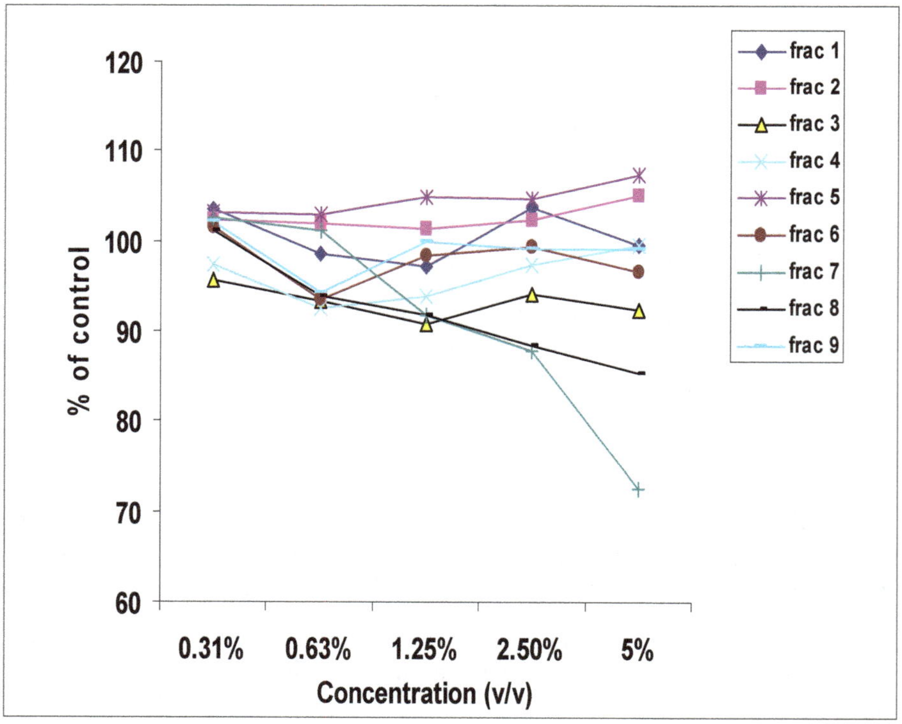

Fig. 2. Antiproliferative effects of 9 SEC-HPLC fractions on MCF-7 cells. Cell proliferation was analyzed in 96-well plate using a CellTiter 96® Aqueous One Solution Cell Proliferation Assay kit. Values were graphed as Mean±SD, n=4.

Fraction 7 was also tested with HMEC cells, and no antiproliferative effects were observed (Figure 3). Fraction 7 was further analyzed with RP-HPLC, which showed the presence of about 11 peaks in Fraction 7 (Figure 4). SEC-HPLC Fraction 7 was also analyzed via MALDI-TOF, which indicated that the peak masses ranged from 659 to 2074 Da. (Figure 5).

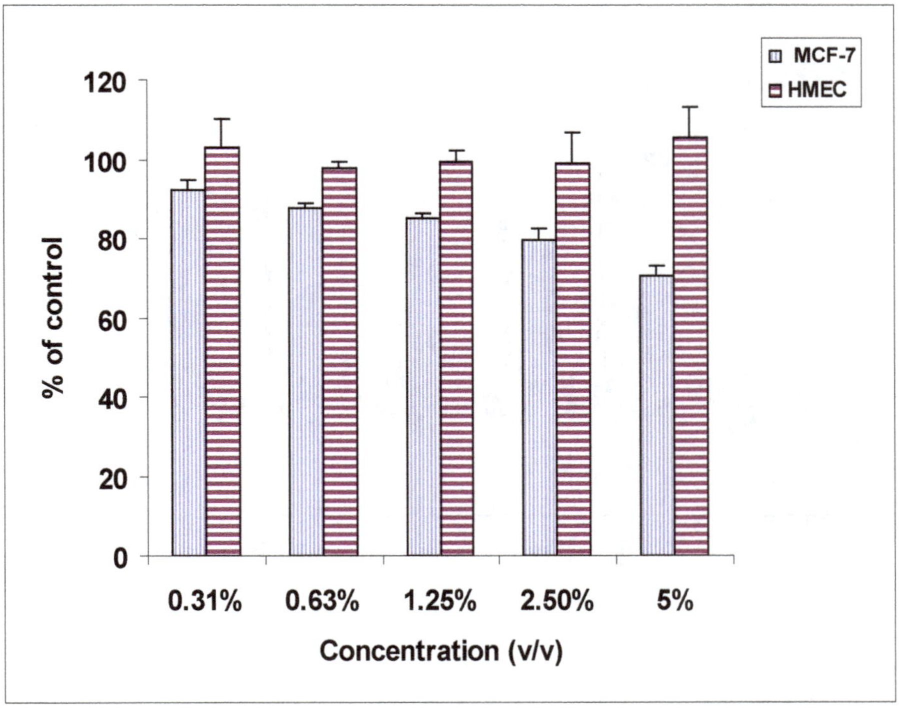

Fig. 3. Antiproliferative effects of SEC-HPLC Fraction 7 on MCF-7 and HMEC cells. Cell proliferation was analyzed in 96-well plate using a CellTiter 96® Aqueous One Solution Cell Proliferation Assay kit. Values were graphed as Mean+SD, n=4.

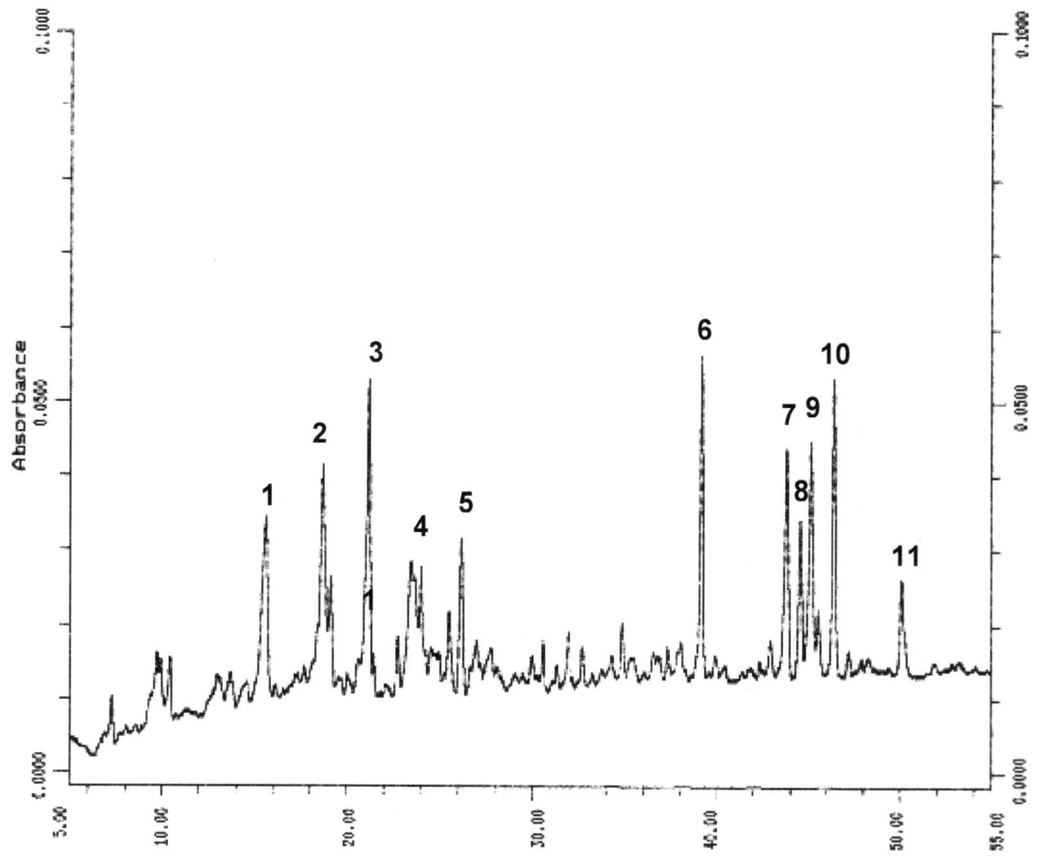

Fig. 4. Elution profile of SEC-HPLC Fraction 7 of kefir mother culture using RP-HPLC. A Prosphere 300 C4, 5 μm, 250 mm x 4.6 mm column was used. After the column was equilibrated with buffer A (0.1% TFA in water) at a flow rate of 1 ml per min, the fractions were eluted with a linear gradient of Buffer A (0.1% TFA in water) and Buffer B (60% of acetonitrile in 0.1% TFA: 40% of 0.1% TFA in water) as follows: 0 to 60 min, 0 to 90% B; and 61 to 65 min, 90 to 0% B. Absorbance was monitored at channel A 210 nm and channel B 280 nm. The retention times of the peaks 1 to 11 are 15.4, 18.6, 21.1, 23.3, 26.1, 39.1, 43.7, 44.5, 45.2, 46.3, and 50.1 min, respectively.

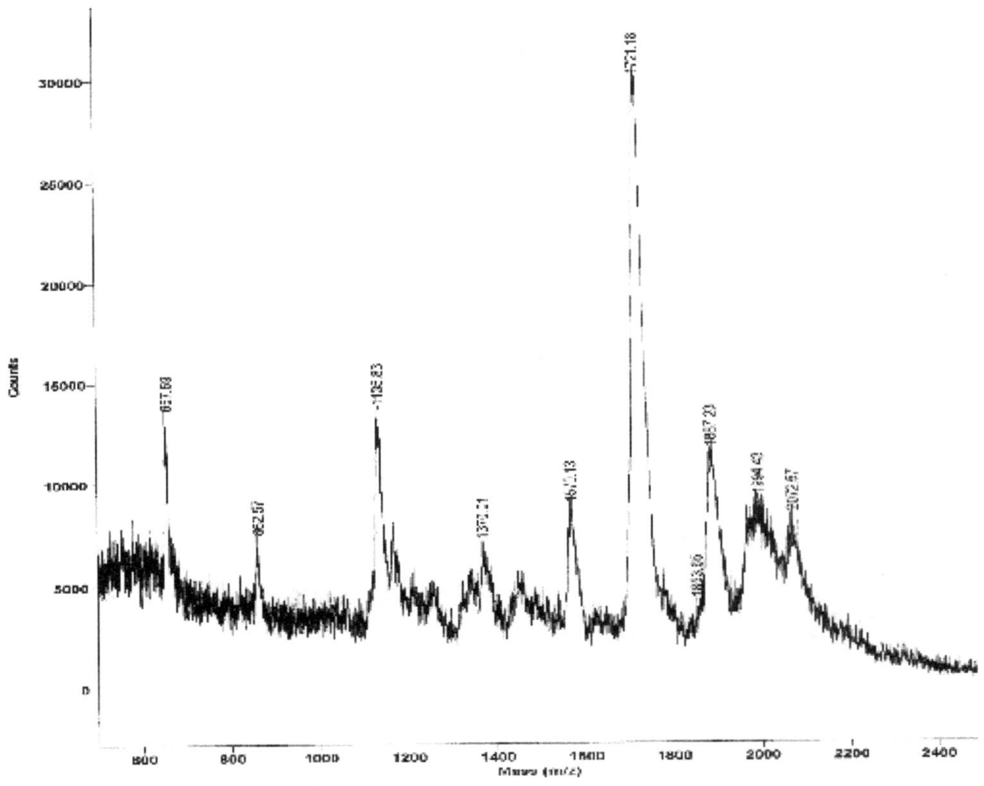

Fig. 5. Mass spectrogram of SEC-HPLC Fraction 7 of kefir mother culture analyzed by a MALDI-TOF mass spectrometer with a laser at 337 nm and an acceleration voltage of 20.000 V.

A preparative C4 column was utilized to obtain sufficient amounts of mother culture kefir fractions of MWCO less than 3000 Da for more extensive structure analysis and cell culture studies. The average nitrogen content of the lyophilized filtrate of MWCO less than 3000 Da was 0.58%. Five g of the lyophilized MWCO less than 3000 Da fractions was dissolved in 20 ml of water. Ten milliliters of reconstituted solution were loaded on the column, and 100 fractions were collected in 1 min intervals (Figure 6).

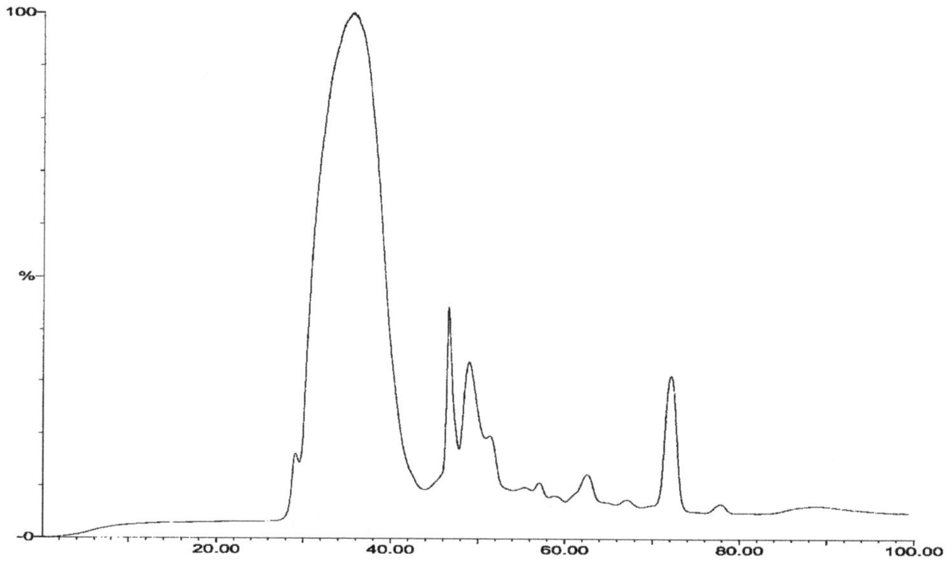

Fig. 6. Elution profile of MWCO less than 3000 Da fraction of kefir mother culture extract analyzed by preparative RP-HPLC. Appropriate amount of samples were loaded on a C4 preparative column (300 Å, 5 μm, 300 mm x 50 mm) (Vydac Company, Herperia, CA) and separated with Waters Delta Prep 4000 HPLC system. After the column was equilibrated with buffer A at a flow rate of 13 ml, the fractions were eluted with a linear gradient of Buffer A (0.6% acetic acid in water) and Buffer B (0.6% acetic acid in acetonitrile) as follows: 0 to 70 min, 0 to 60% B; 70 to 80 min, 60 to 70% B; 80 to 100 min, 70 to 80% B; 100 to 105 min, 80 to 0% B. The absorbance was measured at 210 nm. A total of 100 fractions were collected between 0 and 100 min, with samples taken at 1-min intervals.

The peptide concentration of each preparative HPLC fraction is shown in Figure 7, Fractions 28 to 58, 62 to 64, and 72 to 74 were screened for antiproliferative effects on MCF-7 cells with three concentrations of 0.4%, 2% and 10% (Figure 8).

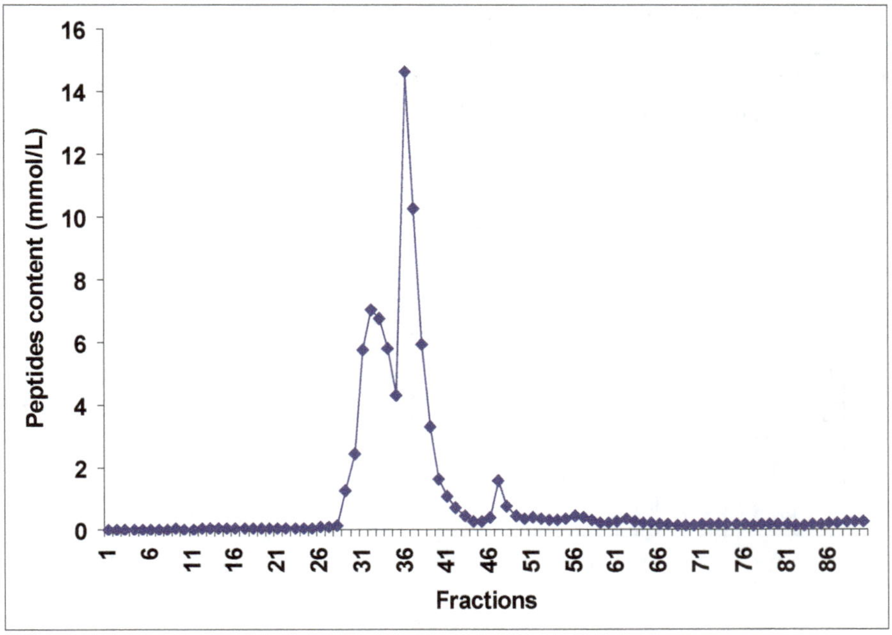

Fig. 7. Peptide concentrations in preparative RP-HPLC fractions. One hundred fractions obtained from preparative RP-HPLC were freeze-dried and then reconstituted with nanopure water to certain concentration. Peptide concentrations were determined in triplicates by OPA method. Mean values were plotted.

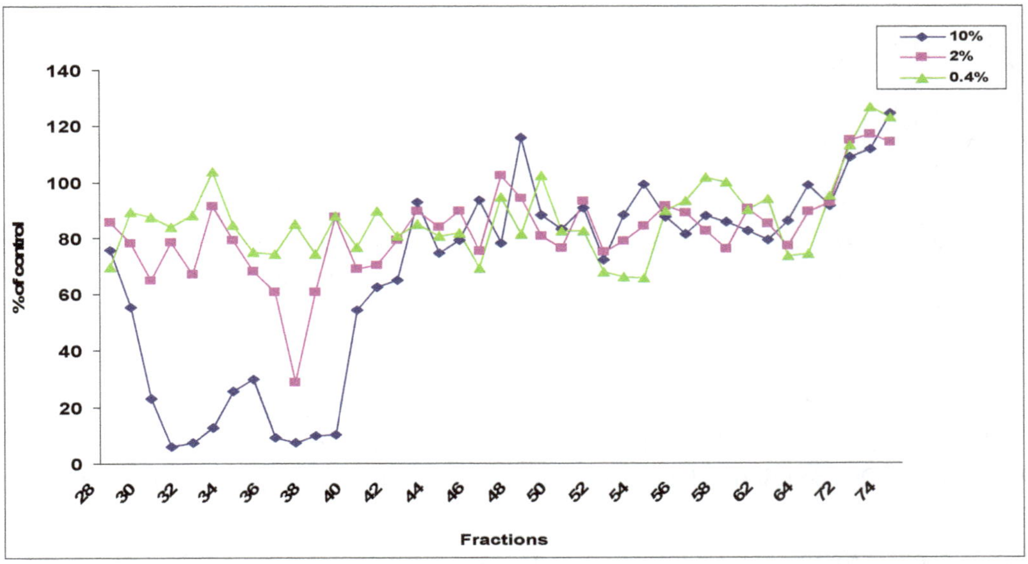

Fig. 8. Antiproliferative effects of fractions of preparative RP-HPLC on MCF-7 cells. Cell proliferation was analyzed in 96-well plate using a CellTiter 96® Aqueous One Solution Cell Proliferation Assay kit. Each fraction was diluted at three concentrations and was run in quadruplicate. Mean values were plotted.

Fractions 29 to 41, 62 were found to have antiproliferative effects on MCF-7 cells. These fractions were further screened for antiproliferative effects with serial dilution. A dose dependent antiproliferative effect was observed when MCF-7 cells were treated with fractions 29, 30, 34, and 37, while not on HMEC cells (Figure 9).

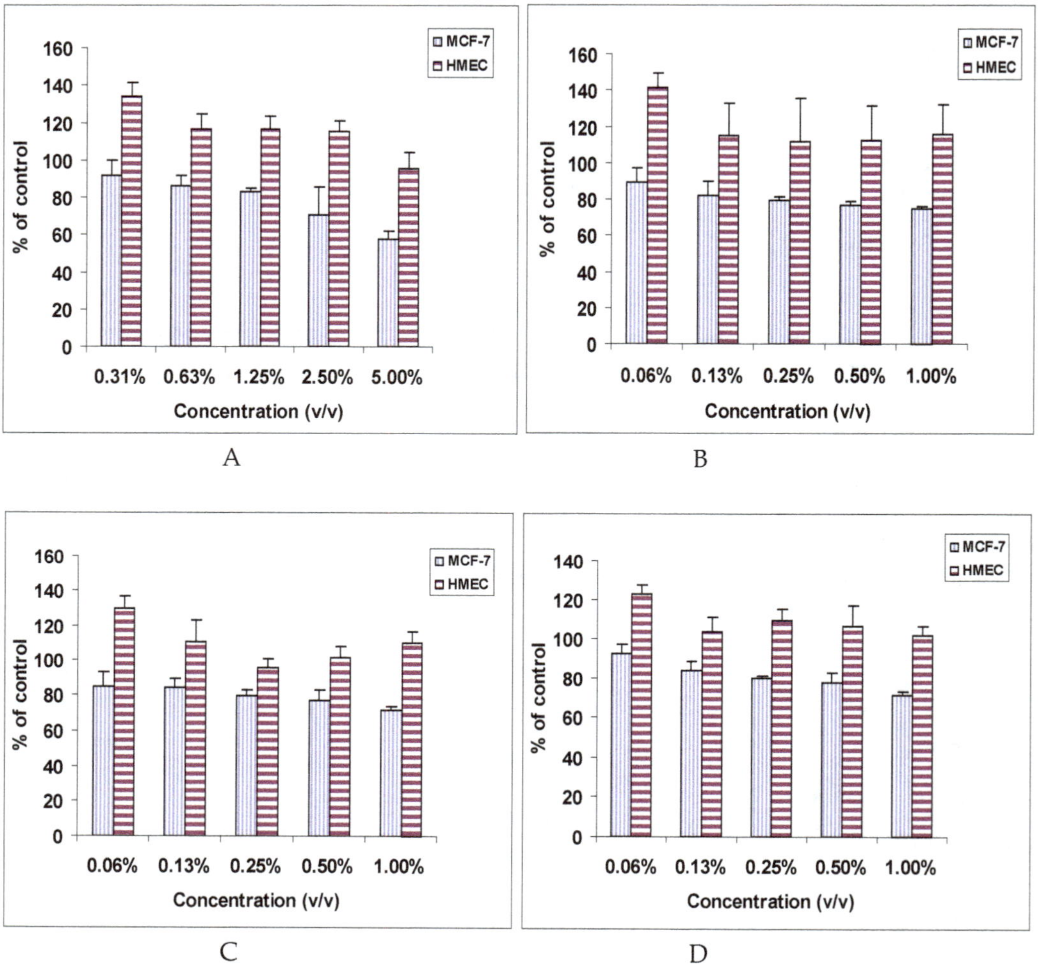

Fig. 9. Dose effect of preparative RP-HPLC Fraction 29 (A), 30 (B), 34 (C), and 37 (D) on MCF-7 and HMEC cells. Cell proliferation was analyzed in 96-well plate using a CellTiter 96® Aqueous One Solution Cell Proliferation Assay kit. Values were graphed as Mean±SD, n=4.

Tamoxifen is a commonly used medication for breast cancer patients. In this study, only the dosage above 0.2 μM/l showed antiproliferative effects on MCF-7 cells. The effective dose reported here was higher than the value reported by Doisneau-Sixou *et al.* (2003). RP-HPLC Fraction 30 of kefir mother culture extract significantly increased MCF-7 cell susceptibility to tamoxifen (Figure 10). A dose dependent antiproliferative effect was also observed.

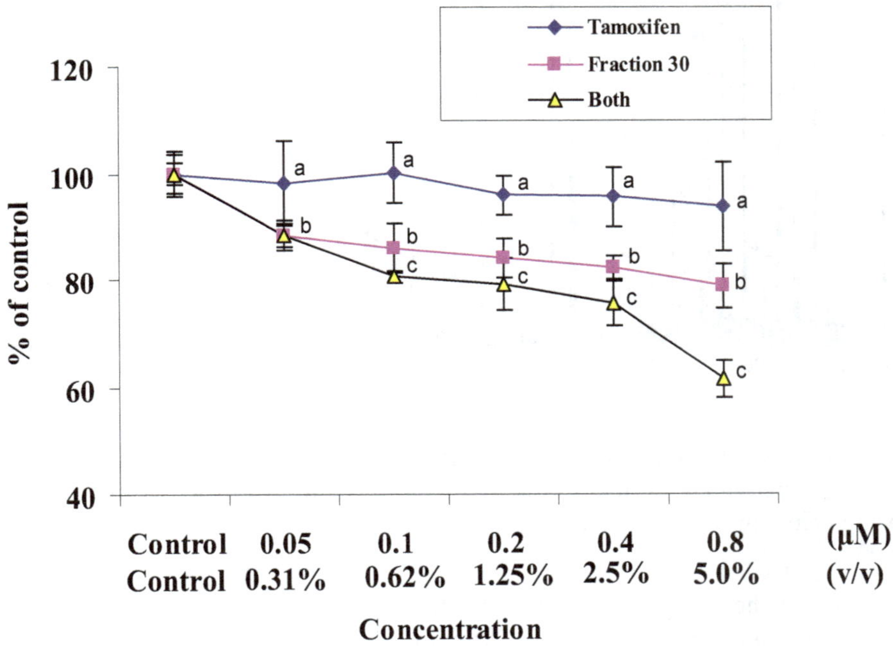

Fig. 10. Antiproliferative effect of RP-HPLC Fraction 30 of kefir alone or in combination with tamoxifen on MCF-7 cells. Means±SD (n=4) with the same letter are not significantly different at $P < 0.05$ for comparison among treatments at the same dose level.

Electrospray mass spectrometry was used to determine the molecular weight profile of the active Fractions 29, 30, 34, and 37. Figure 11 is the ESI-mass spectrum of HPLC fraction 30. The spectrum represents a typical molecular ion profile of the active HPLC fractions (29, 30, 34 and 37). The similarity in the molecular ion profile of the active fractions indicated that the active component(s) is spread over HPLC Fractions 30 to 37. The spectrum showed mainly singly charged molecular ions with m/z ratios ranging from 300 to 900. The peaks appearing below m/z 300 were found to be fragments of the peaks with m/z ranging from 300 to 900.

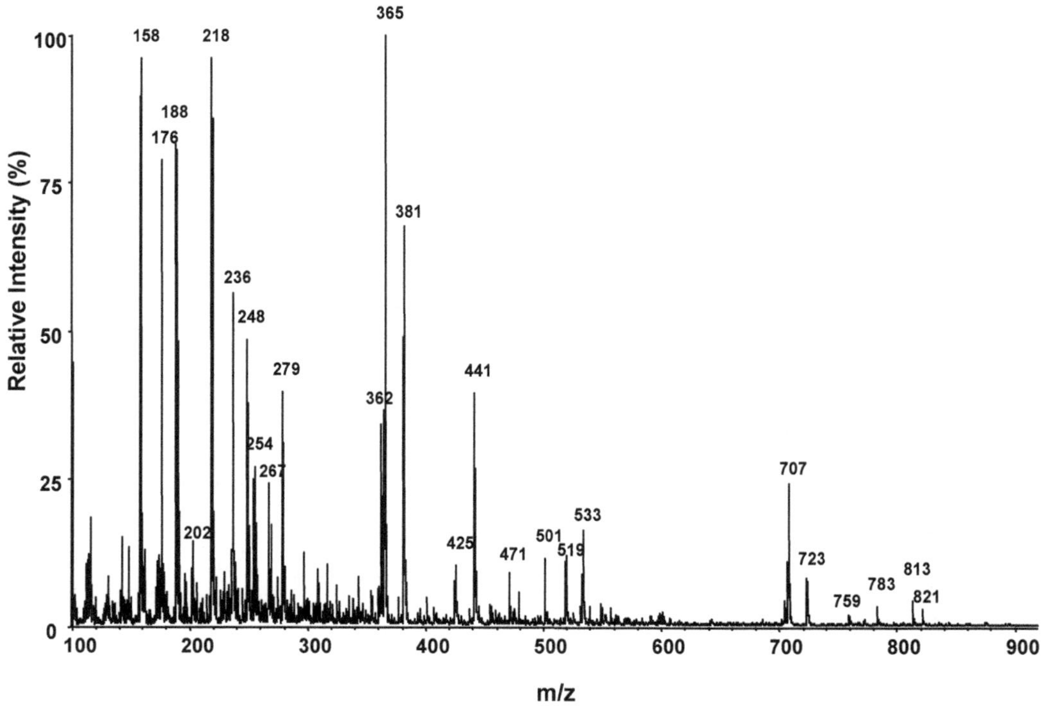

Fig. 11. Mass spectrum of HPLC Fraction 30 done by electrospray mass spectrometry. The mainly singly charged molecular ions with m/z ratios range from 300 to 900. The peaks appearing below m/z 300 were found to be fragments of the peaks with m/z ranging from 300 to 900.

To characterize the composition and chemical structure of the active components in the HPLC fractions, molecular ions ranging from m/z 300 to 900 were subjected to collision ion dissociation (CID) tandem mass spectrometry. Figure 12A, showed the CID spectrum of the molecular ion at m/z 821. Fragmentation of the molecular ion at m/z 821 produced a neutral loss of 342 mass units, which corresponds to the loss of a lactose moiety. It also produced a series of neutral loses of 60 mass units, which correspond to the loss of acetic acid moieties. The neutral loss of 60 atomic mass units may also be derived from sugar cleavage products (Figure 13). The CID spectrum of the molecular ion at m/z 813 (Figure 12B) also produced a neutral loss of 342 (lactose) and neutral losses of 120 atomic mass units, which may be derived from fragmentation of lactose (Figure 13). A neutral loss of 162, which corresponds to the loss of a hexose moiety (glucose or galactose), is also observed. This was also observed at m/z 759. The fragmentation patterns of the molecular ions at m/z 821 and 813 indicate that they have similar structural features. The molecular ions with m/z 707 (Figure 12E) and 723 (Figure 12D) represent sodium and potassium ion dimmers of lactose, respectively. The peaks at m/z at 365 and 381 represent the sodium and potassium ions of lactose respectively (Figure 14).

Another interesting feature about the fragmentation pattern of with m/z ranging from 707 to 823 is that they fragmented into common fragment ions at m/z 261 and 98. Further isolation and fragmentation (MS-MS) of the ion at m/z 261 showed that its major product ion is the ion at m/z 98. Further isolation and fragmentation of the ion at m/z 98 produced two ions at m/z 54 and 39. The tandem mass spectrometric analysis of the molecular ion of the active HPLC fraction show that most of the peaks produced a stable product ion at m/z 98, but the ion at 98 could not be ascribed to known structure peptide. Analysis of the fragmentation pattern of the molecular ion at m/z 759 (Figure 12C), however, revealed that the molecular ion could be derived from the interaction between serine and lactose.

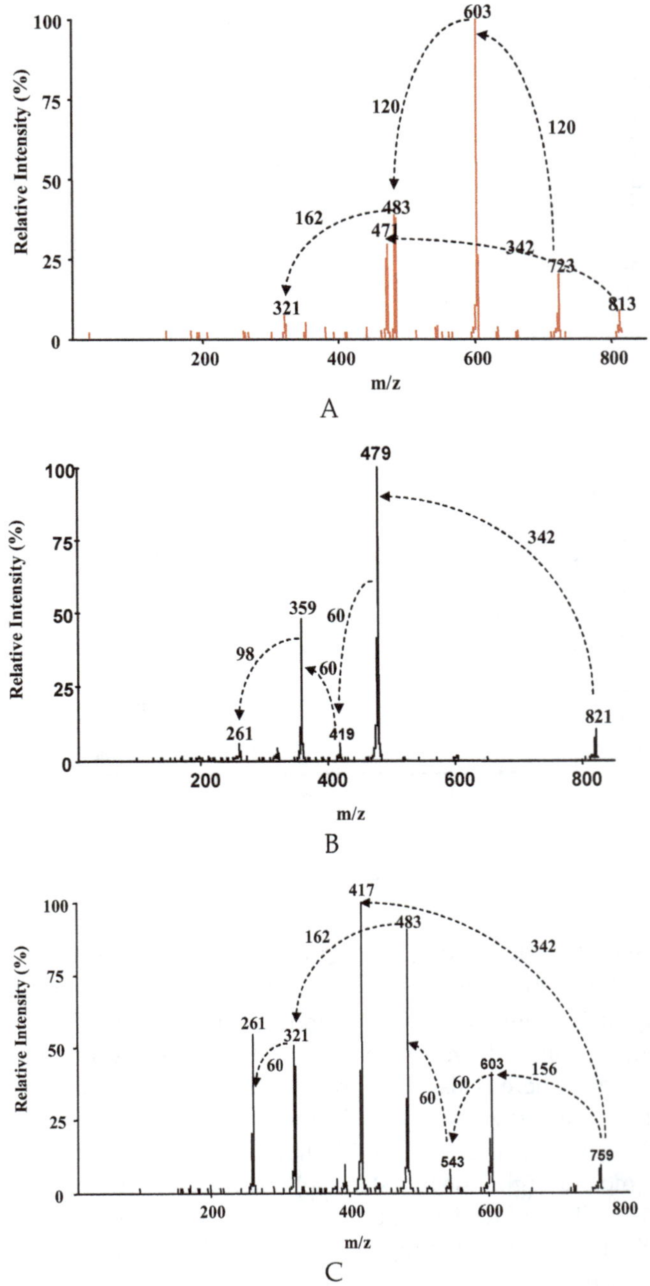

Fig. 12. (Continued)

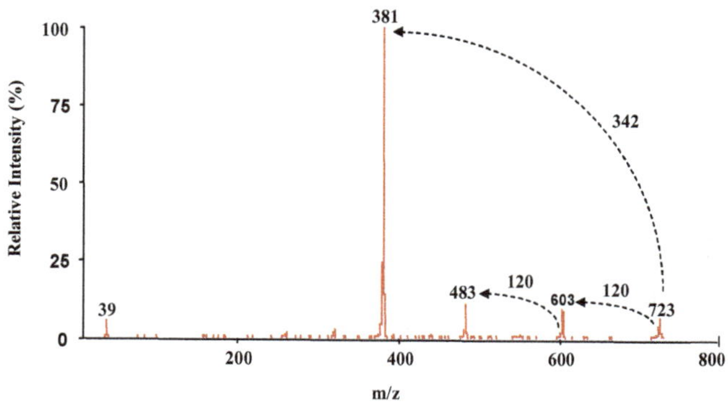

D

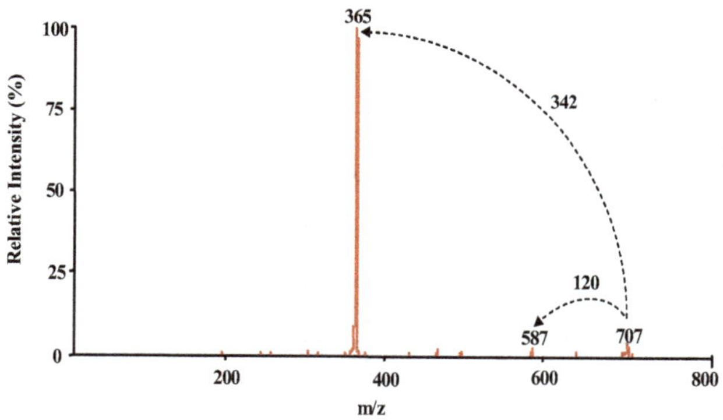

E

Fig. 12. Spectrum of molecular ion at m/z = 821 (A), m/z=813 (B), m/z= 759 (C), m/z=723 (D), and m/z=707 (E) done by collision ion dissociation (CID) tandem mass spectrometry. As indicated in Figure A, fragmentation of the molecular ion at m/z 821 produced a neutral loss of 342 and 60 mass units, which corresponds to the loss of a lactose moiety and acetic acid moiety respectively. There is also a neutral loss of 98, which could not be ascribed to a known structure. Ion at m/z =261 was also observed. Fragmentation of the molecular ion at m/z 813 produced a neutral loss of 342 and 120 mass units, which might be derived from lactose and hexose moieties (glucose or galactose) respectively. Fragmentation of the molecular ion at m/z 759 produced a neutral loss of 342 and serial loss of 60 mass units. Fragmentation of the molecular ion at m/z=723 produced neutral losses of 342 and 120 atomic mass unit. The main fragment is the ion at m/z 365 with the neutral loss of 342 (lactose) from m/z 707.

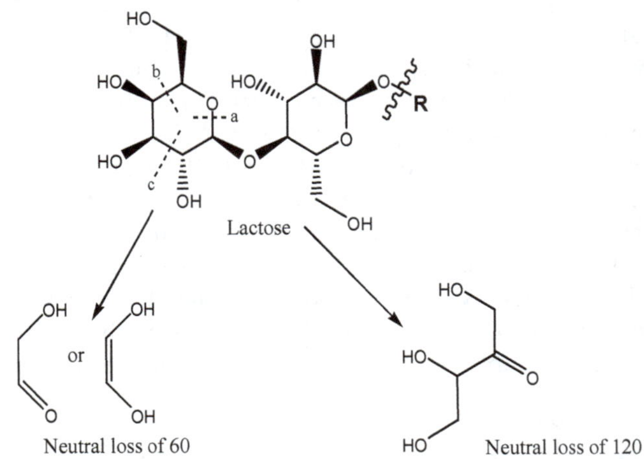

Fig. 13. Scheme 1: Generation of neutral loss of 60 and 120 atomic mass unit from fragmentation of lactose. Fragmentation at "a" and "b" will generate a neutral loss of 60 and fragmentation at "a" and "c" will generate a neutral loss of 120 atomic mass unit. They can be derived from fragmentation of acetic acid and lactose.

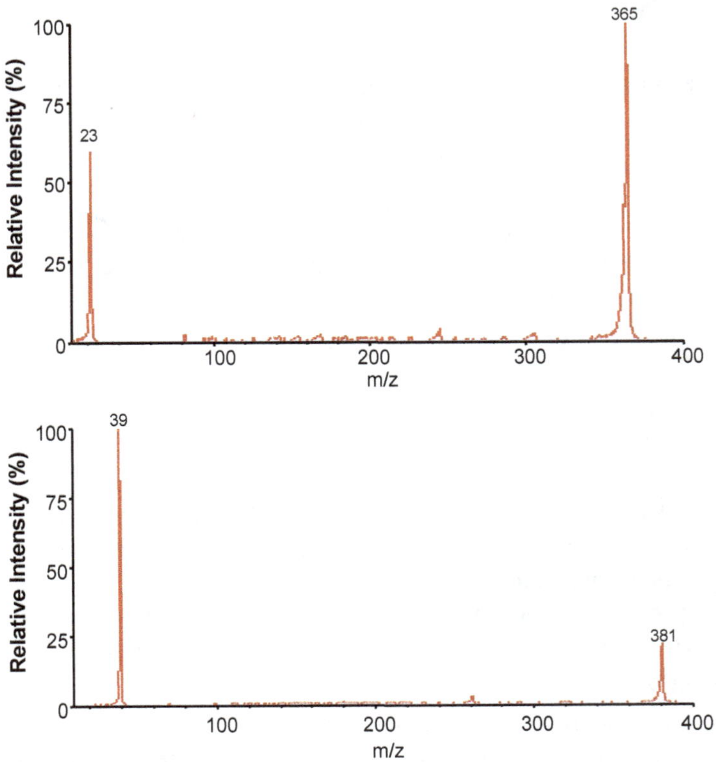

Fig. 14. Spectrum of molecular ion at m/z 365 and 381 done by collision ion dissociation (CID) tandem mass spectrometry. The peaks at m/z at 365 and 381 represent the sodium and potassium ions of lactose respectively.

A possible scheme for the generation of the ion at m/z 759 is presented in Scheme 2 (Figure 15). The proposed structure agrees with the fragmentation pattern. This interaction may be due to chemical reactions. The interaction between the amino group of serine and the reducing end of lactose is likely a chemical reaction similar to the Maillard reaction, and the interaction between the hydroxyl groups of lactose and the carboxyl group of serine is a simple esterification reaction. The reactions, particularly the esterification reaction may also be driven biochemically by esterases. The active fraction likely still contains a mixture of chemicals as suggested by the results of RP-HPLC (Figure 16). The exact molecular structure of these compounds is not known. However, results of the extensive MS analysis suggested that the compounds are possibly complex polymers that have lactose as the backbone structure. The proposed structure shown in Scheme 2 is a product with two lactose units linked by a serine. A more complex molecule with linkage with acetic acid is also possible.

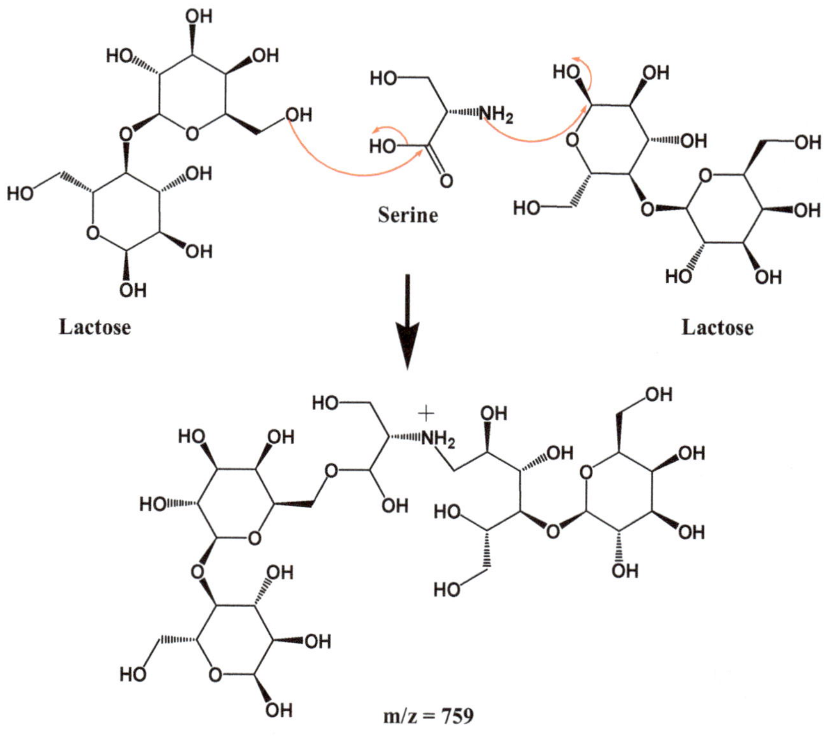

Fig. 15. Scheme 2: A possible interaction for the generation of the ion at m/z 759. As shown in the scheme, the interaction between the amino group of serine and the reducing end of lactose is likely a chemical reaction similar to the Maillard reaction, and the interaction between the hydroxyl groups of lactose and the carboxyl group of serine is a simple esterification reaction. The reactions, particularly the esterification reaction may also be driven biochemically by esterases.

The isolated bioactive fraction showed antiproliferative effects on cancer cells while not on normal cells. As indicated in the RP-HPLC chromatograph, the isolated fractions such as Fraction 30 are likely composed of multiple components that may be acting either singly or synergistically to exert the antiproliferative effects. Although the presence of peptides was suggested in the fractions as determined by the OPA methodology, the MS data did not support the presence of known peptide structures. The failure to identify any known peptides is likely due to the limitation of the OPA method, which can only detect the presence of primary amines and thus the primary amines in peptides cannot be differentiated from other amine containing compounds.

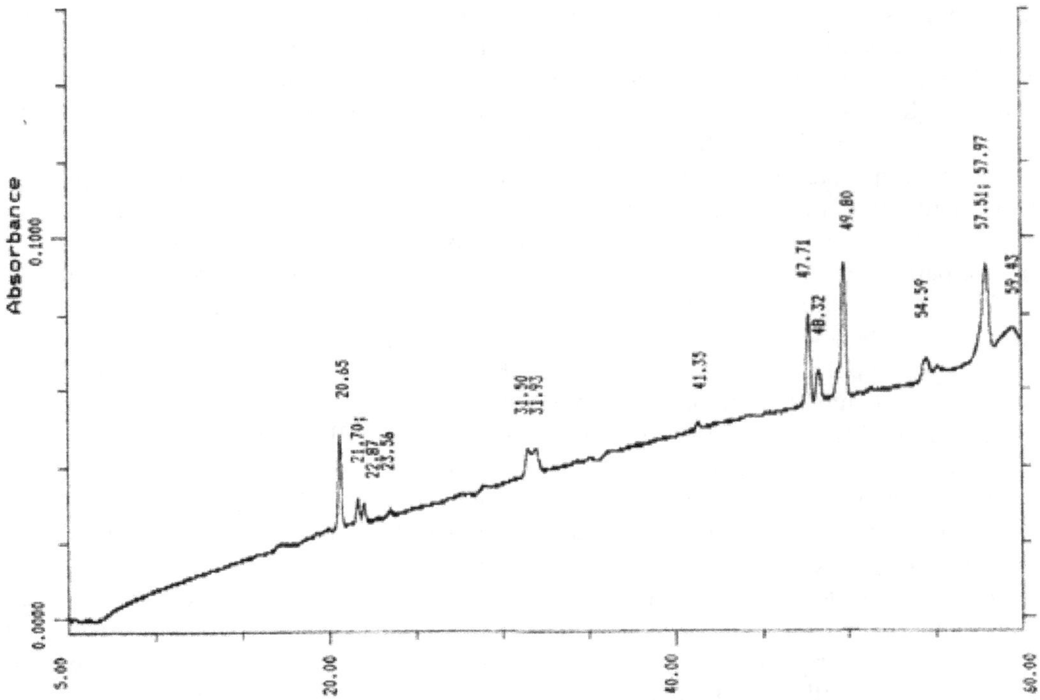

Fig. 16. Chromatograph of preparative HPLC Fraction 30 done by RP-HPLC. 50 µl of reconstituted preparative HPLC Fraction 30 which showed antiproliferative effect on MCF-7 cells was injected into a Prosphere 300 C4 column (5 µm, 250 mm x 4.6 mm) (Alltech Associate, Inc. Deerfield, IL 60015, USA) on Beckman HPLC System and eluted with a linear gradient of Buffer A (0.1% TFA in water) and Buffer B (60% of acetonitrile in 0.1% TFA: 40% of 0.1% TFA in water) as follows: 0 to 60 min, 0 to 90% B; and 61 to 65 min, 90 to 0% B. Absorbance was monitored at channel A 210 nm.

4. Conclusion

Due to the complex mixture of components in the specific fractions and the whole kefir extracts, the antiproliferative role of specific components such as proteins, peptides, organic acids and some small molecules, such as free amino acids, oligosaccharides and their interactions has been unclear. One of the main components of the bioactive antiproliferative kefir fractions is composed of lactose and acetic acid, possibly an end product of fermentation of the milk protein and sugar by the kefir bacteria and yeast. The lactose polymer suggests that the active component may be fragments of previously isolated polysaccharides termed as kefirans (Kooiman, 1968). Kefiran is a water-soluble polysaccharide consisted of approximately equal proportions of D-glucose and D-galactose (Kooiman, 1968; Micheli *et al.*, 1999). Kefiran has been reported to have antitumor activity

(Shiomi *et al.*, 1982; Murofushi *et al.*, 1983). It was also shown to be one of the substances having few or no side effect(s) in functioning to retard tumor growth in vivo.

It is noteworthy that one of the proposed novel bioactive structures contains serine and glucose or galactose; hence, it is conceivable that this molecule could be a sphingolipid compound. The ceramide component of sphingolipids is derived from serine and sphingolipids such as cerebrosides, which contain either a glucose or galactose. Sphingolipids such as gangliosides are sphingosine compounds that contain several glucose or galactose units. Also, lower molecular weight ceramide moieties have been detected in dairy gangliosides (Colarow *et al.*, 2003) and cultured dairy products have been shown to be a rich source of gangliosides (Kathleen *et al.*, 2000). Ceramide is derived from sphingomyelin (SpM) and can act as an intracellular second messenger for tumor necrosis factor-alpha, IL-1beta, and other cytokines. Ceramide has also been implicated in the acquired drug resistance that often characterizes breast cancer cells (Liu *et al.*, 1999). C2 and C6 ceramides are cell permeable ceramide analogs that have been shown to induce cell apoptosis (Fillet *et al.*, 2003). Osada *et al.* (1993) demonstrated that kefir contains an active substance, which enhances IFN-beta secretion of a human osteosarcoma line MG-63 treated with a chemical inducer, poly I: poly C. The active substance in the fermented milk was identified to be SpM. SpM from fermented milk (F-SpM) was a mixture of four molecular species of SpMs having C21-, C22-, C23- and C24-fatty acids. F-SpM enhanced the IFN secretion 14 times; SpMs from other food sources also enhanced IFN secretion but more moderately (2-3 times). We have observed a synergistic effect when MCF-7 cells were treated with ceramide analogs in the presence of extract of mother culture (data not shown). The putative sphingolipid component(s) in kefir that we have detected may have acted synergistically with the ceramide analogs leading to apoptosis of MCF-7 cells. In support of this concept, SpM has been shown to enhance the ceramide formation and ceramide-induced apoptosis in concert with the chemotherapeutic agent, gemcitabine, in human pancreatic cancer cells (Modrak *et al.*, 2004). Modification of ceramide metabolism also increases MCF-7 cells sensitivity to cytotoxics (Lucci *et al.*, 1999).

In summary, we have isolated the bioactive components from kefir mother culture that show antitumor cell proliferative effects. The MS data indicate that the isolated compounds are likely SpM complexes such as gangliosides that might have anti-tumor activities that are similar to that of ceramide. The biological functions of these ceramide-like compounds warrant further studies. The appearance of multiple components in the isolated bioactive antitumor fractions suggests the possibility that such components may be acting both independently and synergistically to exert the antiproliferative effects. Instead of searching for single compound in kefir, a mixture or a combination of components may be the best approach to have the highest potency for antitumor properties. The potential of using the kefir extract as co-drug for chemotherapy should be explored. In that regard, RP-HPLC Fraction 30 increased significantly the susceptibility of MCF-7 cells to tamoxifen, a commonly used anti-breast cancer drug. These results thus provide the rationale for future research to explore the potential of using kefir extracts as co-drugs for breast cancer chemotherapy and/or a functional food used for prevention of breast cancer.

5. Acknowledgments

This study was supported in part by grants from Liberty Brand Products, Inc. and a Natural Science and Engineering Research of Canada grant to S.K. and H.M.C. The authors thank the contribution of Dr. Kobi Yeboah for the mass spectrometry analysis. S.K. owns shares in KCLM Research in Nutrition Inc., which holds an exclusive option to license the intellectual property rights to the anticancer properties of kefir and kefir extracts.

6. References

Biffi, A.; Coradini, D., Larsen, R., Riva, L. & Di Fronzo, G. (1997). Antiproliferative Effect of Fermented Milk on the Growth of a Human Breast Cancer Cell Line. *Nutrition and Cancer*, Vol.28, No.1, (January 1997), pp. 93-99, ISSN 0163-5581

Bradford, M.M. (1976). A Rapid and Sensitive Method for the Quantitation of Microgram Quantities of Protein Utilizing the Principle of Protein-Dye Binding. *Analytical Biochemistry*, Vol.72, No. 1-2, (May 1976), pp. 248–254, ISSN 0003-2697

Cevikbas, A.; Yemni, E., Ezzedenn, F.W. & Yardimici, T. (1994). Antitumoral Antibacterial and Antifungal Activities of Kefir and Kefir Grain. *Phytotherapy Research*, Vol.8, No.2, (March 1993) pp. 78-82, ISSN 0951-418X

Chen, C.; Chan, H.M., & Kubow, S. (2007). Kefir Extracts Suppress In Vitro Proliferation of Estrogen-Dependent Human Breast Cancer Cells But Not Normal Mammary Epithelial Cells. *Journal of Medicinal Food*, Vol.10, No.3, (September 2007), pp. 416-422, ISSN 1096-620X

Church, F.C.; Swaisgood, H.E., Porter, D.H. & Catinani, G.L. (1983). Spectrophotometric Assay Using *O*-Phthaldialdehyde for Determination of Proteolysis in Milk and Isolation Milk Proteins. *Journal of Dairy Science*, Vol.66, No.6, (June 1983), pp. 1219-1227

Colarow, L.; Turini, M., Teneberg, S. & Berger, A. (2003). Characterization and Biological Activity of Gangliosides in Buffalo Milk. *Biochimica et Biophysica Acta (BBA) - Molecular and Cell Biology of Lipids*, Vol.1631, No.1, (February 2003), pp. 94-106, ISSN 0006-3002

Dillehay, D.L.; Webb, S.J., Schmelz, E.-M. & Merrill, A.H.Jr. (1994). Dietary Sphingomyelin Inhibits 1,2-Dimethylhydrazine-Induced Colon Cancer in CF1 Mice. *Journal of Nutrition*, Vol.124, No.5, (May 1994), pp. 615–620, ISSN 0022-3166

Doisneau-Sixou, S.F.; Cestac, P., Faye, J.C., Favre, G. & Sutherland, R. (2003). Additive Effects of Tamoxifen and the Farnesyl Transferase Inhibitor FTI-277 on Inhibition of MCF-7 Breast Cancer Cell-Cycle Progression. *International Journal of Cancer*, Vol.106, No.5, (September 2003), pp. 789-798, ISSN 0020-7136

Fillet, M.; Bentires-Alj, M., Deregowski, V., Greimers, R., Gielen, J., Piette, J., Bours, V. & Merville, M.P. (2003). Mechanisms Involved in Exogenous C2- and C6-Ceramide-Induced Cancer Cell Toxicity. *Biochemical Pharmacology*, Vol.65, No.10, (May 2003), pp. 1633-1642, ISSN 0006-2952

Furukawa, N.; Matsuoka, A., Takahashi, T. & Yamanaka, Y. (2000). Anti-Metastatic Effect of Kefir Grain Components on Lewis Lung Carcinoma and Highly Metastatic B16 Melanoma in Mice. *Journal of Agriculture Science Tokyo Nogyo Daigaku*, Vol.45, No.1, (January 2000), pp. 62-70, ISSN 0375-9202

Garrote, G.L.; Abraham, A.G. & Antoni, G.L. (2000). Inhibitory Power of Kefir: The Role of Organic Acids. *Journal of Food Protection*, Vol.63, No.3, (March 2000), pp. 364-369, ISSN 0362-028X

Guzel-Seydim, Z.B.; Seydim, A.C. & Greene, A.K. (2003). Comparison of Amino Acid Profiles of Milk, Yogurt and Turkish Kefir. *Milchwissenschaft*, Vol.58, No.3 (March 2003), pp. 158-160, ISSN 0026-3788

Kathleen, H.; Moore A., Ettinger, C. & Melvin, T.Y. (2000). Variation in Ganglioside Content of Bovine Dairy Products. *Journal of Food Composition and Analysis,* Vol.13, No.5 (March 2000), pp. 783-790, ISSN 0889-1575

Kooiman, P. (1968). The Chemical Structure of Kefiran, the Water-Soluble Polysaccharide of the Kefir Grain. *Carbohydrate Research,* Vol.7, No.2, (June 1968), pp. 200-211

Liu, Y.-Y.; Han, T.-Y., Giuliano, A.E., Ichikawa, S., Hirabayashi, Y. & Cabot, M.C. (1999). Glycosylation of Ceramide Potentiates Cellular Resistance to Tumor Necrosis Factor-Alpha-Induced Apoptosis. *Experimental Cell Research,* Vol.252, No.2 (November 1999), pp. 464-470, ISSN 0014-4827

Lucci, A.; Han, T.Y., Liu, Y.Y., Giuliano, A.E. & Cabot, M.C. (1999). Modification of Ceramide Metabolism Increases Cancer Sensitivity to Cytotoxics. *International Journal of Oncology,* Vol.15, No. 3, (September 1999), pp. 541-546, ISSN 1019-6439

Mesner, P.W. Jr.; Budihardjo, I.I. & Kaufmann, S.H. (1997). Chemotherapy-Induced Apoptosis. *Advances in Pharmacology,* Vol.41, pp. 461-499

Micheli, L.; Uccelletti, D., Paleschi, C. & Crescenzi, V. (1999). Isolation and Characterization of a Lactobacillus Strain Producing the Exopolysacchsride Kefiran. *Applied Microbiology and Biotechnology,* Vol.34, No.1 (December 1999), pp. 137-143, ISSN 0175-7598

Modrak, D.E.; Cardillo, T.M., Newsome, G.A., Goldenberg, D.M. & Gold, D.V. (2004). Synergistic Interaction Between Sphingomyelin and Gemcitabine Potentiates Ceramide-Mediated Apoptosis in Pancreatic Cancer. *Cancer Research,* Vol. 64, No.22, (November 2004), pp. 8405-8410, ISSN 0008-5472

Murofushi, M.; Shiomi, M. & Aibara, K. (1983). Effect of Orally Administered Polysaccharide from Kefir Grain on Delayed-Type Hypersensitivity and Tumor Growth in Mice. *Japanese Journal of Medical Science and Biology,* Vol.36, No.1 (February 1983), pp. 49-53, ISSN 0021-5112

Osada, K.; Nagira, K., Teruya, K., Tachibana, H., Shirahata, S. & Murakami, H. (1993). Enhancement of Interferon-Beta Production with Sphingomyelin from Fermented Milk. *Biotherapy,* Vol.7, No.2, (February 1993), pp. 115-123, ISSN 0921-299X

Parvez, S.; Malik, K.A., Ah, Kang. S. & Kim, H.Y. (2006). Probiotics and Their Fermented Food Products are Beneficial for Health. Journal of Applied Microbiology, Vol.100, No.6, (June 2006), pp. 1171-1185, ISSN 1364-507

Ronco, A.L., Stefani, E. & Dattoli, R. (2002). Dairy Foods and Risk of Breast Cancer: A Case-Control Study in Montevideo, Uruguay. *European Journal of Cancer Prevention.* Vol.11, No.5, (October 2002), pp. 457-463, ISSN 0959-8278

Schonberg, S. & Kordan H.E. (1995). The Inhibitory Effects of Conjugated Dienoic Derivatives (CLA) of Linoleic Acid on the Growth of Human Tumor Cell Lines is in Part Due to Increased Lipid Peroxidation. *Anticancer research,* Vol.15, No.4, (July-August 1995), pp. 1241-1246, ISSN 0250-7005

Shiomi, M.; Sasaki, K., Murofushi, M. & Aibara, K. (1982). Antitumor Activity in Mice of Orally Administered Polysaccharide from Kefir Grain. *Japanese Journal of Medical Science and Biology,* Vol.35, No.2 (April 1982), pp. 75-80, ISSN 0021-5112

Svensson, M.; Sabharwal, H., Mossberg, A.K., Lipniunas, P., Leffler, H., Svanborg, C. & Linse, S. (1999). Molecular characterization of alpha-lactalbumin folding variants that induce apoptosis in tumor cells. *Journal of Biological Chemistry,* Vol.274, No.10 (March 1999), pp. 6388-6396, ISSN 0021-9258

11

Experimental Therapeutics for the Treatment of Triple Negative Breast Cancer

Julian Dzeyk, Babasaheb Yadav and Rhonda J. Rosengren
University of Otago
New Zealand

1. Introduction

Triple negative breast cancers (TNBCs) are defined as tumors that do not express the estrogen receptor (ER), the progesterone receptor (PR) and the HER2 isoform of the epidermal growth factor receptor (EGFR)(Foulkes et al., 2010). They account for approximately 10-17% of all breast cancers (Reis-Filho & Tutt, 2008). Clinically, they are more prevalent among young African and African-American women (Reis-Filho & Tutt, 2008). TNBCs are poorly differentiated, highly malignant, more aggressive and have a poor outcome (Chen & Russo, 2009). They are also characterized by early recurrence and a high rate of visceral metastasis (Conte & Guarneri, 2009). Moreover, the peak risk of recurrence occurs within three years of diagnosis and the mortality rates are increased for five years after diagnosis (Kwan et al., 2009). The molecular changes associated with TNBCs have been characterized by various immunohistochemistry and gene expression profiling studies. Specifically, they include *p53* mutation, overexpression of Ki67 and EGFR, and dysfunction in the BRCA1 pathway (Rowe et al., 2009). It is estimated that EGFR is expressed in 60% of TNBCs (Arslan et al., 2009). In addition, TNBCs have an over expression of cytokeratins 5, 6, 14, and 17, smooth muscle actin, P-cadherin and c-kit (Irvin & Carey, 2008, Venkitaraman, 2010).

2. Naturally-derived experimental therapies

2.1 Epigallocatechin gallate

TNBCs have limited treatment options due to the lack of a specific therapeutic target, such as hormonal or antibody therapy as well as a diverse biology and treatment sensitivity (Arslan et al., 2009). Therefore, there is an urgent need for novel therapeutic agents for the management of TNBC. Accordingly, naturally-derived compounds are under investigation and provide a source of experimental drugs from which novel therapies could develop. One of these natural agents is epigallocatechin gallate (EGCG, Figure 1). It is the most abundant and active catechin obtained from green tea (*Camellia sinensis*) (Graham, 1992), as it has shown anti-tumorigenic activity in a variety of cancer models including TNBC cell lines such as MDA-MB-231 and MDA-MB-468 cells. Specifically, EGCG inhibited the proliferation of MDA-MB-468 and MDA-MB-231 cells with inhibitory concentrations (IC_{50}) of 30 and 80 μg/ml, respectively (Kavanagh et al., 2001, Masuda et al., 2002). Mechanisms for the cytotoxic effect of EGCG include induction of apoptosis as well as the modulation of various cell signaling proteins involved in cell survival, proliferation and death. Specifically, EGCG (20-60 μg/ml) caused 20-54% of MDA-MB-468 cells to become apoptotic after 72 h (Roy et al., 2005), while 25 μM caused 12% of MDA-MB-231 cells to undergo apoptosis after 36 h (Stuart et al., 2007). Even though EGCG causes cells to undergo cell cycle arrest in the G1 phase, this is not a mechanistic driver of apoptosis in TNBC cells, as the significant increase in apoptosis precedes the increase in G1 arrest (Stuart et al, 2007). Therefore, other mechanisms drive apoptosis.

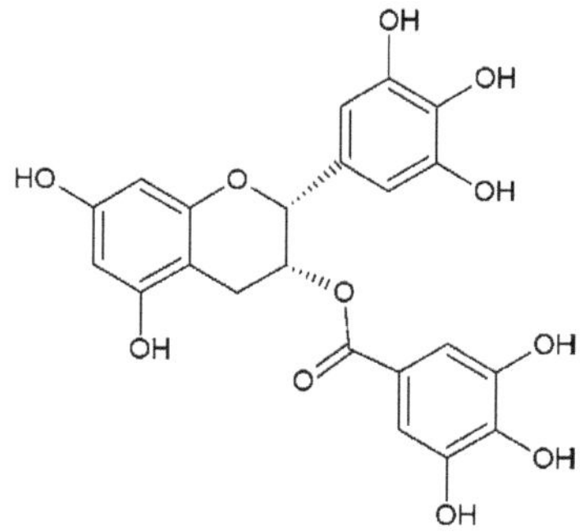

Fig. 1. Chemical structure of (-)-epigallocatechin gallate.

The cell surface epidermal growth factor receptor is over-expressed in 45-70% of TNBC cells and is associated with poor prognosis of patients (Bosch et al., 2010, Koenders et al., 1991). EGFR activation via growth fator binding causes dimerization and subsequent auto-phosphorylation of specific tyrosine residues at the intracellular C-terminal end of the receptor. Through conserved protein binding domains (SH2, SH3) that interact with the phospho-tyrosine residues of EGFR, intracellular signaling cascades such as the mitogen activated kinase (MAPK) pathway, C-Jun N-terminal kinase (JNK) pathway and the phosphoinosital-3-kinase/Akt (PI3K/Akt) pathway can be activated (Casalini et al., 2004). Of particular importance for breast cancer is the PI3K/Akt pathway which is associated with phosphatase and tensin homolog (PTEN) inactivation, commonly found to be dysregulated in cancers (DeGraffenried et al., 2004). The protein product (phosphatase) of the tumor suppressor gene PTEN is involved in cell cycle regulation, preventing cells from growing and dividing excessively (Chu & Tarnawski, 2004). In a gene expression analysis of 106 breast cancer patients it was shown that there was a 34% decrease in PTEN and a corresponding 29% increase in EGFR expression, but only in patients with triple-negative breast tumors (Andre et al., 2009). A further study with 11 TNBC patients provided evidence that low PTEN expression is associated with increased activation of Akt. Although it should be noted that the Spearman correlation between Akt and PTEN expression was 0.593, and may therefore suggest that Akt could be activated and affected by multiple mechanisms (Berrada et al., 2010). In MDA-MB-468 cells, EGCG treatment (30 μg/ml) for 72 h inhibited the phosphorylation and therefore the activation of EGFR, Akt and STAT3 in the presence and absence of TGF-α (Masuda *et al.* 2007).

Using scintillation proximity assays, EGCG inhibited all four (PI3Kα, PI3Kβ, PI3Kγ, and PI3Kδ) class I PI3K isoforms (Van Aller et al., 2011). In particular EGCG was potent towards the PI3Kα isoform with a K_i value of 380 nM. Additionally, mTOR was inhibited with a K_i of 320 nM. Further analysis showed inhibition of both PI3K and mTOR occurred via competition with ATP binding to these proteins (Van Aller et al., 2011). This was confirmed by molecular modeling studies where the structure of PI3Kγ complexed with myricetin (PDB:1E90) was used to dock with EGCG. Myricetin, a structurally related flavonoid, is an ATP competitive inhibitor of PI3K with an IC_{50} of 1.8 μM (Walker et al., 2000). Except for the chromandiol moiety of EGCG which was flipped by 180° compared to the chromone moiety of myricetin, the binding mode of EGCG is similar to that of myricetin, further supporting the notion that EGCG is a PI3K inhibitor by competing with ATP binding (Van Aller et al., 2011). Since the mTOR (C2 isoform) is one of the 3-phosphoinositide-dependent kinases responsible for the activation/phosphorylation of Akt at Ser473, the effects of EGCG on phospho-Akt was examined in MDA-MB-231 cells. EGCG inhibited Akt phosphorylation in a concentration-dependent manner with IC_{50} values below 1 μM, which was consistent with a direct inhibition of mTOR and PI3K by EGCG (Van Aller et al., 2011).

The anti-apoptotic Bcl-2 protein family is important for mitochondrial and endoplasmic reticulum membrane permeability as well as transduction and integration of apoptotic signals upon homo- and heterodimerization (Adams & Cory, 1998). Another protein from the Bcl-2 family, Bax, is classified as pro-apoptotic protein, which directs the release of cytochrome c. The expression ratio of Bax/Bcl-2 is a determining factor for apoptosis in biochemical studies (Adams & Cory, 1998). In MDA-MB-468 cells, EGCG (20-60 μg/ml) for 48 h caused a dose-dependent 1-to-3-fold increase in the expression ratio of Bax and Bcl-2 (Roy et al., 2005). This indicated that the apoptosis inducing effects of EGCG are transmitted via reductions in anti-apoptotic signals by reducing Bcl-2 protein and increasing pro-apoptotic signals mediated by Bax (Roy et al., 2005). Western blotting of other important pro-apoptotic signaling proteins provided further verification of the underlying mechanism by which EGCG induces apoptosis. It was shown that treatment of MDA-MB-468 cells with EGCG (20 μg/ml) for 48 h elevated the expression of cytochrome c (2-fold), Apaf-1 (7-fold), caspase 3 as well as poly(ADP-ribose) polymerase (PARP) (Roy et al., 2005). Similar observations were also made in MDA-MB-231 cells, which were treated with 50 or 80 μg/ml for 24 h. The protein expression ratio of Bax and Bcl-2, as visualized by Western blotting, showed a dose-dependent relationship. The full length PARP protein (116 kDa) was also degraded into the cleaved, inactive 85 kDa form by the proteolytic caspase-3, which is an integral part of mitochondrial-regulated apoptosis (Thangapazham et al., 2007a).

Another potential target for cancer chemoprevention is the ribonucleoprotein telomerase (synthesizes the cap-telomere-end, 5'-TTAGGG-3', of eukaryotic chromosomes), as it is expressed in ~85% of human cancers (75% of breast carcinoma *in situ* and 88% in ductal and lobulal breast carcinomas (Shay & Bacchetti, 1997)). In contrast, after embryonic development, telomerase is barely detectable in normal human somatic cells (Cunningham et al., 2006). The action of EGCG on telomerase activity has also been assessed in MDA-MB-231 cells and MCF10A non-cancerous breast cells. Using a conventional gel-based PCR method, the relative mRNA levels of human telomerase reverse transcriptase (*hTERT*; the key catalytic subunit of telomerase (Cunningham et al., 2006)) were measured in both cell lines after treatment with 40 μM of EGCG for 3, 6, 9 or 12 days. EGCG was found to time-dependently inhibit *hTERT* expression (~40 and ~50% decrease after 9 and 12 days, respectively) in MDA-MB-231 but not MCF10A cells (Meeran et al., 2011). Since *hTERT* is an epigenetically regulated gene (Cunningham et al., 2006), the activity of epigenetic-modulating enzymes such as DNA methyltransferases (DNMTs), histone acetyltransferases (HATs), and histone deacetylases (HDACs) was assessed in order to determine the mechanism under which EGCG influences *hTERT* mRNA levels. Specifically, in MDA-MB-231 cells EGCG (40 μM) treatment for 9 days decreased both DNMT and HAT activity by

~40%, while HDAC activity was unaffected (Meeran et al., 2011). The authors suggested that the observed effects might be due to direct binding of EGCG to the active site of DNMTs and inhibition of HATs. Additionally, treatment with EGCG (40 µM) reduced methylation to ~60%. This indicated that the inhibition of DNMT expression following EGCG treatment could be a contributing factor in the facilitation of *hTERT* promoter demethylation, which would lead to transcriptional repression of *hTERT* expression (Meeran et al., 2011).

An intricate part of tumor growth, invasion and metastasis is the process of new blood vessel formation, referred to as angiogenesis. A key mediator required for this process is vascular endothelial growth factor (VEGF), which is expressed at 34% higher levels in TNBC patients compared to hormone-sensitive tumors (Andre et al., 2009). Angiogenesis is also stimulated by other pro-angiogenic factors such as basic fibroblast growth factor and hypoxia-inducible factor (Schneider & Miller, 2005). Therefore, VEGF targeting anti-angiogenic agents such as bevacizumab have been beneficial in the treatment of TNBC patients (Carey et al., 2010). Matrix metalloproteinases (MMPs) also play an important role in the progression of invasive and metastatic breast cancer (Schneider & Miller, 2005). Targeting various markers such as MMPs that inhibit the rapid growth and metastasis has emerged as one of the strategies for treatment of highly proliferative TNBCs (Greenberg & Rugo, 2010). The inhibition of angiogenesis is yet another critical component to the plethora of effects elicited by EGCG. Specifically, EGCG (40 µg/ml) significantly decreased VEGF peptide levels by 85% and VEGF mRNA levels by 75% compared to control in MDA-MB-231 cells (Sartippour et al., 2002). Effects of the drug were also assessed on VEGF promoter activity and results showed that EGCG (40 µg/ml) reduced promoter activity by ~30% (Sartippour et al., 2002). EGCG also decreased VEGF production in MDA-MB-468 cells by 55% as well as NFκB activity by 4-fold compared to control (Masuda et al., 2007). The effect of protein kinase C has also been examined, as this protein has been shown to be a modulator of VEGF expression (Hossain et al., 2000). Using Western blotting, it was shown that protein kinase C levels decreased by ~70% upon EGCG treatment compared to control (Sartippour et al., 2002). In a Boyden chamber assay, to assess the anti-metastatic potential of EGCG using MDA-MB-231, cells it was shown that treatment with 80 µg/ml for 24 h caused a 28% reduction in cell invasiveness. Furthermore, EGCG decreased the expression of matrix metalloproteinase-9 (MMP-9) 5-fold using microarray experiments. This was confirmed using RT-PCR, which also showed a down-regulation of MMP-9 at the transcriptional level (Thangapazham et al., 2007a). Thus, EGCG suppresses angiogenesis in TNBC via a variety of mechanisms.

An important prognostic markers for breast cancer is Met, a transmembrane receptor for the hepatocyte growth factor (HGF). Importantly, it also has been assessed as one of the targets of EGCG. High levels of Met are correlated with a lower patient survival rate, which led researchers to postulate that EGCG may affect HGF signaling via Met. Using Western blotting in MDA-MB-231 cells, it was shown that 1 h pre-treatment with EGCG (0.6-30 µM) followed by 15 min of exposure to HGF (30 ng/ml), significantly blocked HGF-induced Met, AKT and ERK phosphorylation (Bigelow & Cardelli, 2006). A Boyden chamber assay using MDA-MB-231 cells showed that the observed ~7-fold increase in invading cells by HGF was decreased to ~2-fold by EGCG (5 µM) (Bigelow & Cardelli, 2006). Therefore the modulation of Met by EGCG also contributes to its anti-cancer action in TNBC cells.

The anticancer activity of EGCG is also evident *in vivo*, as isolated EGCG and/or a mixture of green tea polyphenols have suppressed TNBC growth *in vivo*. Specifically, in a MDA-MB-231 xenograft model tumor volume after 10 weeks of treatment was reduced by 45% in EGCG treated mice and by 61% in green tea polyphenol (GTP) treated mice compared to control (Thangapazham et al., 2007b). GTP and EGCG treatment increased the number of apoptotic cells by 3.5 and 2.6-fold, respectively. This study showed that GTP was slightly more effective than pure EGCG in reducing the tumor incidence, volume and number of apoptotic cells. However, this may be related to the dose given (~3 mg/mouse GTP vs. 1 mg/mouse EGCG) (Thangapazham et al., 2007b). These findings are supported by earlier *in vivo* studies with EGCG or green tea extracts (GTE) (Kavanagh et al. 2001, Sartippour et al., 2001). Specifically, 0.62, 1.25, 2.5 g/l of GTE dose-dependently prevented tumor growth, with a 90% reduction in tumor volume in the 2.5g/l treatment group compared to control (Sartippour et al., 2001). Using immunohistochemistry it was also shown that GTE decreased the overall microvessel density by ~50% in the treated animals compared to control (Sartippour et al., 2001). Importantly, these studies and many others demonstrated that the *in vitro* anticancer effects of EGCG translate into tumor suppression *in vivo*.

2.2 Curcumin

Curcumin (Figure 2), obtained from the roots and rhizomes of the perennial plant *Curcuma longa*, is cytotoxic towards both ER positive and TNBC cells (Verma et al., 1997). For example, curcumin (10 μM) inhibited the proliferation of MDA-MB-468 and MDA-MB-231 cells, with IC_{50} values of 1 μM and 16.25 μg/ml, respectively (Squires et al., 2003). Mechanisms for the cytotoxic effect of curcumin include G2/M cell cycle arrest, induction of apoptosis as well as the modulation of various cell signaling proteins involved in cell survival, proliferation and death. Specifically, cell cycle studies demonstrated that curcumin (20 μM) treatment for 24 h increased the proportion of MDA-MB-231 cells in the G2/M phase by 164% (Chiu & Su, 2009, Fang et al., 2011). Furthermore, curcumin (20 μM) increased the proportion of MDA-MB-468 cells in the G2/M phase by 143% (Squires et al., 2003). Thus, in contrast to EGCG, G2/M phase arrest is one of the drivers of curcumin-mediated apoptosis.

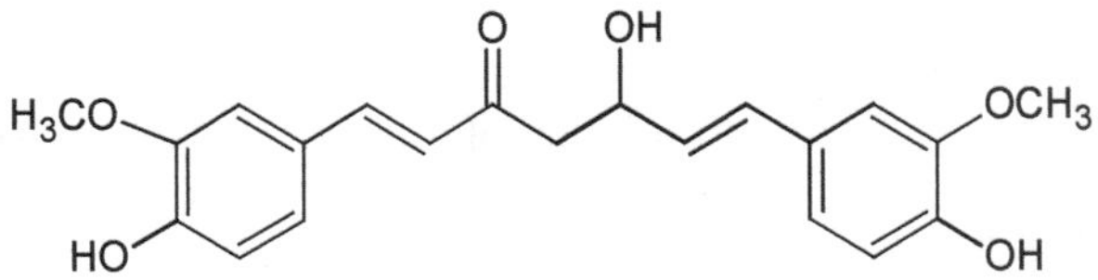

Fig. 2. Chemical structure of curcumin.

The cell cycle is promoted by activation of cyclin dependent kinases, which are positively regulated by cyclins and negatively by cyclin dependent kinase inhibitors (CDKIs) (Malumbres & Barbacid, 2009). Cyclin D1 regulates cell cycle progression through G1-phase of the cell cycle by activating CDK4 and CDK6. Cyclin D1 is a proto-oncogene which is overexpressed in ER negative breast cancers and is a predictor of poor prognosis (Umekita et al., 2002), while cyclin E along with CDK2 regulates the entry of cells from late G1 to S phase. Cyclin E overexpression is associated with poor prognosis and high proliferation in ER negative breast cancer patients (Potemski et al., 2006). CDKIs, p21 and p27 belong to Cip/Kip family of proteins and their decreased expression has been correlated with poor prognosis in breast cancer patients (Catzavelos et al., 1997, Pellikainen et al., 2003). It is reported that altered expression of proteins regulating the cell cycle makes TNBC more sensitive to cytotoxic therapy (Rouzier et al., 2005). Studies have demonstrated that curcumin modulates the expression of cyclins, CDKs and CDKIs in breast cancer cells.

Specifically, curcumin decreased the expression of cyclin D1 and increased levels of p21 expression in MDA-MB-231 cells (Liu et al., 2009) and this was followed by the induction of apoptosis (Chiu & Su, 2009).

Curcumin induces apoptosis in most, if not all, breast cancer cell lines and this occurs mainly via a mitochondrial-dependent pathway (Karunagaran et al., 2005). In most cells, curcumin induces a loss of mitochondrial membrane potential, opening of the transition pore, release of cytochrome c, caspase-9 activation, caspase-3 activation and subsequent cleavage of PARP all of which lead to DNA fragmentation and apoptosis (Aggarwal et al., 2003, Ravindran et al., 2009). Down regulation of anti-apoptotic proteins (Bcl-2 and Bcl-XL) and upregulation of pro-apoptotic proteins (Bad and Bax) also leads to curcumin induced apoptosis in many cancer cells including breast cancer (Ravindran et al., 2009). Curcumin-induced apoptosis via inhibition of reactive oxygen species (ROS) has also been shown. ROS regulate intracellular signaling pathways in various cancer cells including breast cancer (Waris & Ahsan, 2006). Higher production of ROS and glutathione depletion cause oxidative stress, loss of cell function and ultimately leads to apoptosis. Curcumin causes rapid depletion of glutathione (GSH) which results in an increase in the production of ROS and induction of apoptosis (Shehzad et al., 2010). Additionally, curcumin induced apoptosis in MDA-MB cells through the generation of ROS originating from glutathione depletion by buthioninesulfoximine thereby further sensitizing the tumor cells to curcumin (Syng-Ai et al., 2004).

The induction of apoptosis and modulation of the cell cycle result from the effect of curcumin on various intracellular pathways. Curcumin inhibits epidermal growth factor stimulated phosphorylation of EGFR and further inhibits downstream ERK1/2, JNK, and Akt activity in MDA-MB-468 cells (Squires et al., 2003). NFκB is a transcription factor that regulates various genes involved in both proliferation and apoptosis and aberrant NFκB expression is implicated in different types of breast cancers (Wu & Kral, 2005). Furthermore, it is constitutively activated in ER negative breast cancers and its inhibition suppresses cell growth and induces cell death (Biswas et al., 2001, Schlotter et al., 2008). For example, 5 μg/ml of curcumin reduced the expression of nuclear NFκB in MDA-MB-231 cells (Liu et al., 2009). Also, curcumin abolished paclitaxel induced NFκB activation in MDA-MB-435 breast cancer cells (Aggarwal et al., 2005). Modulation of the Wnt/β-catenin pathway by curcumin has been shown to play a role in the inhibition of cell proliferation and induction of apoptosis in MDA-MB-231 breast cancer cells (Prasad et al., 2009). The Wnt/β-catenin pathway is an important pathway as it is associated with worse overall survival in TNBC (Khramtsov et al., 2010).

Curcumin is an inhibitor of angiogenesis, as 50 μM suppressed the transcription levels of VEGF and b-FGF in MDA-MB-231 cells (Shao et al., 2002). Additionally, curcumin downregulated post-transcriptional levels of both HIF-1□α and HIF-1□β in MDA-MB-231 cells (Thomas et al., 2008). Curcumin also inhibited the invasive potential of MDA-MB-231 cells via down regulation of MMP-2, MMP-3 and MMP-9 and up regulation of tissue inhibitor metalloproteinase (TIMP-1, 2) which regulates tumor cell invasion (Boonrao et al., 2010, Shao et al., 2002). In another study, the anti-invasive properties of curcumin were mediated through inhibition of RON tyrosine kinase receptor (Narasimhan & Ammanamanchi, 2008). Curcumin also inhibits integrin α (6) β (4), a laminin adhesion receptor in MDA-MB-231 cells and thus inhibits cell motility and invasion (Kim et al., 2008). Recently, it was shown that curcumin induces upregulation of maspin, a serine protease inhibitor and thus inhibits invasion of MDA-MB-231 cells (Prasad et al., 2009). Furthermore, curcumin inhibited migration of MDA-MB-231 cells through the down regulation of protein expression of the transcription factor, NFκB (Chiu & Su, 2009). Lastly, curcumin also reduced the expression of the two prometastatic cytokines, CXCL1 and -2, which in turn reduces expression of the chemotactic receptor CXCR4 along with other metastasis-promoting genes (Bachmeier et al., 2008).

The anti-metastatic effect of curcumin has also been studied in various *in vivo* models. Dietary administration of curcumin (2%) significantly decreased the incidence of breast cancer metastasis to the lung in an MDA-MB-231 xenograft model. They also observed that curcumin significantly suppressed the expression of NFκB, COX2 and MMP-9 (Aggarwal et al., 2005). In another study, curcumin decreased lung metastasis in a mouse xenograft model. MDA-MB-231 cells were inoculated into nude mice by intercardiac injection and the treatment group was fed with 1% dietary curcumin. After 5 weeks of treatment, 21% of animals from the curcumin treatment group were metastasis free compared with the control group who all had metastasis (Bachmeier et al., 2007). Many other studies have used chemical carcinogens such as dimethylbenzanthracene or diethylstilbestrol to show that curcumin inhibits mammary carcinogenesis. However, none of these models are representative of TNBC. Nevertheless, curcumin elicits a plethora of effects in TNBC and importantly, as with EGCG, anticancer activity is retained *in vivo*. Both compounds also modulated many different cell signaling pathways that cumulate in a strong apoptotic response (Figure 3).

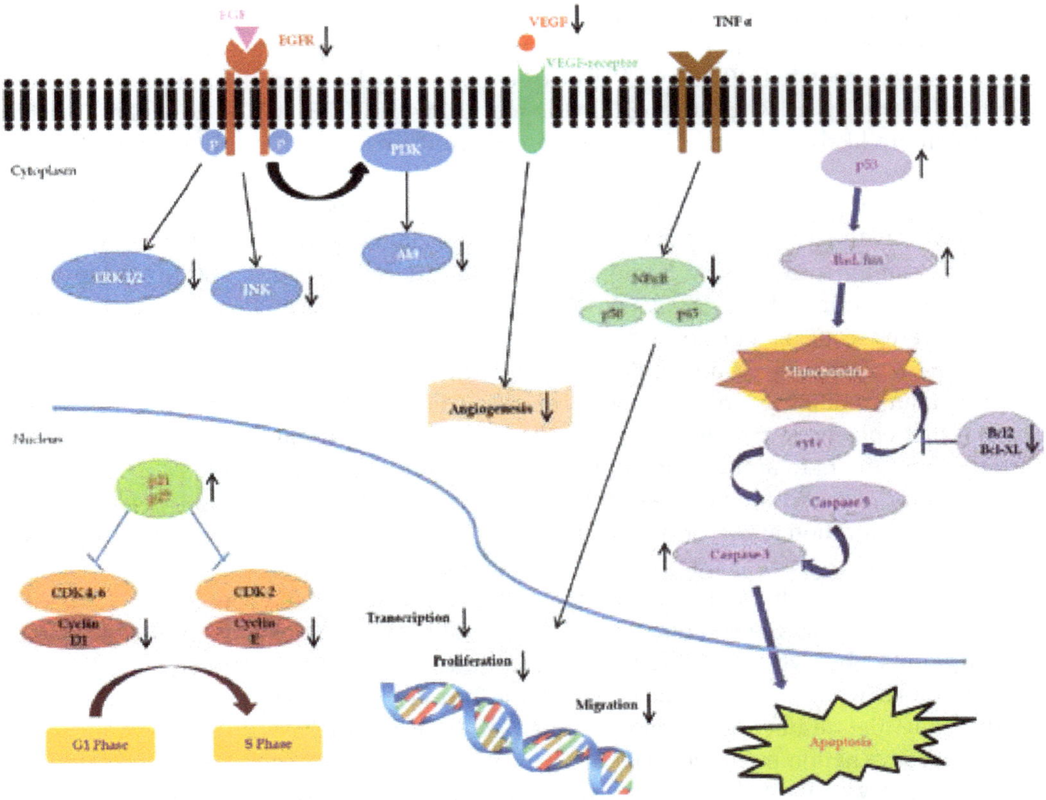

Fig. 3. Schematic diagram of intracellular cell signaling cascades activated following auto-phosphorylation of the EGFR. Arrows indicate an increase or decrease in the protein expression/activity following treatment with either EGCG or curcumin in models of TNBC.

3. Improving naturally derived compounds

3.1 Combination studies

Initial studies with EGCG or curcumin demonstrated that these natural compounds had promise as potential treatments for TNBC. However, both compounds have also been used in various combination studies in order to improve their efficacy. This was achieved in MDA-MB-231 cells where EGCG (20 μM) in combination with paclitaxel (1 μM) reduced cell viability by ~80% after 24 h compared to control (Luo et al., 2010). Treatment of just paclitaxel reduced cell viability by ~40%, whereas EGCG on its own had no effect compared to control. These results suggested that EGCG may act synergistically with paclitaxel to enhance its anti-carcinogenic effects (Luo et al., 2010). Other studies have also shown synergistic effects by using EGCG in combination with other known breast cancer treatments. One such study showed that the selective estrogen receptor modulator (SERM), tamoxifen in combination with EGCG elicited synergistic cytotoxicity as well as earlier and enhanced apoptosis in MDA-MB-231 cells (Chisholm et al., 2004, Stuart et al., 2007). This effect was further analyzed in an *in vivo* xenograft model. Specifically, mice were treated with either tamoxifen (75 μg/kg), EGCG (25 mg/kg) or a combination of the two for 10 weeks. Results showed that the tumor volume in the EGCG + tamoxifen treatment group was 75% smaller compared to vehicle or tamoxifen (Scandlyn et al., 2008). Combination treated mice also had significantly smaller tumors compared to EGCG treatment. Tumor suppression was not through the up-regulation of the ER in MDA-MB-231 cells (Scandlyn et al., 2008). Instead EGFR and its activated form were reduced by ~78% compared to control. Similar reductions in mTOR and CYP1B1 expression were also found in tumors from EGCG + tamoxifen treated mice, indicating that the reductions of EGFR, mTOR as well as CYP1B1 expression are likely to be important mechanistic contributors to the suppression of tumor growth (Scandlyn et al., 2008).

Highly interesting was the finding that EGCG at the specific concentration of 10 μM in combination with 10 ng/ml of trichostatin A (TSA; a histone deacetylase inhibitor) increased estrogen receptor-α expression 6-fold in MDA-MB-231 cells (Li et al., 2010). Using CHiP assays it was confirmed that EGCG and TSA increased histone acetyl transferase activity 5-fold compared control. Furthermore, the combination of EGCG, TSA and tamoxifen in MDA-MB-231 cells, caused a significant ~60% reduction in cell viability, which was more effective than combining tamoxifen with either EGCG or TSA (Li et al., 2010). These results showed that epigenetic modifications induced by EGCG + TSA may be useful in sensitizing ER-negative tumors to anti-hormonal therapy. However, it should be noted that the EGCG concentration required for the observed 6-fold increase in ER-α expression was exactly 10 μM, any concentration above or below did not have any effect on ER-α expression (Li et al., 2010). Additionally, a similar effect *in vivo* has not been reported.

Combining EGCG with another SERM, raloxifene, has also shown synergistic cytotoxicity. In MDA-MB-231 cells the combination of EGCG (25 μM) and raloxifene (5 μM) decreased the cell number by ~28% compared to control. Individually, both compounds at the same concentrations were not cytotoxic towards the cancer cells (Stuart & Rosengren, 2008). Additionally, the number of apoptotic cells after 48 h was 34% higher compared to control following combination treatment. The mechanism of action was further assessed by protein expression analysis and the results showed that the protein expression of EGFR, Akt, mTOR and S-6-kinase were decreased by 22, 31, 41 and 46%, respectively (Stuart et al., 2010) after 18 h of treatment. Thus these two compounds elicit a strong response in pathways downstream of the EGFR.

Interestingly, combination of the two naturally derived compounds curcumin and EGCG was effective in both *in vitro* and *in vivo* models of TNBC. In MDA-MB-231 cells these two compounds (EGCG at 25 μM and curcumin at 3 μM) increased apoptotic cells and G2 arrest 2.6-fold compared to curcumin alone (Somers-Edgar et al., 2008). This effect was only observed in TNBC cells and not in MCF-7 cells. Importantly, this *in vitro* effect translated to tumor suppression *in vivo*. Specifically, curcumin (200 mg/kg) and EGCG (25 mg/kg) significantly suppressed MDA-MB-231 xenograft tumor volume by 49% compared to vehicle control after 10 weeks of treatment (Somers-Edgar et al., 2008). This was in part driven by a 78% decrease in VEGFR-1 protein expression in tumors. Tumor suppression has also been shown in other combination studies with curcumin. Specifically, when curcumin was combined with paclitaxel in an MDA-MB-231 xenograft model, there was a significant reduction in tumor growth following combination treatment compared to either agent alone. Mechanistic studies showed that the combination decreased the expression of MMP-9 and increased apoptosis in the tumors of treated mice. Interestingly, the dose of paclitaxel was much lower (7 mg/kg) than previously reported as a single treatment (Kang et al., 2009). Success has also been shown using *in vitro* combination studies. Specifically, when curcumin was combined with piperine the two drugs worked synergistically to inhibit breast cancer stem cell self-renewal without affecting normal cells. The authors showed that this effect was mediated by the inhibition of mammosphere formation via the Wnt signaling pathway (Kakarala et al., 2010). Synergistic growth inhibition and the induction of apoptosis in MDA-MB-231 cells also occurred following the combination of curcumin and xanthorrhizol (Cheah et al., 2009). These studies all illustrate that the naturally derived compounds EGCG and curcumin can also be used in combination in order to increase the potency of these compounds and/or potentially sensitize cancer cells to the effects of other chemotherapeutic agents.

3.2 Novel drug delivery of natural compounds

Various novel drug delivery systems such as nanoparticles, liposomes, micells, adjuvants and phospholipid complexes have been developed in order to specifically target cancer cells in order to improve efficacy and bioavailability, while reducing toxicity. (Anand et al., 2008). Nanoparticles can improve the biodistribution of drugs, as they are able to act as carriers of anti-cancer drugs by selectively using the unique pathophysiology of tumors, such as their enhanced vascular permeability and extensive angiogenesis (Figure 4) (Cho et al., 2008). The term nanochemoprevention was recently introduced, combining nanotechnology with chemoprevention using EGCG as an encapsulated agent in polylactic acid-polyethylene glycol nanoparticles. The safety and improved efficacy of such gelantin nanoparticles has resulted in increased accumulation within the tumor and prolonged *in vivo* circulation (Vlerken et al., 2007). This is very important, as a downfall of both EGCG and curcumin is their low bioavailability (Siddiqui et al., 2009). To ensure that EGCG contained in such nanoparticles was functionally similar to free EGCG, it was essential to first test these nanoparticles *in vitro*. To accomplish this, MDA-MB-231 cells were treated with empty gelatin nanoparticles (5 μM), nanoparticles with EGCG (1 and 5 μM), or free EGCG (5 μM) for 30 min or 5 h. This was followed by the addition of HGF (30 ng/ml) and lysate preparation for Western blotting. The analysis showed that 5 μM free EGCG was able to block HGF-induced Met, AKT and ERK activation. On the other hand both the nanoparticles with and without EGCG did not inhibit HGF-induced signalling after pre-incubation of 30 min. However, at the 5 h time-point the gelatin coated nanoparticle containing EGCG blocked HGF-induced signalling, therefore demonstrating that EGCG activity was retained but released slowly (Shutava et al., 2009).

Recently, curcumin nanoparticles have shown enhanced bioavailability and greater cytotoxicity against breast cancer cells. For example, silk fibroin-derived curcumin nanoparticles (< 100 nm) exhibited higher uptake, intracellular residence time and efficacy against HER2 positive MDA-MB-453 breast cancer cells (Gupta et al., 2009). In another study, curcumin-PLGA nanoparticle formulation elicited an enhanced inhibitory effect on the growth of MDA-MB-231 cells compared with curcumin alone (Yallapu et al., 2010). Furthermore, curcumin-PLGA-PEG nanoparticles showed a concentration-dependent anti-proliferative effect toward MDA-MB-231 cells. It was observed that curcumin nanoparticle formulation had a higher bioavailability and longer half-life in rats compared to curcumin. Specifically, after intravenous administration of curcumin or curcumin-nanoparticle (2.5 mg/kg), the serum levels of curcumin were almost twice as high in the curcumin-nanoparticle treated rats (Anand et al., 2010). Curcumin (Cur-OEG) nanoparticles have also been studied for their anticancer effect in both *in vitro* and *in vivo* models of breast cancer. Curc-OEG nanoparticles showed broad *in vitro* antitumor activity toward several human cancer cells with an IC_{50} value of 1.4 µg/ml in MDA-MB-468 cells. These particles showed safety and efficacy *in vivo*, as a single 25 mg/kg intravenous injection of Curc-OEG nanoparticles was non-toxic to the mice and exhibited improved bioavailability and significant tumor suppression after 48 h in an MDA-MB-468 xenograft model.

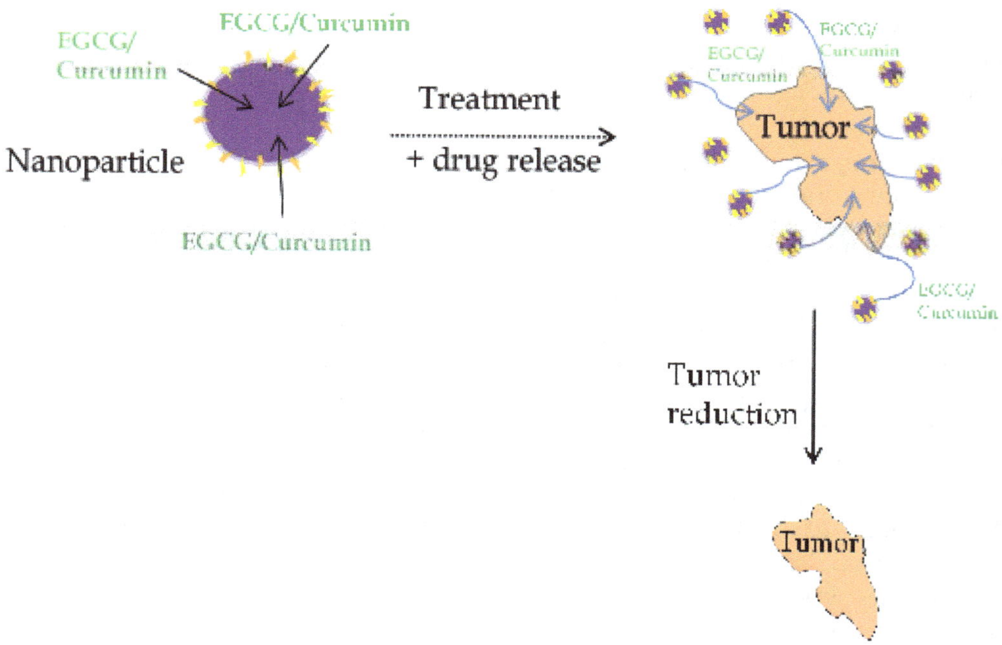

Fig. 4. Schematic of the principles of nanoparticle drug delivery. Nanoparticles, commonly consist of various different polymers and polyelectrolytes, encapsulate the drug of interest and following administration show enhanced bioavailability and accumulation within the tumor. Subsequently the drug is released (blue errors) from the nanoparticle and taken up by the tumor.

Injectable sustained release poly(D,L-lacctide-co-glycolide (PLGA)-microparticles of curcumin for breast cancer chemoprevention have also been formulated. These PLGA-microparticles exhibited enhanced bioavailability compared to curcumin in mice. Specifically, a single dose of subcutaneously injected PLGA-microparticles sustained curcumin levels in the blood for a month whereas single or multiple i.p. injections of curcumin resulted in a shorter half-life (Shahani et al., 2010). In addition, the curcumin concentration was 10–30-fold higher in the lungs and brain than in the blood. Furthermore, curcumin inhibited the growth of tumors in an MDA-MB-231 mouse xenograft model by 49% compared to the mice treated with blank PLGA-microparticles (Shahani et al., 2010). Mechanisms for this effect were attributed to the down regulation of the markers of angiogenesis, metastasis and proliferation. Specifically, the curcumin PLGA-microparticles treated group showed smaller and less well developed CD31 positive microvessels compared to curcumin alone. Furthermore, treatment with curcumin PLGA-microparticles decreased the relative VEGF expression in tumors by 78%, compared with control (Shahani et al., 2010). Additionally, the relative expression of MMP-9 in tumors from the curcumin PLGA-microparticle treated group was decreased 57% compared to control, while Ki-67 and cyclin D1 were decreased by 45% and 52%, respectively. There was also a 2.5-fold increase in the number of apoptotic cells compared to blank PLGA-microparticle treatment (Shahani et al., 2010). Since repeated systemic dosing of curcumin had no effect on tumor cell proliferation, apoptosis, or the relative cyclin D1 expression, the study concluded that sustained release microparticles of curcumin are more effective than repeated systemic injections of curcumin for breast cancer chemoprevention. Thus, significant improvement in the selectivity and potency of both EGCG and curcumin can be achieved through the use of nanomedicine.

3.3 Prodrugs, analogues and synthetic derivatives

Even though preclinical research shows promising results *in vitro* and *in vivo* with natural polyphenolic compounds such as EGCG and curcumin, clinical trials have shown limited success commonly due to inefficient delivery and bioavailability of these agents (Siddiqui et al., 2009). Thus, bioavailability is one of the major downfalls of these compounds. Additional strategies for improving these compounds include the synthesis of prodrugs, analogues and synthetic derivatives. All of these techniques aim to produce a compound with greater stability, bioavailability and ultimately efficacy.

Various studies have shown that biotransformation reactions, in particular methylation but potentially also glucuronidation and sulfate conjugation, modify the hydroxyl groups of EGCG, resulting in reduced biological activities (Landis Piwowar et al., 2007, Okushio et al., 1999). To prevent this, one group has synthesized novel fluoro-substituted EGCG pro-drug analogues by eliminating the reactive hydroxyl groups and replacing them with either peracetate groups (Pro-EGCG) or one or two fluorine(s) at the meta-position (Pro-F-EGCG2) or the meta- and para-positions on the phenyl ring (Pro-F-EGCG4) (Figure 5)(Yang et al., 2010). These analogues (50 mg/kg) were given daily via subcutaneous injections for 31 days to mice bearing MDA-MB-231 xenografts. Tumor growth was suppressed by ~63% by Pro-EGCG compared to control, whereas Pro-F- EGCG2 and Pro-F-EGCG4 were slightly more effective as tumor growth was reduced by ~67% and ~70%, respectively, compared to control (Yang et al., 2010). As an indicator of apoptosis, PARP cleavage (65 kDa) was found to a greater extent in tumors from mice treated with the fluorosubstituted analogues. Furthermore, the TUNEL assay showed apoptotic cells in the tumors of the animals treated with Pro-F-EGCG2 or Pro-F-EGCG4 but not in untreated control group. Cells with apoptotic nuclei were also shown in the treated animals. The proteasomal chymotrypsin-like activity was reduced by 33% and 42% in animals treated with Pro-F-EGCG2 or Pro-F-EGCG4, respectively, compared to control. Additionally, it was shown using Western blotting, that the proteasome substrates p27 and Bax were increased in EGCG-analogue treated animals indicating that the proteasome activation may be a cellular target of the EGCG analogues (Yang et al., 2010). Therefore, prodrugs of EGCG are emerging as an experimental therapy with potential for clinical translation.

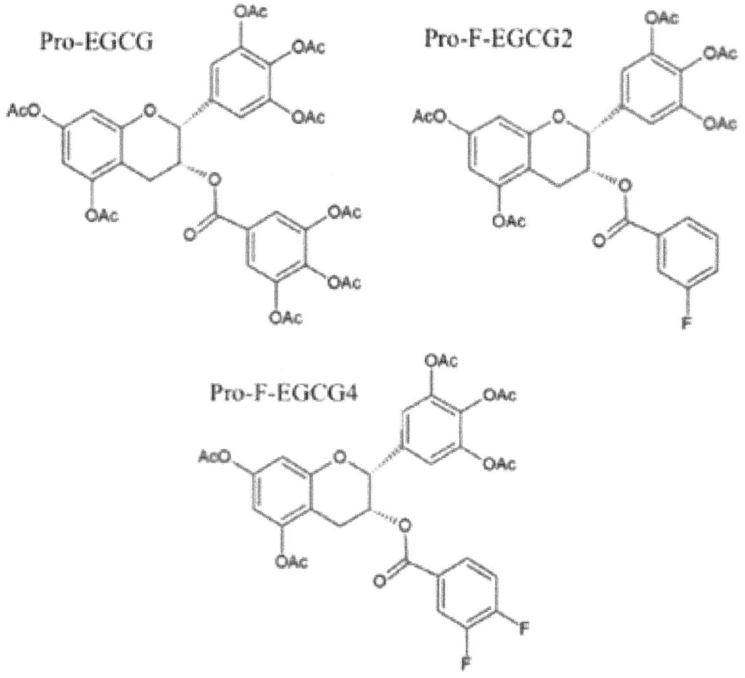

Fig. 5. Chemical structures of EGCG analogues (Yang et al., 2010).

Development of curcumin analogues has developed as a strategy to enhance bioavailability and selectivity towards cancer cells. Modification of the aromatic rings and β-diketone moiety of curcumin has led to different curcumin analogues with improved activities (Table 1)(Mosley et al., 2007). The first-generation curcumin derivatives were the cyclohexanones, which exhibited enhanced activity and stability in biological medium compared to curcumin. For example, the cyclohexanone-containing curcumin derivative 2,6-bis ((3-methoxy-4-hydroxyphenyl) methylene)-cyclohexanone (BMHPC) was cytotoxic toward ER-negative breast cancer cells (IC50 of 5.0 μM) and displayed anti-angiogenic properties in human and murine endothelial cell lines (Adams et al., 2004). These results led the authors to further synthesize several fluorinated derivatives, one of which (EF-24)(Table 1) exhibited potent cytotoxicity toward MDA-MB-231 cells (IC50 of 0.8 μM) (Adams et al., 2005). Moreover, EF-24 induced breast tumor regression in athymic nude mice. Specifically, tumor weight following 20 mg/kg was decreased by ~30% compared to control, whereas 100 mg/kg decreased tumor weight by 55%. Interestingly, no toxicity was observed at a dose of 100 mg/kg, which was well below maximum tolerated dose (MTD) of 200 mg/kg (Adams et al., 2005). Mechanistic studies were also performed in MDA-MB-231 cells. Specifically, EF-24

(10 μM) inhibited cell proliferation by 70-80% and arrested cells in the G2/M phase of the cell cycle. Additionally, EF24 (20 μM) increased the percentage of early apoptotic cells to 25.3 % after 72 h. Similarly, the cell population in late apoptosis increased to 45.6%. In addition, EF-24 increased intracellular ROS levels by 55% at 48 h (Adams et al., 2005). Further mechanistic studies demonstrated that EF-24 inhibited the pro-angiogenic transcription factor, HIF-1□α □at the posttranscriptional level by a VHL-dependent but proteasome-independent mechanism in MDA-MB-231 cells (Thomas et al., 2008). The therapeutic potential of EF-24 by using coagulation factor VIIa (fVIIa) as a carrier for targeted delivery of EF-24 to the tissue factor (TF) expressed in tumor cells and vascular endothelial cells and thus showed its anti-angiogenic and anti-cancer activity in breast cancer cells. They demonstrated that EF-24-FFRck-fVIIa conjugate significantly decreased the viability of the TF-expressing MDA-MB-231 and HUVEC cells in a concentration dependent manner. Furthermore, the administration of 5 intravenous injections of the EF-24-FFRck-fVIIa conjugate (containing 50 μM of EF-24) for two weeks significantly reduced the tumor size in MDA-MB-231 breast cancer xenografts. Moreover, the tumor cells showed activation of caspase 3 as a marker of apoptosis (Shoji et al., 2008).

Another set of curcumin analogues (FLLL 11 and FLLL 12)(Table 1) produced by exchanging the β-diketone moiety for an α β unsaturated ketone, exhibited more potent antitumor activity than curcumin in various ER positive and ER negative human breast cancer cells (Lin et al., 2009). The IC_{50} values for FLLL11 and FLLL12 ranged from 9 to 48 fold lower than curcumin. Furthermore, both the analogues at 10 μM inhibited STAT3, Akt and HER2/Neu pathways and induced apoptosis. The apoptosis was mediated via activation of cleaved PARP and caspase 3. These analogues were also effective in combination with doxorubicin as they exhibited a synergistic anti-proliferative effect in MDA-MB-231 breast cancer cells. In addition, the compounds inhibited anchorage independent growth and cell migration in MDA-MB-231 cells (Lin et al., 2009). In another study, Li et al, synthesized two series of monoketone curcumin analogues namely, heptadienone and pentadienone series and investigated their anti-cancer properties *in vitro*. Among the 24 compounds that were synthesized, compound 23 (Table 1) was the most potent analogue with IC_{50} values in sub-micromolar range in MDA-MB-231 cells (Fuchs et al., 2009). Various 1,5-diarylpentadienon containing curcumin analogues with an alkoxy substitution on aromatic rings at each of the positions 3 and 5 have also been synthesized (Ohori et al., 2006). One of the analogues, GO-YO30 (Table 1) showed substantially higher cytotoxicity and anchorage independency compared to curcumin in MDA-MB-231 cells. Furthermore, it also inhibited STAT activity in a dose-dependent manner. Interestingly, GO-YO30 induced apoptosis in MDA-MB-231 at concentrations far lower than those required to elicit a comparable effect following curcumin treatment (Hutzen et al., 2009).

Monoketo curcumin analogues with a piperidone ring impart a rigid confirmation that has led to a broad spectrum of antitumor activity. Compound, 8 and 18 (Table 1) bearing the n-alkyl piperidone group showed potent cytotoxic activity towards various breast cancer cells (Youssef & El-Sherbeny, 2005). This structure was recently further modified by replacing the methylene groups and the two carbonyl groups in curcumin by N-methyl-4 piperidone. The resulting compound 5-bis (4-hydroxy-3- methoxybenzylidene)- N - methyl-4-piperidone (PAC) (Table 1) was 5 times more effective than curcumin in inducing apoptosis in ER negative breast cancer cells (MDA-MB-231, BEC114) (Al-Hujaily et al., 2010). Also, it's pro-apoptotic effect was 10 times higher against ER negative breast cancer cells than against ER positive cells (MCF-7, T-47D). Cell cycle analysis revealed that PAC (10 μM) treatment of

MDA-MB-231 cells increased the proportion of cells undergoing G2/M phase arrest by 185%. Furthermore, at 10 μM, PAC induced apoptosis in 55% of MDA-MB-231 cells (Al-Hujaily et al., 2010). PAC exhibited its cytotoxic effect by down regulating the expression of NFκB, survivin and its downstream effectors cyclin D1 and Bcl-2 and subsequently showed up-regulation of p21[WAF1] expression both *in vitro* and *in vivo*. Interestingly, PAC (100 mg/kg/day) suppressed the growth of MDA-MB-231 xenografts (Al-Hujaily et al., 2010). Importantly, the solubility of PAC was 27-fold higher than curcumin and 1 h after the injection, the levels of ^{18}F-PAC in the blood was 5-fold higher than the levels ^{18}F-curcumin. These studies suggested better pharmacokinetics and tissue bio-distribution of PAC compared to curcumin in mice (Al-Hujaily et al., 2010).

Compound Name	Structure	Cell line	IC 50 (μM)
BMHPC	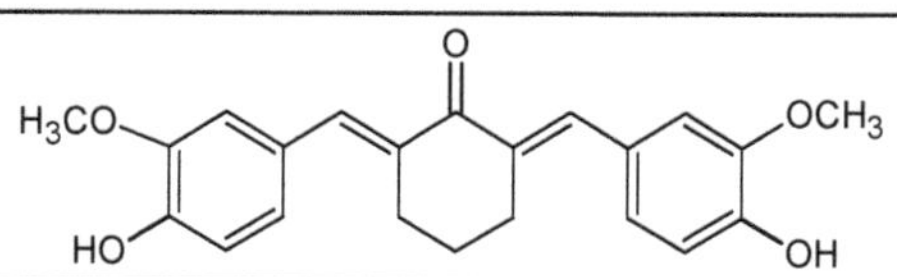	MDA-MB-231	5
EF-24	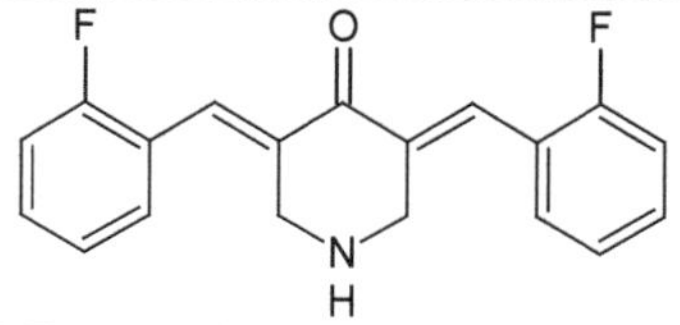	MDA-MB-231	0.8
FLLL11	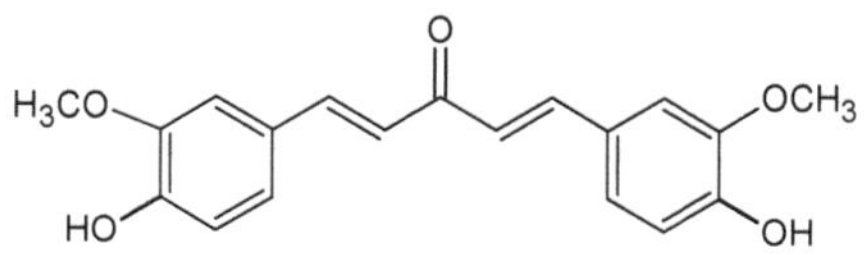	MCF-7 MDA-MB-231 MDA-MB-468 MDA-MB-453 SKBr3	2.4 2.8 0.3 4.7 5.7
FLLL12	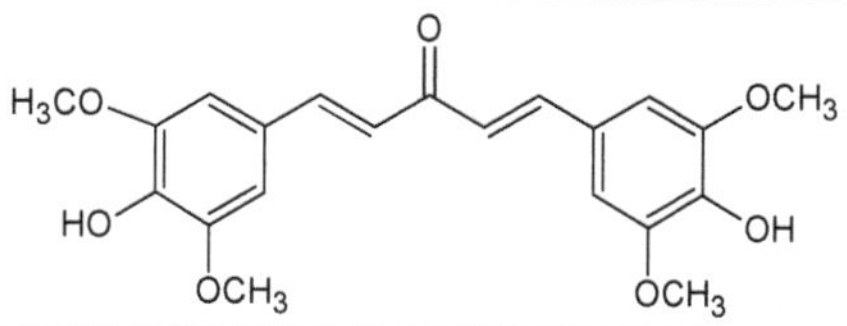	MCF-7 MDA-MB-231 MDA-MB-468 MDA-MB-453 SKBr3	1.7 2.7 0.3 1.3 3.8
GO-YO30	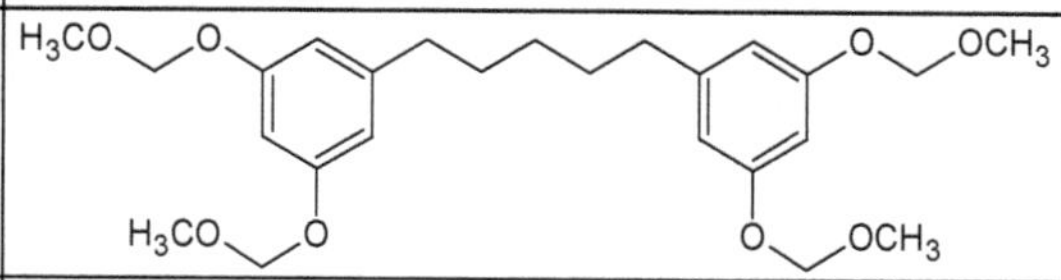	MDA-MB-231	1.2
PAC	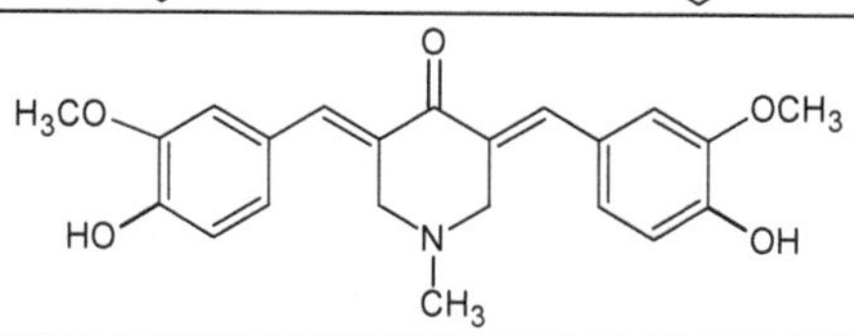	Not known	
RL90	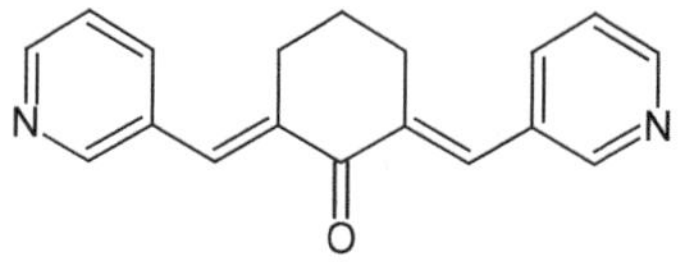	MDA-MB-231 SKBr3	1.54 0.51

Compound Name	Structure	Cell line	IC 50 (μM)
RL91	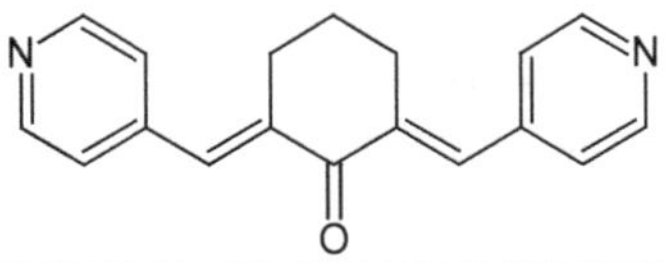	MDA-MB-231 SKBr3	1.10 0.23
B10	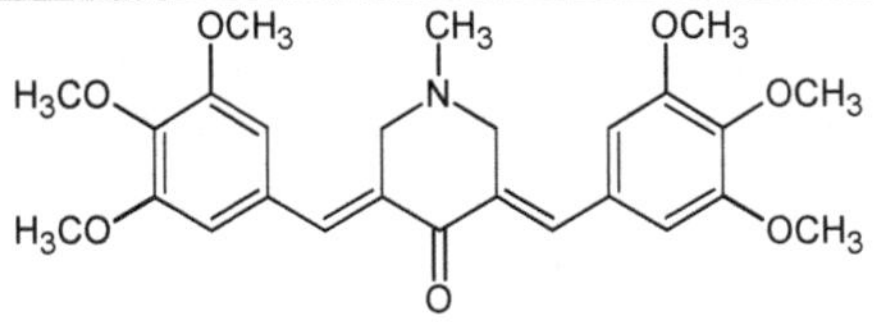	MDA-MB-231 MDA-MB-468 SKBr3	0.3 0.3 0.4
B1	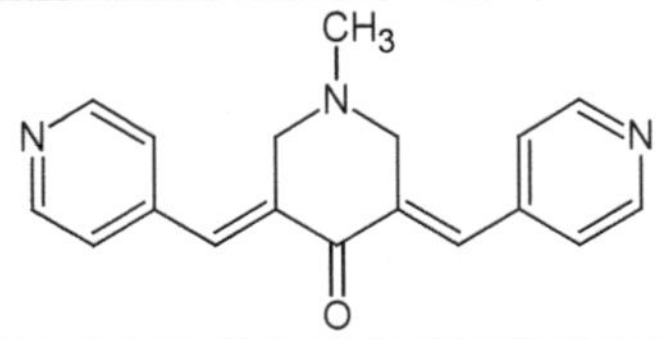	MDA-MB-231 MDA-MB-468 SKBr3	0.8 0.5 0.6
Compound 23	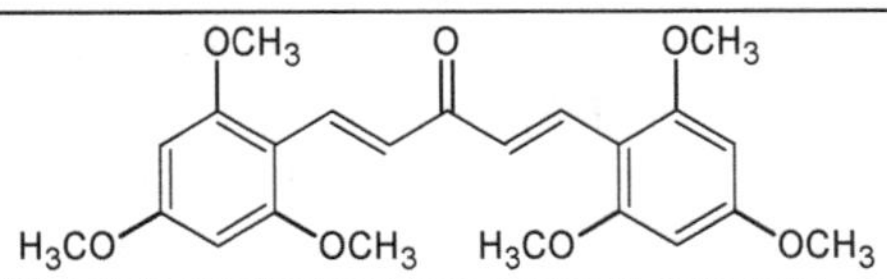	MCF-7 MDA-MB-231	0.4 0.6
Compound 8	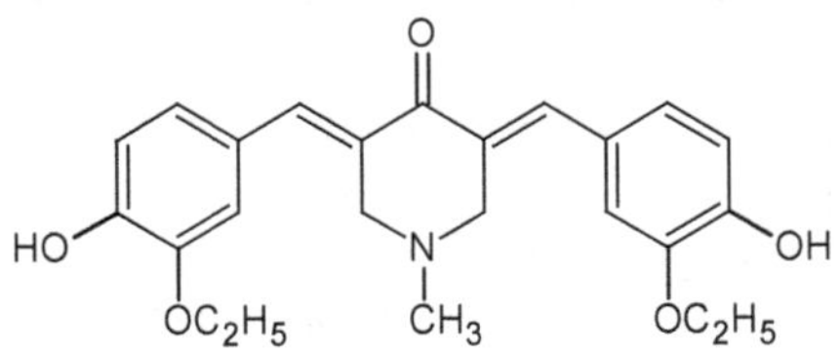	MCF-7 MDA-MB-31 MDA-MB-435 HS-578T BT-549 T-47D	2.3 17.9 6.8 5.4 32.8 15.1
Compound 18	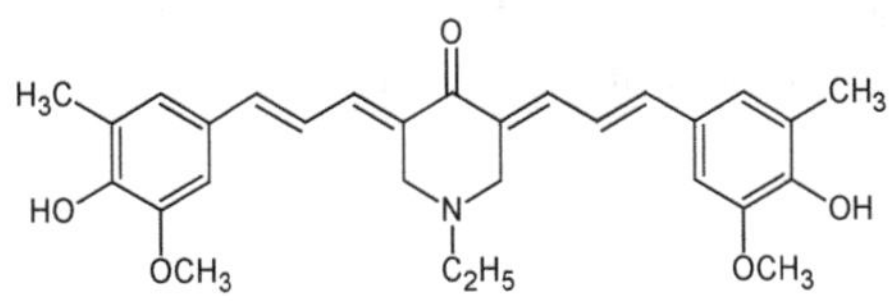	MCF-7 MDA-MB-31 MDA-MB-435 HS-578T BT-549 T-47D	3.3 2.8 3.7 3.8 2.6 2.7

Table 1. Chemical structures of curcumin derivatives and their relative *in vitro* potency.

Second generation curcumin analogues have been synthesized by replacing the phenyl group of cyclohexanone curcumin derivatives with heterocyclic rings. Two analogues, 2,6-bis(pyridin-3-ylmethylene)-cyclohexanone (RL90) and 2,6-bis(pyridin-4-ylmethylene)-cyclohexanone (RL91)(Table 1) showed potent cytotoxic towards ER negative breast cancer cells (MDA-MB-231, SKBr3) and modulated the expression of variety of cell signaling proteins such as EGFR, Akt, HER2, β-catenin and NFκB. Treatment with RL90 and RL91 also showed activation of stress kinases, as evidenced by phosphorylation of both JNK1/2 and p38 MAPK. Furthermore, RL90 and RL91 produced cell cycle arrest at G2/M phase in MDA-MB-231 and SKBr3 cells. Specifically, treatment of MDA-MB-231 cells with RL90 (3 μM) or RL91 (2.5 μM) significantly increased the proportion of cells in G2/M phase by 52 and 49% compared to control, respectively. RL90 and RL91 also increased the proportion of apoptotic cells by 164% and 406% of control, respectively (Somers-Edgar et al., 2011). Thus, these second-generation curcumin derivatives are more potent *in vitro* than first generation derivatives such as BMHPC.

Another set of cyclohexanone analogues of curcumin included modification resulting in N-methylpiperidone, tropinone or cyclopentanone core groups. The aromatic substitutions on these compounds included pyrrole, imidazole, indole flouro-pyridines as well as trimethoxyphenyl and dimethoxyphenyl groups. The resulting compounds were screened for their cytotoxicity in TNBC cells. Among 18 analogues examined, 3,5-bis (pyridine-4-yl)-1-methylpiperidin-4-one (B1) and 3,5-bis (3,4,5-trimethoxybenzylidene)-1-methylpiperidin-4-one (B10) (Table 1) showed potent cytotoxicity towards MBA-MB-231 and MDA-MB-468 cells with IC_{50} values below 1 μM (Yadav et al., 2010). Furthermore, B1 and B10 induced apoptosis in MDA-MB-231 cells. Specifically, B1 (2 μM) significantly increased the proportion of apoptotic cells by 4-fold compared to control at 12 h whereas B 10 (1 μM) was more potent as there was a 10-fold increase in the proportion of apoptotic MDA-MB-231 cells after 24 h (Yadav et al., 2010).

The last set of compounds involves a series of mono-carbonyl analogues of curcumin using three different 5-carbon linkers, namely cyclopentanone, acetone, and cyclohexanone with various substituents on aryl rings. They reported that all the analogues had enhanced stability *in vitro* and improved pharmacokinetic profile *in vivo*. In this study, 500 mg/kg of compound B02 and B33 (Table 1) were orally administered to male Sprague-Dawley rats. The peak plasma concentrations of B02 and B33 were increased to 0.82 μg/ml and 4.1 μg/ml, respectively, compared to curcumin (0.091 μg/ml). This correlated with a decrease in the plasma clearance of both drugs (B02 was 125.4 l/kg/h and B33 38.98 l/kg/h) compared to curcumin (835.2 l/Kg/h). Furthermore, the half-life of B02 was increased 2-fold greater than curcumin and absorption of B33 was rapid. In addition, the analogues with acetone or cyclohexanone spacer groups showed increased cytotoxicity against several tumor cell lines. Interestingly, the analogues in which the benzene ring was replaced by a hetero aromatic ring enhanced the cytotoxic activity of these mono-carbonyl analogues (Liang et al., 2009). Overall, these studies all demonstrated that significant improvement occurs with each successive generation of synthetic analogues.

4. Conclusion

There is a large body of evidence demonstrating that the natural compounds EGCG and curcumin have potent actions in both *in vitro* and *in vivo* models of triple negative breast cancer. While these compounds both have many beneficial actions, they are hindered by poor bioavailability. However, their knowledge base of mechanistic actions have allowed them to be improved by various methods such as; 1) use in combination therapies, 2) imported via specific targeting via nanomedine and 3) improved via chemical modification into prodrugs or new structural analogues. Therefore, it is likely that a novel therapy for triple negative breast cancer will emerge as a synthetic derivative of one of these natural compounds that may ultimately be delivered to the tumor via nanomedicine.

5. References

Adams, B. K., Cai, J., Armstrong, J., Herold, M., Lu, Y. J., Sun, A., Snyder, J. P., Liotta, D. C., Jones, D. P. & Shoji, M. (2005). EF24, a novel synthetic curcumin analog, induces apoptosis in cancer cells via a redox-dependent mechanism. *Anticancer Drugs,* Vol. 16, No. 3, pp. 263-275, 0959-4973

Adams, B. K., Ferstl, E. M., Davis, M. C., Herold, M., Kurtkaya, S., Camalier, R. F., Hollingshead, M. G., Kaur, G., Sausville, E. A., Rickles, F. R., Snyder, J. P., Liotta, D. C. & Shoji, M. (2004). Synthesis and biological evaluation of novel curcumin analogs as anti-cancer and anti-angiogenesis agents. *Bioorg Med Chem,* Vol. 12, No. 14, pp. 3871-3883, 0968-0896

Adams, J. & Cory, S. (1998). The Bcl-2 protein family: arbiters of cell survival. *Science,* Vol. 281, No. 5381, pp. 1322-1326, 0036-8075

Aggarwal, B. B., Kumar, A. & Bharti, A. C. (2003). Anticancer potential of curcumin: preclinical and clinical studies. *Anticancer Res,* Vol. 23, No. 1A, pp. 363-398, 0250-7005

Aggarwal, B. B., Shishodia, S., Takada, Y., Banerjee, S., Newman, R. A., Bueso-Ramos, C. E. & Price, J. E. (2005). Curcumin suppresses the paclitaxel-induced nuclear factor-kappaB pathway in breast cancer cells and inhibits lung metastasis of human breast cancer in nude mice. *Clin Cancer Res,* Vol. 11, No. 20, pp. 7490-7498, 1078-0432

Al-Hujaily, E. M., Mohamed, A. G., Al-Sharif, I., Youssef, K. M., Manogaran, P. S., Al-Otaibi, B., Al-Haza'a, A., Al-Jammaz, I., Al-Hussein, K. & Aboussekhra, A. (2010). PAC, a novel curcumin analogue, has anti-breast cancer properties with higher efficiency on ER-negative cells. *Breast Cancer Res Treat,* Vol. No. pp. 1573-7217

Anand, P., Nair, H. B., Sung, B., Kunnumakkara, A. B., Yadav, V. R., Tekmal, R. R. & Aggarwal, B. B. (2010). Design of curcumin-loaded PLGA nanoparticles formulation with enhanced cellular uptake, and increased bioactivity in vitro and superior bioavailability in vivo. *Biochemical Pharmacology,* Vol. 79, No. 3, pp. 330-338, 1873-2968

Anand, P., Thomas, S. G., Kunnumakkara, A. B., Sundaram, C., Harikumar, K. B., Sung, B., Tharakan, S. T., Misra, K., Priyadarsini, I. K., Rajasekharan, K. N. & Aggarwal, B. B. (2008). Biological activities of curcumin and its analogues (Congeners) made by man and Mother Nature. *Biochem Pharmacol,* Vol. 76, No. 11, pp. 1590-1611, 1873-2968

Andre, F., Job, B., Dessen, P., Tordai, A., Michiels, S., Liedtke, C., Richon, C., Yan, K., Wang, B. & Vassal, G. (2009). Molecular characterization of breast cancer with high-resolution oligonucleotide comparative genomic hybridization array. *Clinical Cancer Research,* Vol. 15, No. 2, pp. 441-451, 1078-0432

Arslan, C., Dizdar, O. & Altundag, K. (2009). Pharmacotherapy of triple-negative breast cancer. *Expert Opin Pharmacother,* Vol. 10, No. 13, pp. 2081-2093, 1744-7666

Bachmeier, B., Nerlich, A. G., Iancu, C. M., Cilli, M., Schleicher, E., Vene, R., Dell'Eva, R., Jochum, M., Albini, A. & Pfeffer, U. (2007). The chemopreventive polyphenol Curcumin prevents hematogenous breast cancer metastases in immunodeficient mice. *Cell Physiol Biochem,* Vol. 19, No. 1-4, pp. 137-152, 1015-8987

Bachmeier, B. E., Mohrenz, I. V., Mirisola, V., Schleicher, E., Romeo, F., Hohneke, C., Jochum, M., Nerlich, A. G. & Pfeffer, U. (2008). Curcumin downregulates the inflammatory cytokines CXCL1 and -2 in breast cancer cells via NFkappaB. *Carcinogenesis,* Vol. 29, No. 4, pp. 779-789, 1460-2180

Berrada, N., Delaloge, S. & André, F. (2010). Treatment of triple-negative metastatic breast cancer: toward individualized targeted treatments or chemosensitization? *Annals of Oncology,* Vol. 21, No. Suppl 7, pp. vii30-vii35, 0923-7534

Bigelow, R. & Cardelli, J. (2006). The green tea catechins,(-)-epigallocatechin-3-gallate (EGCG) and (-)-Epicatechin-3-gallate (ECG), inhibit HGF/Met signaling in immortalized and tumorigenic breast epithelial cells. *Oncology,* Vol. 25, No. 13, pp. 1922-1930, 0950-9232

Biswas, D. K., Dai, S. C., Cruz, A., Weiser, B., Graner, E. & Pardee, A. B. (2001). The nuclear factor kappa B (NF-kappa B): a potential therapeutic target for estrogen receptor negative breast cancers. *Proc Natl Acad Sci U S A,* Vol. 98, No. 18, pp. 10386-10391, 0027-8424

Boonrao, M., Yodkeeree, S., Ampasavate, C., Anuchapreeda, S. & Limtrakul, P. (2010). The inhibitory effect of turmeric curcuminoids on matrix metalloproteinase-3 secretion in human invasive breast carcinoma cells. *Arch Pharm Res,* Vol. 33, No. 7, pp. 989-998, 0253-6269

Bosch, A., Eroles, P., Zaragoza, R., Vina, J. R. & Lluch, A. (2010). Triple-negative breast cancer: molecular features, pathogenesis, treatment and current lines of research. *Cancer Treat Rev,* Vol. 36, No. 3, pp. 206-215, 1532-1967

Carey, L., Winer, E., Viale, G., Cameron, D. & Gianni, L. (2010). Triple-negative breast cancer: disease entity or title of convenience? *Nat Rev Clin Oncol,* Vol. 7, No. 12, pp. 683-692, 1759-4782

Casalini, P., Iorio, M., Galmozzi, E. & Ménard, S. (2004). Role of HER receptors family in development and differentiation. *Journal of Cellular Physiology,* Vol. 200, No. 3, pp. 343-350, 1097-4652

Catzavelos, C., Bhattacharya, N., Ung, Y. C., Wilson, J. A., Roncari, L., Sandhu, C., Shaw, P., Yeger, H., Morava-Protzner, I., Kapusta, L., Franssen, E., Pritchard, K. I. & Slingerland, J. M. (1997). Decreased levels of the cell-cycle inhibitor p27Kip1 protein: prognostic implications in primary breast cancer. *Nat Med,* Vol. 3, No. 2, pp. 227-230, 1078-8956

Cheah, Y. H., Nordin, F. J., Sarip, R., Tee, T. T., Azimahtol, H. L., Sirat, H. M., Rashid, B. A., Abdullah, N. R. & Ismail, Z. (2009). Combined xanthorrhizol-curcumin exhibits synergistic growth inhibitory activity via apoptosis induction in human breast cancer cells MDA-MB-231. *Cancer Cell Int,* Vol. 9, No. pp. 1, 1475-2867

Chen, J. Q. & Russo, J. (2009). ERalpha-negative and triple negative breast cancer: Molecular features and potential therapeutic approaches. *Biochim Biophys Acta,* Vol. 1796, No. 2, pp. 162-175, 0006-3002

Chisholm, K., Bray, B. & Rosengren, R. (2004). Tamoxifen and epigallocatechin gallate are synergistically cytotoxic to MDA-MB-231 human breast cancer cells. *Anti-Cancer Drugs,* Vol. 15, No. 9, pp. 889-897, 0959-4973

Chiu, T. L. & Su, C. C. (2009). Curcumin inhibits proliferation and migration by increasing the Bax to Bcl-2 ratio and decreasing NF-kappaBp65 expression in breast cancer MDA-MB-231 cells. *Int J Mol Med,* Vol. 23, No. 4, pp. 469-475, 1107-3756

Cho, K., Wang, X., Nie, S., Chen, Z. G. & Shin, D. M. (2008). Therapeutic nanoparticles for drug delivery in cancer. *Clin Cancer Res,* Vol. 14, No. 5, pp. 1310-1316, 1078-0432

Chu, E. & Tarnawski, A. (2004). PTEN regulatory functions in tumor suppression and cell biology. *Medical Science Monitor: International Medical Journal of Experimental and Clinical Research,* Vol. 10, No. 10, pp. 235-241, 1234-1010

Conte, P. & Guarneri, V. (2009). Triple-negative breast cancer: current management and future options. *EJC Supplements,* Vol. 7, No. 1, pp. 14-18, 1359-6349

Cunningham, A., Love, W., Zhang, R., Andrews, L. & Tollefsbol, T. (2006). Telomerase inhibition in cancer therapeutics: molecular-based approaches. *Current Medicinal Chemistry,* Vol. 13, No. 24, pp. 2875–2888,

DeGraffenried, L., Fulcher, L., Friedrichs, W., Grünwald, V., Ray, R. & Hidalgo, M. (2004). Reduced PTEN expression in breast cancer cells confers susceptibility to inhibitors of the PI3 kinase/Akt pathway. *Annals of Oncology,* Vol. 15, No. 10, pp. 1510-1516, 0923-7534

Fang, H. Y., Chen, S. B., Guo, D. J., Pan, S. Y. & Yu, Z. L. (2011). Proteomic identification of differentially expressed proteins in curcumin-treated MCF-7 cells. *Phytomedicine,* Vol. No. pp. 1618-095X

Foulkes, W. D., Smith, I. E. & Reis-Filho, J. S. (2010). Triple-negative breast cancer. *N Engl J Med,* Vol. 363, No. 20, pp. 1938-1948, 1533-4406

Fuchs, J. R., Pandit, B., Bhasin, D., Etter, J. P., Regan, N., Abdelhamid, D., Li, C., Lin, J. & Li, P. K. (2009). Structure-activity relationship studies of curcumin analogues. *Bioorg Med Chem Lett,* Vol. 19, No. 7, pp. 2065-2069, 1464-3405

Graham, H. (1992). Green tea composition, consumption, and polyphenol chemistry* 1. *Preventive Medicine,* Vol. 21, No. 3, pp. 334-350, 0091-7435

Greenberg, S. & Rugo, H. S. (2010). Challenging clinical scenarios: treatment of patients with triple-negative or basal-like metastatic breast cancer *Clin Breast Cancer,* Vol. 10, No. pp. S20-29, 1938-0666

Gupta, V., Aseh, A., Rios, C. N., Aggarwal, B. B. & Mathur, A. B. (2009). Fabrication and characterization of silk fibroin-derived curcumin nanoparticles for cancer therapy. *Int J Nanomedicine,* Vol. 4, No. pp. 115-122, 1178-2013

Hossain, M., Bouton, C., Pevsner, J. & Laterra, J. (2000). Induction of vascular endothelial growth factor in human astrocytes by lead: involvement of a protein kinase C/activator protein-1 complex-dependent and hypoxia-inducible factor 1-independent signaling pathway. *Journal of Biological Chemistry,* Vol. 8, No. 275, pp. 27874-27882, 0021-9258

Hutzen, B., Friedman, L., Sobo, M., Lin, L., Cen, L., De Angelis, S., Yamakoshi, H., Shibata, H., Iwabuchi, Y. & Lin, J. (2009). Curcumin analogue GO-Y030 inhibits STAT3 activity and cell growth in breast and pancreatic carcinomas. *Int J Oncol,* Vol. 35, No. 4, pp. 867-872, 1791-2423

Irvin, W. J., Jr. & Carey, L. A. (2008). What is triple-negative breast cancer? *Eur J Cancer,* Vol. 44, No. 18, pp. 2799-2805, 1879-0852

Kakarala, M., Brenner, D. E., Korkaya, H., Cheng, C., Tazi, K., Ginestier, C., Liu, S., Dontu, G. & Wicha, M. S. (2010). Targeting breast stem cells with the cancer preventive compounds curcumin and piperine. *Breast Cancer Res Treat,* Vol. 122, No. 3, pp. 777-785, 1573-7217

Kang, H. J., Lee, S. H., Price, J. E. & Kim, L. S. (2009). Curcumin suppresses the paclitaxel-induced nuclear factor-kappaB in breast cancer cells and potentiates the growth inhibitory effect of paclitaxel in a breast cancer nude mice model. *Breast J*, Vol. 15, No. 3, pp. 223-229, 1524-4741

Karunagaran, D., Rashmi, R. & Kumar, T. R. (2005). Induction of apoptosis by curcumin and its implications for cancer therapy. *Curr Cancer Drug Targets*, Vol. 5, No. 2, pp. 117-129, 1568-0096

Kavanagh, K., Hafer, L., Kim, D., Mann, K., Sherr, D., Rogers, A. & Sonenshein, G. (2001). Green tea extracts decrease carcinogen induced mammary tumor burden in rats and rate of breast cancer cell proliferation in culture. *Journal of Cellular Biochemistry*, Vol. 82, No. 3, pp. 387-398, 1097-4644

Khramtsov, A. I., Khramtsova, G. F., Tretiakova, M., Huo, D., Olopade, O. I. & Goss, K. H. (2010). Wnt/beta-catenin pathway activation is enriched in basal-like breast cancers and predicts poor outcome. *Am J Pathol*, Vol. 176, No. 6, pp. 2911-2920, 1525-2191

Kim, H. I., Huang, H., Cheepala, S., Huang, S. & Chung, J. (2008). Curcumin inhibition of integrin (alpha6beta4)-dependent breast cancer cell motility and invasion. *Cancer Prev Res (Phila)*, Vol. 1, No. 5, pp. 385-391, 1940-6215

Koenders, P. G., Beex, L. V., Geurts-Moespot, A., Heuvel, J. J., Kienhuis, C. B. & Benraad, T. J. (1991). Epidermal growth factor receptor-negative tumors are predominantly confined to the subgroup of estradiol receptor-positive human primary breast cancers. *Cancer Res*, Vol. 51, No. 17, pp. 4544-4548,

Kwan, M. L., Kushi, L. H., Weltzien, E., Maring, B., Kutner, S. E., Fulton, R. S., Lee, M. M., Ambrosone, C. B. & Caan, B. J. (2009). Epidemiology of breast cancer subtypes in two prospective cohort studies of breast cancer survivors. *Breast Cancer Res*, Vol. 11, No. 3, pp. R31, 1465-542X (Electronic)

Landis Piwowar, K., Wan, S., Wiegand, R., Kuhn, D., Chan, T. & Dou, Q. (2007). Methylation suppresses the proteasome inhibitory function of green tea polyphenols. *Journal of Cellular Physiology*, Vol. 213, No. 1, pp. 252-260, 1097-4652

Li, Y., Yuan, Y., Meeran, S. & Tollefsbol, T. (2010). Synergistic epigenetic reactivation of estrogen receptor- (ER) by combined green tea polyphenol and histone deacetylase inhibitor in ER -negative breast cancer cells. *Molecular Cancer*, Vol. 9, No. 1, pp. 274-286, 1476-4598

Liang, G., Shao, L., Wang, Y., Zhao, C., Chu, Y., Xiao, J., Zhao, Y., Li, X. & Yang, S. (2009). Exploration and synthesis of curcumin analogues with improved structural stability both in vitro and in vivo as cytotoxic agents. *Bioorg Med Chem*, Vol. 17, No. 6, pp. 2623-2631, 1464-3391

Lin, L., Hutzen, B., Ball, S., Foust, E., Sobo, M., Deangelis, S., Pandit, B., Friedman, L., Li, C., Li, P. K., Fuchs, J. & Lin, J. (2009). New curcumin analogues exhibit enhanced growth-suppressive activity and inhibit AKT and signal transducer and activator of transcription 3 phosphorylation in breast and prostate cancer cells. *Cancer Sci*, Vol. 100, No. 9, pp. 1719-1727, 1349-7006

Liu, Q., Loo, W. T., Sze, S. C. & Tong, Y. (2009). Curcumin inhibits cell proliferation of MDA-MB-231 and BT-483 breast cancer cells mediated by down-regulation of NFkappaB, cyclinD and MMP-1 transcription. *Phytomedicine*, Vol. 16, No. 10, pp. 916-922, 1618-095X

Luo, T., Wang, J., Yin, Y., Hua, H., Jing, J., Sun, X., Li, M., Zhang, Y. & Jiang, Y. (2010). (-)-Epigallocatechin gallate sensitizes breast cancer cells to paclitaxel in a murine model of breast carcinoma. *Breast Cancer Research,* Vol. 12, No. 1, pp. R8-18, 1465-5411

Malumbres, M. & Barbacid, M. (2009). Cell cycle, CDKs and cancer: a changing paradigm. *Nat Rev Cancer,* Vol. 9, No. 3, pp. 153-166, 1474-1768

Masuda, M., Suzui, M., Lim, J. T. E., Deguchi, A., Soh, J. W. & Weinstein, I. B. (2002). Epigallocatechin 3 gallate decreases VEGF production in head and neck and breast carcinoma cells by inhibiting EGFR related pathways of signal transduction. *Journal of Experimental Therapeutics and Oncology,* Vol. 2, No. 6, pp. 350-359, 1533-869X

Meeran, S., Patel, S., Chan, T. & Tollefsbol, T. (2011). A Novel Prodrug of Epigallocatechin-3-gallate: Differential Epigenetic hTERT Repression in Human Breast Cancer Cells. *Cancer Prevention Research,* epub ahead of print, 1940-6207

Mosley, C. A., Liotta, D. C. & Snyder, J. P. (2007). Highly active anticancer curcumin analogues. *Adv Exp Med Biol,* Vol. 595, No. pp. 77-103, 0065-2598

Narasimhan, M. & Ammanamanchi, S. (2008). Curcumin blocks RON tyrosine kinase-mediated invasion of breast carcinoma cells. *Cancer Res,* Vol. 68, No. 13, pp. 5185-5192, 1538-7445

Ohori, H., Yamakoshi, H., Tomizawa, M., Shibuya, M., Kakudo, Y., Takahashi, A., Takahashi, S., Kato, S., Suzuki, T., Ishioka, C., Iwabuchi, Y. & Shibata, H. (2006). Synthesis and biological analysis of new curcumin analogues bearing an enhanced potential for the medicinal treatment of cancer. *Mol Cancer Ther,* Vol. 5, No. 10, pp. 2563-2571, 1535-7163

Okushio, K., Suzuki, M., Matsumoto, N., Nanjo, F. & HARA, Y. (1999). Methylation of tea catechins by rat liver homogenates. *Bioscience, Biotechnology, and Biochemistry,* Vol. 63, No. 2, pp. 430-432, 0916-8451

Pellikainen, M. J., Pekola, T. T., Ropponen, K. M., Kataja, V. V., Kellokoski, J. K., Eskelinen, M. J. & Kosma, V. M. (2003). p21WAF1 expression in invasive breast cancer and its association with p53, AP-2, cell proliferation, and prognosis. *J Clin Pathol,* Vol. 56, No. 3, pp. 214-220, 0021-9746

Potemski, P., Kusinska, R., Watala, C., Pluciennik, E., Bednarek, A. K. & Kordek, R. (2006). Cyclin E expression in breast cancer correlates with negative steroid receptor status, HER2 expression, tumor grade and proliferation. *J Exp Clin Cancer Res,* Vol. 25, No. 1, pp. 59-64, 0392-9078

Prasad, C. P., Rath, G., Mathur, S., Bhatnagar, D. & Ralhan, R. (2009). Potent growth suppressive activity of curcumin in human breast cancer cells: Modulation of Wnt/beta-catenin signaling. *Chem Biol Interact,* Vol. 181, No. 2, pp. 263-271, 1872-7786

Ravindran, J., Prasad, S. & Aggarwal, B. B. (2009). Curcumin and cancer cells: how many ways can curry kill tumor cells selectively? *AAPS J,* Vol. 11, No. 3, pp. 495-510, 1550-7416

Reis-Filho, J. S. & Tutt, A. N. (2008). Triple negative tumours: a critical review. *Histopathology,* Vol. 52, No. 1, pp. 108-118, 1365-2559

Rouzier, R., Perou, C. M., Symmans, W. F., Ibrahim, N., Cristofanilli, M., Anderson, K., Hess, K. R., Stec, J., Ayers, M., Wagner, P., Morandi, P., Fan, C., Rabiul, I., Ross, J. S., Hortobagyi, G. N. & Pusztai, L. (2005). Breast cancer molecular subtypes respond differently to preoperative chemotherapy. *Clin Cancer Res,* Vol. 11, No. 16, pp. 5678-5685, 1078-0432

Rowe, D. L., Ozbay, T., O'Regan, R. M. & Nahta, R. (2009). Modulation of the BRCA1 protein and induction of apoptosis in triple negative breast cancer cell lines by the polyphenolic compound curcumin. *Breast Cancer,* Vol. 3, No. pp. 61-75, 1178-2234

Roy, A., Baliga, M. & Katiyar, S. (2005). Epigallocatechin-3-gallate induces apoptosis in estrogen receptor–negative human breast carcinoma cells via modulation in protein expression of p53 and Bax and caspase-3 activation. *Molecular cancer therapeutics,* Vol. 4, No. 1, pp. 81-90, 1535-7163

Sartippour, M., Heber, D., Ma, J., Lu, Q., Go, V. & Nguyen, M. (2001). Green tea and its catechins inhibit breast cancer xenografts. *Nutrition and Cancer,* Vol. 40, No. 2, pp. 149-156, 0163-5581

Sartippour, M., Shao, Z., Heber, D., Beatty, P., Zhang, L., Liu, C., Ellis, L., Liu, W., Go, V. & Brooks, M. (2002). Green tea inhibits vascular endothelial growth factor (VEGF) induction in human breast cancer cells. *Journal of Nutrition,* Vol. 132, No. 8, pp. 2307-2311, 0022-3166

Scandlyn, M., Stuart, E., Somers-Edgar, T., Menzies, A. & Rosengren, R. (2008). A new role for tamoxifen in oestrogen receptor-negative breast cancer when it is combined with epigallocatechin gallate. *British Journal of Cancer,* Vol. 99, No. 7, pp. 1056-1063, 0007-0920

Schlotter, C. M., Vogt, U., Allgayer, H. & Brandt, B. (2008). Molecular targeted therapies for breast cancer treatment. *Breast Cancer Research,* Vol. 10, No. 4, pp. 211, 1465-542X

Schneider, B. P. & Miller, K. D. (2005). Angiogenesis of breast cancer. *J Clin Oncol,* Vol. 23, No. 8, pp. 1782-1790, 0732-183X

Shahani, K., Swaminathan, S. K., Freeman, D., Blum, A., Ma, L. & Panyam, J. (2010). Injectable sustained release microparticles of curcumin: a new concept for cancer chemoprevention. *Cancer Research,* Vol. 70, No. 11, pp. 4443-4452, 1538-7445

Shao, Z. M., Shen, Z. Z., Liu, C. H., Sartippour, M. R., Go, V. L., Heber, D. & Nguyen, M. (2002). Curcumin exerts multiple suppressive effects on human breast carcinoma cells. *Int J Cancer,* Vol. 98, No. 2, pp. 234-240, 0020-7136 (

Shay, J. & Bacchetti, S. (1997). A survey of telomerase activity in human cancer. *European Journal of Cancer,* Vol. 33, No. 5, pp. 787-791, 0959-8049

Shehzad, A., Wahid, F. & Lee, Y. S. (2010). Curcumin in cancer chemoprevention: molecular targets, pharmacokinetics, bioavailability, and clinical trials. *Arch Pharm (Weinheim),* Vol. 343, No. 9, pp. 489-499, 1521-4184

Shoji, M., Sun, A., Kisiel, W., Lu, Y. J., Shim, H., McCarey, B. E., Nichols, C., Parker, E. T., Pohl, J., Mosley, C. A., Alizadeh, A. R., Liotta, D. C. & Snyder, J. P. (2008). Targeting tissue factor-expressing tumor angiogenesis and tumors with EF24 conjugated to factor VIIa. *J Drug Target,* Vol. 16, No. 3, pp. 185-197, 1061-186X

Shutava, T., Balkundi, S., Vangala, P., Steffan, J., Bigelow, R., Cardelli, J., O'Neal, D. & Lvov, Y. (2009). Layer-by-layer-coated gelatin nanoparticles as a vehicle for delivery of natural polyphenols. *ACS nano,* Vol. 3, No. 7, pp. 1877-1885, 1936-0851

Siddiqui, I., Adhami, V., Bharali, D., Hafeez, B., Asim, M., Khwaja, S., Ahmad, N., Cui, H., Mousa, S. & Mukhtar, H. (2009). Introducing nanochemoprevention as a novel approach for cancer control: proof of principle with green tea polyphenol epigallocatechin-3-gallate. *Cancer Research,* Vol. 69, No. 5, pp. 1712, 0008-5472

Somers-Edgar, T. J., Scandlyn, M. J., Stuart, E. C., Le Nedelec, M. J., Valentine, S. P. & Rosengren, R. J. (2008). The combination of epigallocatechin gallate and curcumin suppresses ER alpha-breast cancer cell growth in vitro and in vivo. *Int J Cancer,* Vol. 122, No. 9, pp. 1966-1971, 1097-0215

Somers-Edgar, T. J., Taurin, S., Larsen, L., Chandramouli, A., Nelson, M. A. & Rosengren, R. J. (2011). Mechanisms for the activity of heterocyclic cyclohexanone curcumin derivatives in estrogen receptor negative human breast cancer cell lines. *Invest New Drugs,* Vol. 29, No. 1, pp. 87-97, 1573-0646

Squires, M. S., Hudson, E. A., Howells, L., Sale, S., Houghton, C. E., Jones, J. L., Fox, L. H., Dickens, M., Prigent, S. A. & Manson, M. M. (2003). Relevance of mitogen activated protein kinase (MAPK) and phosphotidylinositol-3-kinase/protein kinase B (PI3K/PKB) pathways to induction of apoptosis by curcumin in breast cells. *Biochem Pharmacol,* Vol. 65, No. 3, pp. 361-376, 0006-2952

Stuart, E., Jarvis, R. & Rosengren, R. (2010). In vitro mechanism of action for the cytotoxicity elicited by the combination of epigallocatechin gallate and raloxifene in MDA-MB-231 cells. *Oncology Reports,* Vol. 24, No. 3, pp. 779-785, 1021-335X

Stuart, E., Larsen, L. & Rosengren, R. (2007). Potential mechanisms for the synergistic cytotoxicity elicited by 4-hydroxytamoxifen and epigallocatechin gallate in MDA-MB-231 cells. *International Journal of Oncology,* Vol. 30, No. 6, pp. 1407-1412, 1019-6439

Stuart, E. & Rosengren, R. (2008). The combination of raloxifene and epigallocatechin gallate suppresses growth and induces apoptosis in MDA-MB-231 cells. *Life Sciences,* Vol. 82, No. 17, pp. 943-948, 0024-3205

Syng-Ai, C., Kumari, A. L. & Khar, A. (2004). Effect of curcumin on normal and tumor cells: role of glutathione and bcl-2. *Mol Cancer Ther,* Vol. 3, No. 9, pp. 1101-1108, 1535-7163

Thangapazham, R., Passi, N. & Maheshwari, R. (2007a). Green tea polyphenol and epigallocatechin gallate induce apoptosis and inhibit invasion in human breast cancer cells. *Cancer Biology & Therapy,* Vol. 6, No. 12, pp. 1938-1943, 4974

Thangapazham, R., Singh, A., Sharma, A., Warren, J., Gaddipati, J. & Maheshwari, R. (2007b). Green tea polyphenols and its constituent epigallocatechin gallate inhibits proliferation of human breast cancer cells in vitro and in vivo. *Cancer Letters,* Vol. 245, No. 1-2, pp. 232-241, 0304-3835

Thomas, S. L., Zhong, D., Zhou, W., Malik, S., Liotta, D., Snyder, J. P., Hamel, E. & Giannakakou, P. (2008). EF24, a novel curcumin analog, disrupts the microtubule cytoskeleton and inhibits HIF-1. *Cell Cycle,* Vol. 7, No. 15, pp. 2409-2417, 1551-4005

Umekita, Y., Ohi, Y., Sagara, Y. & Yoshida, H. (2002). Overexpression of cyclinD1 predicts for poor prognosis in estrogen receptor-negative breast cancer patients. *Int J Cancer,* Vol. 98, No. 3, pp. 415-418, 0020-7136

Van Aller, G., Carson, J., Tang, W., Peng, H., Zhao, L., Copeland, R., Tummino, P. & Luo, L. (2011). Epigallocatechin gallate (EGCG), a major component of green tea, is a dual phosphoinositide-3-kinase/mTOR inhibitor. *Biochemical and Biophysical Research Communications,* Vol. 406, No. 2, pp. 194-199, 0006-291X

Venkitaraman, R. (2010). Triple-negative/basal-like breast cancer: clinical, pathologic and molecular features. *Expert Rev Anticancer Ther,* Vol. 10, No. 2, pp. 199-207, 1744-8328

Verma, S. P., Salamone, E. & Goldin, B. (1997). Curcumin and genistein, plant natural products, show synergistic inhibitory effects on the growth of human breast cancer

MCF-7 cells induced by estrogenic pesticides. *Biochem Biophys Res Commun,* Vol. 233, No. 3, pp. 692-696, 0006-291X

Vlerken, L., Vyas, T. & Amiji, M. (2007). Poly (ethylene glycol)-modified nanocarriers for tumor-targeted and intracellular delivery. *Pharmaceutical Research,* Vol. 24, No. 8, pp. 1405-1414, 0724-8741

Walker, E., Pacold, M., Perisic, O., Stephens, L., Hawkins, P., Wymann, M. & Williams, R. (2000). Structural determinants of phosphoinositide 3-kinase inhibition by wortmannin, LY294002, quercetin, myricetin, and staurosporine. *Molecular Cell,* Vol. 6, No. 4, pp. 909-919, 1097-2765

Waris, G. & Ahsan, H. (2006). Reactive oxygen species: role in the development of cancer and various chronic conditions. *J Carcinog,* Vol. 5, No. pp. 14, 1477-3163

Wu, J. T. & Kral, J. G. (2005). The NF-kappaB/IkappaB signaling system: a molecular target in breast cancer therapy. *J Surg Res,* Vol. 123, No. 1, pp. 158-169, 0022-4804

Yadav, B., Taurin, S., Rosengren, R. J., Schumacher, M., Diederich, M., Somers-Edgar, T. J. & Larsen, L. (2010). Synthesis and cytotoxic potential of heterocyclic cyclohexanone analogues of curcumin. *Bioorg Med Chem,* Vol. 18, No. 18, pp. 6701-6707, 1464-3391

Yallapu, M. M., Gupta, B. K., Jaggi, M. & Chauhan, S. C. (2010). Fabrication of curcumin encapsulated PLGA nanoparticles for improved therapeutic effects in metastatic cancer cells. *J Colloid Interface Sci,* Vol. 351, No. 1, pp. 19-29, 1095-7103

Yang, H., Sun, D., Chen, D., Cui, Q., Gu, Y., Jiang, T., Chen, W., Wan, S. & Dou, Q. (2010). Antitumor activity of novel fluoro-substituted (-)-epigallocatechin-3-gallate analogs. *Cancer Letters,* Vol. 292, No. 1, pp. 48-53, 0304-3835

Youssef, K. M. & El-Sherbeny, M. A. (2005). Synthesis and antitumor activity of some curcumin analogs. *Arch Pharm (Weinheim),* Vol. 338, No. 4, pp. 181-189, 0365-6233

Permissions

All chapters in this book were first published by InTech Open; hereby published with permission under the Creative Commons Attribution License or equivalent. Every chapter published in this book has been scrutinized by our experts. Their significance has been extensively debated. The topics covered herein carry significant findings which will fuel the growth of the discipline. They may even be implemented as practical applications or may be referred to as a beginning point for another development.

The contributors of this book come from diverse backgrounds, making this book a truly international effort. This book will bring forth new frontiers with its revolutionizing research information and detailed analysis of the nascent developments around the world.

We would like to thank all the contributing authors for lending their expertise to make the book truly unique. They have played a crucial role in the development of this book. Without their invaluable contributions this book wouldn't have been possible. They have made vital efforts to compile up to date information on the varied aspects of this subject to make this book a valuable addition to the collection of many professionals and students.

This book was conceptualized with the vision of imparting up-to-date information and advanced data in this field. To ensure the same, a matchless editorial board was set up. Every individual on the board went through rigorous rounds of assessment to prove their worth. After which they invested a large part of their time researching and compiling the most relevant data for our readers.

The editorial board has been involved in producing this book since its inception. They have spent rigorous hours researching and exploring the diverse topics which have resulted in the successful publishing of this book. They have passed on their knowledge of decades through this book. To expedite this challenging task, the publisher supported the team at every step. A small team of assistant editors was also appointed to further simplify the editing procedure and attain best results for the readers.

Apart from the editorial board, the designing team has also invested a significant amount of their time in understanding the subject and creating the most relevant covers. They scrutinized every image to scout for the most suitable representation of the subject and create an appropriate cover for the book.

The publishing team has been an ardent support to the editorial, designing and production team. Their endless efforts to recruit the best for this project, has resulted in the accomplishment of this book. They are a veteran in the field of academics and their pool of knowledge is as vast as their experience in printing. Their expertise and guidance has proved useful at every step. Their uncompromising quality standards have made this book an exceptional effort. Their encouragement from time to time has been an inspiration for everyone.

The publisher and the editorial board hope that this book will prove to be a valuable piece of knowledge for researchers, students, practitioners and scholars across the globe.

List of Contributors

Di Benedetto Melanie
INSERM U940/CSPBAT, Université P13, France

Shiro Koizume and Yohei Miyagi
Molecular Pathology & Genetics Division, Kanagawa Cancer Center Research Institute, Japan

Weimin Fan
Program of Innovative Cancer Therapeutics, First Affiliated Hospital of Zhejiang University College of Medicine, Hangzhou, China
Department of Pathology and Laboratory Medicine, Medical University of South Carolina, Charleston, USA

Meihua Sui
Program of Innovative Cancer Therapeutics, First Affiliated Hospital of Zhejiang University College of Medicine, Hangzhou, China
Center for Bionanoengineering, Department of Chemical and Biological Engineering, Zhejiang University, Hangzhou, China

Joerg Kumbrink and Kathrin H. Kirsch
Department of Biochemistry, Boston University School of Medicine, Boston, MA, USA

Chong-Zhi Wang, Guang-Jian Du and Chun-Su Yuan
Tang Center for Herbal Medicine Research and Department of Anesthesia & Critical Care, The Pritzker School of Medicine, University of Chicago, Chicago, U.S.A.

Grey A. Wilkinson, Adam N. Elwi and Sung-Woo Kim
University of Calgary, Canada

Sylvia Shabaya and Rita Nahta
Emory University, USA

Graziella Joanitti, Sonia Freitas and Ricardo Azevedo
University of Brasilia, Brazil

Weena Jiratchariyakul
Department of Pharmacognosy, Faculty of Pharmacy, Mahidol University, Bangkok, Thailand

Tanawan Kummalue
Department of Clinical Pathology, Faculty of Medicine Siriraj Hospital, Mahidol University, Bangkok, Thailand

Chujian Chen
School of Dietetics and Human Nutrition, Macdonald Campus of McGill University, Ste-Anne-de-Bellevue, Quebec, Canada
School of Public Health, Nantong University, Nantong, Jiangsu, People's Republic of China

Hing Man Chan
Community Health Program, University of Northern British Columbia, Prince George, British Columbia, Canada

Stan Kubow
School of Dietetics and Human Nutrition, Macdonald Campus of McGill University, Ste-Anne-de-Bellevue, Quebec, Canada

Julian Dzeyk, Babasaheb Yadav and Rhonda J. Rosengren
University of Otago, New Zealand

Index

www.ingramcontent.com/pod-product-compliance
Lightning Source LLC
LaVergne TN
LVHW062234200926
848484LV00006B/1543
* 9 7 9 8 8 8 7 4 0 5 0 7 0 *